# THE BMA GUIDE TO
# BACK CARE

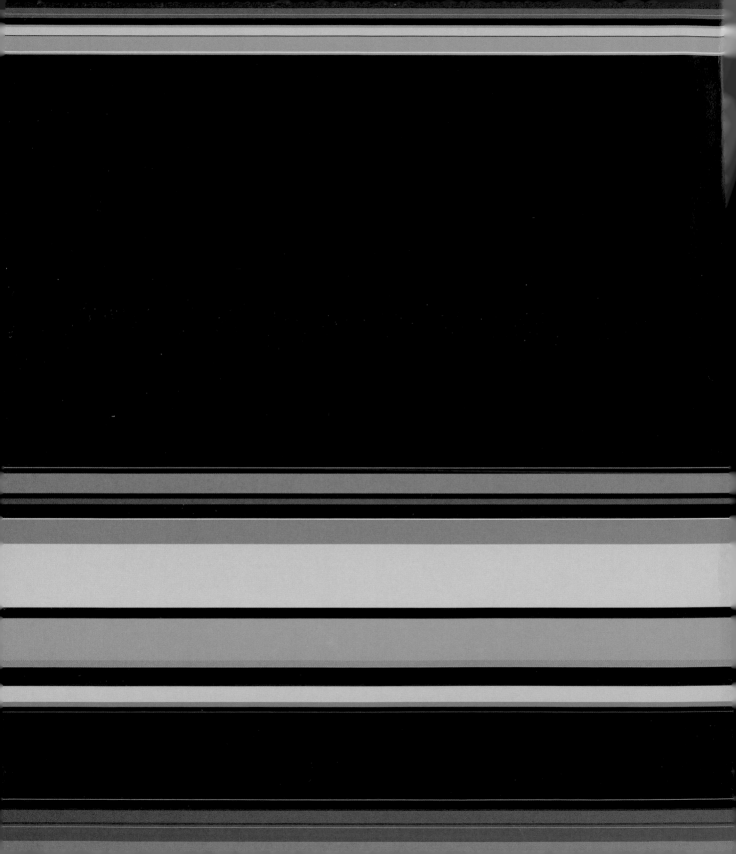

# THE BMA GUIDE TO
# BACK CARE

Project Editors    Corinne Masciocchi,
Hannah Bowen, Cécile
Landau, Scarlett O'Hara

Project Art Editors    Phil Gamble,
Yen Mai Tsang

Production Editor    Joanna Byrne

Production Controller    Sophie Argyris

Jacket Designer    Mark Cavanagh

Managing Editor    Stephanie Farrow

Managing Art Editor    Lee Griffiths

Illustrators    Philip Wilson, Debbie
Maizels, Mark Walker,
Debajyoti Dutta, Phil
Gamble, Darren Awuah

First published in Great Britain in 2011 by
Dorling Kindersley Limited
80 Strand, London WC2R 0RL
Penguin Group (UK)

2 4 6 8 10 9 7 5 3 1
001-179160-August/2011

The information in this book is designed
to help you make informed decisions about
your health, diet, fitness, and exercise/
rehabilitation programme. It is not intended as
a substitute for professional advice from doctors,
specialists, and/or physiotherapists. If you suspect
that you have an injury or other medical problem,
you should seek the approval of your doctor,
specialist, and physiotherapist before you begin
any form of exercise. Neither the publisher nor
anyone else involved in the preparation of this
book is engaged in rendering professional
advice or services to the individual reader.
For further advice on safety, see page 224.

A CIP catalogue record for this book
is available from the British Library.

ISBN 978-1-4053-6429-4

Printed and bound in Singapore by
Star Standard Industries Pte. Ltd.
Discover more at www.dk.com

# CONTENTS

# ABOUT THIS BOOK

**Opening with an introduction** to back and neck anatomy, this book profiles a range of back and neck conditions, their causes, and the treatment options available. The following chapters offer advice on preventing problems using a range of simple strategies and how to cope with pain and adapt your behaviour. The closing section provides a range of rehabilitation exercises which can also be used as part of a fitness programme.

## BACK AND NECK ANATOMY

This section provides an insight into the anatomy of your back and neck, explaining the complex structure of your spine and how it functions with the nerves, muscles, and ligaments surrounding it.

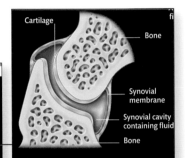

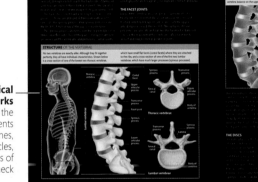

**Anatomical artworks**
help to illustrate the individual elements of the bones, nerves, muscles, and ligaments of your back and neck

**Facet joint structure**
The articular processes of a facet joint are lined with protective cartilage. The synovial membrane surrounding the joint secretes a lubricating fluid that assists movement.

**Detailed breakdowns**
of the structures in your back and neck build up a full anatomical profile

## DIAGNOSIS AND TREATMENT

Opening with three symptoms diagnosis charts, this section profiles a range of neck and back conditions with information on prognoses and therapy options, along with sample medical and physiotherapy treatment tables.

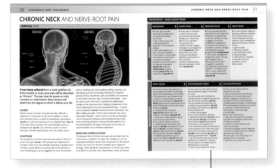

**Treatment tables**
provide examples of the treatments and therapies your doctor and physiotherapist may suggest at different stages of your rehabilitation

## CAUSES OF BACK AND NECK PAIN

This section provides further information on the medical causes of the back and neck conditions outlined in the previous chapter, with comprehensive profiles and fully annotated anatomical artworks.

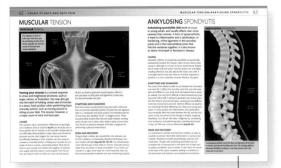

**Anatomical illustrations**
show at a glance how each of the various causes affect the bones, nerves, muscles, and ligaments of your back and neck

## WHERE TO FIND HELP

This section gives you an insight into the process of diagnosis, and provides useful details of the wide range of medical and complementary treatment options now available to sufferers of back and neck pain.

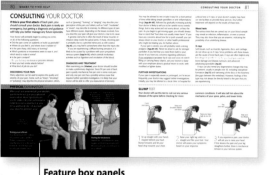

**Feature box panels**
describe the types of treatment you may be given by each of the various healthcare practitioners

## BACK AND NECK MAINTENANCE

Explaining the role your back and neck play in most bodily movements, this section discusses key risk factors and offers guidance on various strategies you can use to reduce your risk of developing problems in the first place.

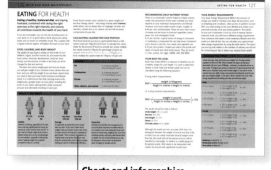

**Charts and infographics**
make key facts and figures clear and easy to digest

## STRATEGIES FOR PREVENTING PAIN

This section shows you the ideal postures and movements for a range of common day-to-day activities at home and work, in order to help reduce your chances of developing back or neck pain, or aggravating an existing condition.

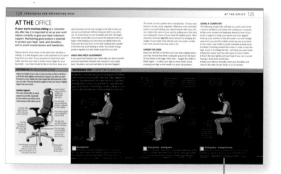

**Annotated illustrations**
present key information on equipment and body positions

## STRATEGIES FOR COPING WITH PAIN

This section arms you with helpful advice on coping with the often debilitating effects of back and neck conditions, along with a range of strategies to help you manage your pain effectively on a more long-term basis.

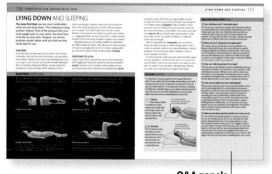

**Q&A panels**
provide clear answers to the key issues that patients tend to raise when they are undergoing treatment

## REHABILITATION EXERCISES

In this section, clear instructions and illustrations guide you through a comprehensive range of exercises that your physiotherapist may recommend to you as part of a rehabilitation programme.

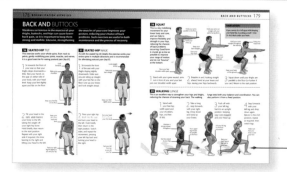

**Step-by-step artworks**
guide you through each exercise in a practical, user-friendly manner

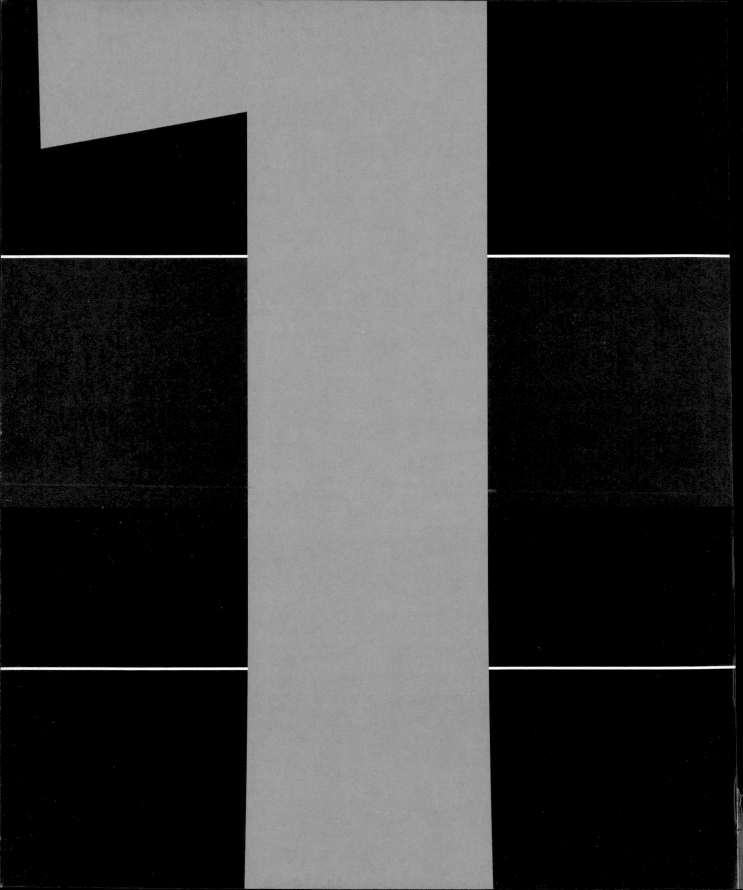

# BACK AND NECK ANATOMY

**This chapter gives an overview** of basic anatomy, helping you to understand the structure of your back and neck, and how your body functions. Detailed anatomical diagrams examine the spine and explain how it links up with the nerves, muscles, and ligaments that surround it.

# THE SPINE

**Your spine is the central support** system for your entire body, assisting with nearly all movement, while supporting and protecting your spinal cord. It must be firm enough to support your body weight when standing, yet flexible and strong enough to anchor your body, while helping your upper and lower limbs to move smoothly.

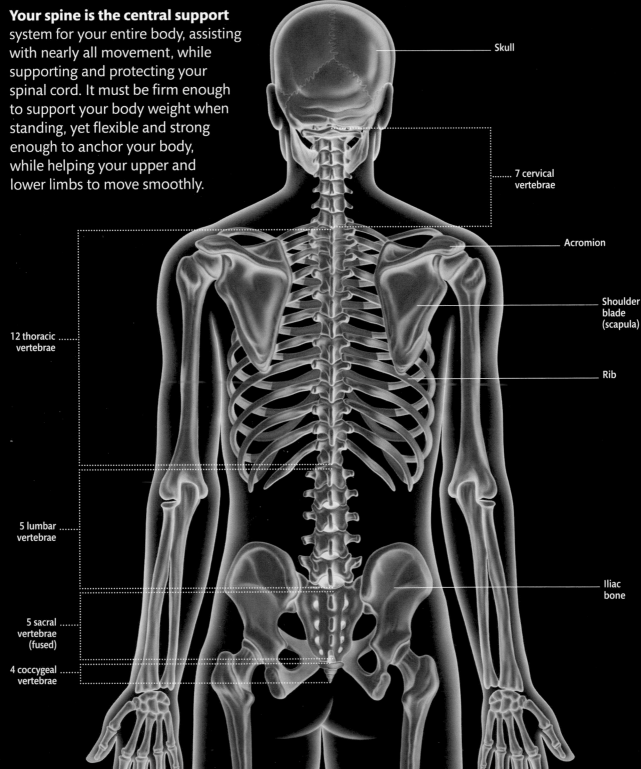

Skull

7 cervical vertebrae

Acromion

Shoulder blade (scapula)

Rib

12 thoracic vertebrae

5 lumbar vertebrae

5 sacral vertebrae (fused)

4 coccygeal vertebrae

Iliac bone

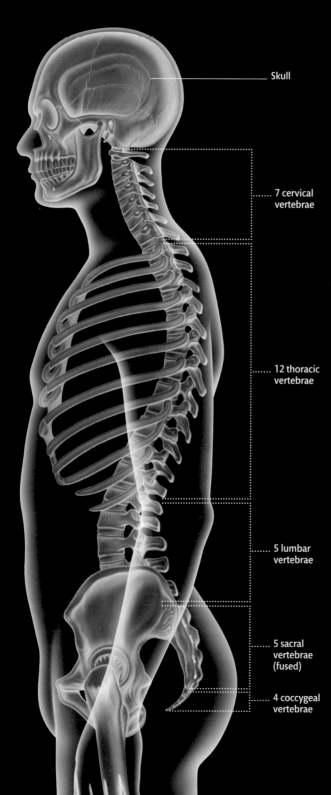

Skull

7 cervical vertebrae

12 thoracic vertebrae

5 lumbar vertebrae

5 sacral vertebrae (fused)

4 coccygeal vertebrae

## THE SPINAL COLUMN

Your spine is a column of up to 34 bones called vertebrae. All but 10 of these vertebrae are movable and they are divided into three groups: seven cervical (neck), 12 thoracic (mid-back), and five lumbar (lower back). The remaining 10 vertebrae are located at the base of the spine; five of these are fused together to form a triangular-shaped bone – the sacrum, which sits between your two iliac bones to form your pelvis. Below this there are three to five (most people have four) fused or partially mobile segments which form your coccyx, the rudimentary "tail" inherited from early human ancestors.

### The cervical spine

The seven cervical vertebrae, or neck bones, provide the main support for your skull and allow you to rotate and nod your head. The spine is a mobile structure and can bend and rotate in almost any direction. The cervical region is the most mobile section of the spine.

### The thoracic spine

Each of the 12 thoracic vertebrae of the mid-back is joined to a rib on either side, with the resulting ribcage surrounding and protecting your heart, lungs, and liver. When you inhale fully, the thoracic spine extends slightly as the ribs rise; when you exhale, the thoracic spine flexes. When you twist your upper body, it rotates around your thoracic spine.

### The lumbar spine

When you are upright – during most of your waking hours – the five lumbar vertebrae must bear the bulk of your weight and provide a flexible link between the upper and lower parts of your body.

### The sacral spine

Below the five lumbar vertebrae, the five sacral vertebrae fuse together to form a bone called the sacrum. This bone is noticeably different in men and women, with the sacrum being longer and narrower in men than it is in women. The sacral vertebrae are connected to the vertebrae at the end of the spine – known as the coccygeal vertebrae – by a joint called the sacrococcygeal symphysis. Together, the coccygeal vertebrae form the coccyx, or tail bone.

## THE VERTEBRAE

The main part of a vertebra is more or less cylindrical, with a flat surface at the top and bottom, and a small hole running vertically through each, towards the back edge. When your vertebrae are aligned, these form a channel – the spinal or neural canal – that contains and protects your spinal cord.

The back of each vertebra has seven projections, called processes. These are arranged in three pairs with an odd one out – the spinous process. Your spinous processes are the knobbly bits that run all the way down your spine.

The spinous process sits in between the six paired processes (three on either side). Two of the pairs – the upper articular processes and the lower articular processes – act as joints,

linking your vertebrae and strengthening your spine. Your back muscles are attached to the remaining pair, the transverse processes, and also to the spinous process, all of which provide anchorage as your muscles contract and relax.

## THE FACET JOINTS

Each of the vertebrae in your spinal column meets at a facet joint. It is here that the lower articular processes of the first vertebra link up, or "articulate", with the upper articular processes of the second. The surfaces of these processes are smooth and flat, like the facets of a diamond – hence the reason that the joints are called facet joints, as well as being known as posterior joints.

### STRUCTURE OF THE VERTEBRAE

No two vertebrae are exactly alike. Although they fit together perfectly, they all have individual characteristics. Shown below is a cross-section of one of the lowest two thoracic vertebrae,

which have small flat facets (costal facets) where they are attached to the ribs, and a cross-section of one of the first two lumbar vertebrae, which have much larger processes (spinous processes).

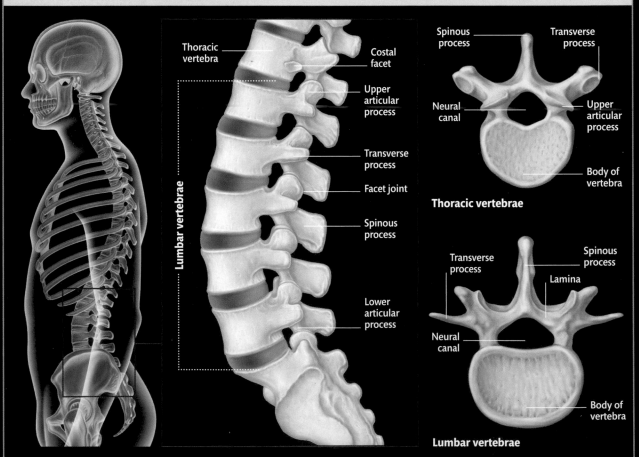

Thoracic vertebrae

Lumbar vertebrae

## SPINAL JOINTS

The joints between your vertebrae are each made up of two main elements: the first is a facet joint in which the lower processes of one vertebra balance on the upper processes of the vertebra beneath it to form a fulcrum (**» below**); the second is a flexible disc that works like a mouldable ball bearing, allowing your spine to twist and bend, while also acting as a shock absorber.

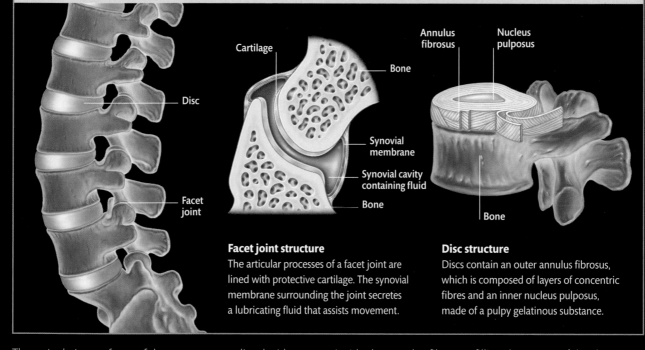

**Facet joint structure**
The articular processes of a facet joint are lined with protective cartilage. The synovial membrane surrounding the joint secretes a lubricating fluid that assists movement.

**Disc structure**
Discs contain an outer annulus fibrosus, which is composed of layers of concentric fibres and an inner nucleus pulposus, made of a pulpy gelatinous substance.

The articulating surfaces of the processes are lined with cartilage, while the joint itself is covered by the synovial membrane, which not only forms a protective capsule around the joint, but also produces synovial fluid – a lubricating liquid that fills the cavity, helping to reduce friction within the joint. It is important to note that you should perform regular and repetitive movement to maintain the health of this cartilage and keep your facet joints working efficiently.

### THE DISCS

The flat surfaces at the top and bottom of the main body of your vertebrae are covered in a thin layer of cartilage known as an end plate. A cartilage pad, called a disc, is positioned between these two end plates, separating each vertebra in your spinal column from the vertebrae above and below it, enabling you to move and twist your body. The outer layers of this disc are made up of bands of tough fibrous cartilage, which form what is known as the annulus fibrosus. The annulus fibrosus then blends with the end plate cartilage, which coats the flat surfaces of each vertebra.

Inside the annulus fibrosus, filling the centre of the disc, is a pulpy gelatinous substance. This gel – the nucleus pulposus – allows the disc to mould and reshape itself like a liquid ball bearing. This means that, in addition to acting as a joint, the disc is able to perform a second, equally essential, role as a shock-absorbing cushion between each vertebra.

A healthy disc is extremely strong – much stronger, in fact, than a vertebra. This great strength means that a disc is capable of absorbing considerable forces, or shocks. The disc is also able to absorb compressive and jarring forces with a high degree of efficiency because it can adapt its shape, distributing the strain across its surface more evenly. However, discs are more vulnerable to stresses that are caused by twisting motions – in extreme cases, such movements can cause the outer layers of the disc to rupture. The annulus fibrosus contains a number of pain-sensitive nerves, and the pain associated with a "slipped disc" – a misnomer, since a disc cannot slip, but herniates or ruptures – is often the result of an injured disc pressing on the dural sheath or a nerve, or even from a tear in the fibres of the annulus fibrosus itself.

# THE SPINAL CANAL AND NERVES

**When your vertebrae** are stacked up to form the spinal column, the holes that run through them form a continuous channel called the spinal canal. This both contains and protects the spinal cord, a cluster of nerve fibres that links the brain with all the nerves in the body, carrying signals back and forth.

**The spinal cord**
The spinal cord runs down from the brain stem, along the spinal canal as far as the first or second lumbar vertebra. A cluster of fine nerve fibres – the cauda equina – hangs down from the base of the cord.

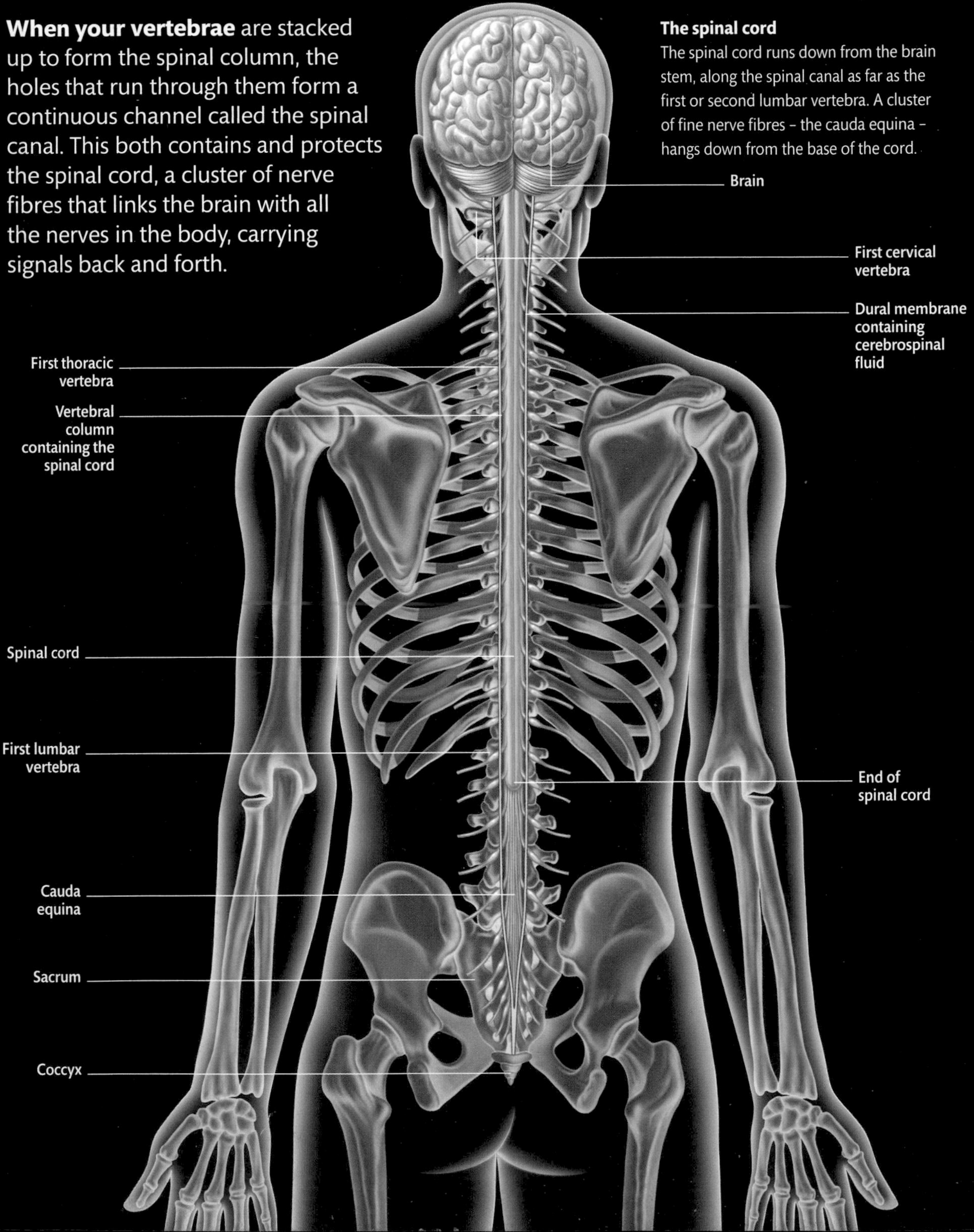

Brain

First cervical vertebra

Dural membrane containing cerebrospinal fluid

First thoracic vertebra

Vertebral column containing the spinal cord

Spinal cord

First lumbar vertebra

End of spinal cord

Cauda equina

Sacrum

Coccyx

## THE SPINAL CORD

The spinal cord is a densely packed bundle of nerve fibres, which links the brain with the vast network of nerves that are responsible for controlling all the movements and sensations of your body. It runs from the base of the skull down to either the first or second lumbar vertebra, depending on the individual. Below this point, nerve fibres extend from the base of the cord in strands, forming what is known, owing to its appearance, as the cauda equina, meaning horse's tail.

The three membranes, or meninges, that protect the brain also surround and protect the spinal cord along its entire length. The outermost of these membranes forms a sheath called the dura, which extends as far as the second of the sacrum's five fused bones. At the points where the pairs of nerve roots emerge from the spinal cord through the gaps in the vertebral column – known as foramina – pairs of dural-root sleeves project from the dural sheath to enclose and protect them.

The dural sheath is extremely responsive to pressure throughout its entire length. Both the dural sheath and root sleeves are quite mobile, but bending or stretching movements can cause the nerve-root sleeve to rub against a protruding disc – if this happens, stretching your leg can cause significant pain, as the nerve becomes irritated.

Inside the dural sheath, between the two inner meninges, lies the cerebrospinal fluid. This clear fluid bathes the spinal cord and is the same as the fluid that surrounds the brain, protecting it from injury. It acts as an extra shock absorber to protect the sensitive spinal cord from shocks.

## HOW NERVES STIMULATE YOUR MUSCLES

The human nervous system is made up of millions of nerve fibres, which transmit electrical impulses to and from the brain. This system allows the brain to control the functioning of the rest of the body. Nerve fibres can be divided into two main types: sensory fibres, which send out signals or messages relating to sensations, such as pain or change of temperature, to the brain; and motor fibres, which relay messages concerned with movement from the brain to the muscles. The movement of the bundles of fibres that make up the muscles – whether they are contracting or expanding – is controlled by impulses from the nerves.

Whenever you decide to bend your arm, for example, the brain sends out a message that is transmitted along the appropriate nerves to your biceps – the muscle in your upper arm. This signal makes the muscle fibres in your biceps contract, which pulls your forearm up, causing your arm to bend at the elbow.

Electrical signals sent from the brain via the nervous system are also responsible for controlling all of the vital bodily functions that keep us alive, such as our heartbeat, breathing, and digestion – all of which involve muscular activity that we are barely ever aware of: this is called the autonomic nervous system. The autonomic nervous system is comprised of sympathetic fibres – which are involved in fight and flight responses, such as increased heart rate – and parasympathetic fibres, which are involved in functions that occur while the body is at rest, such as salivation.

### SPINAL NERVES

These nerves branch off and emerge in pairs from either side of the spinal cord through the foramina, or the gaps in the spinal column between the vertebrae and the facet joints.

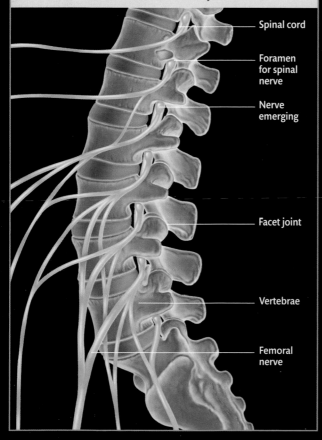

- Spinal cord
- Foramen for spinal nerve
- Nerve emerging
- Facet joint
- Vertebrae
- Femoral nerve

# MUSCLES AND LIGAMENTS

**The muscles of the back** are built up in layers around the skeleton. These muscles are involved with stabilizing and moving the torso.

**The muscles of the back**
The smaller muscles, shown on the right of the diagram, are mainly concerned with postural adjustment. Layered over these are the larger muscles, shown on the left, which are involved with controlling movement.

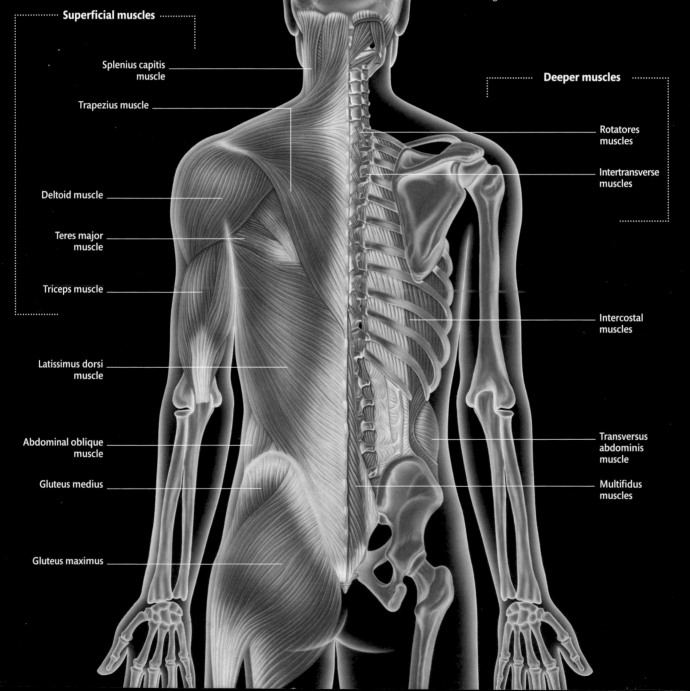

Superficial muscles

Splenius capitis muscle

Trapezius muscle

Deltoid muscle

Teres major muscle

Triceps muscle

Latissimus dorsi muscle

Abdominal oblique muscle

Gluteus medius

Gluteus maximus

Deeper muscles

Rotatores muscles

Intertransverse muscles

Intercostal muscles

Transversus abdominis muscle

Multifidus muscles

## THE MUSCLES

Around each spinal joint is a group of muscles. Each end of every muscle is firmly attached to a different bone, either directly or by means of a tough band of fibrous tissue called a tendon. The deeper layers are made up of small muscles that are mainly involved with fine postural adjustment; on top of these are some larger muscles, which are mostly concerned with assisting the movement of the trunk. Muscles usually function in pairs: when a muscle contracts, the opposite muscle relaxes.

### The stabilizers

Close to the joints between the vertebrae are clusters of small muscles that contract to allow for subtle alterations of movement. These muscles are known as the stabilizers because of their central role in controlling the positioning of the spine.

### The mobilizers

These long, strong muscles are superficially visible and control the major movements of the trunk. At the back are the erector spinae ("spine raisers") muscles. They lengthen when you bend over and contract strongly on straightening, exerting significant compressive force on the spine.

Across the front and sides of the body are abdominal muscles that help to support your spine by maintaining pressure inside the abdomen and chest. For example, when a weightlifter holds his breath before attempting to lift a heavy weight, he is tensing his abdominal muscles. The transversus abdominis (the deepest layer) works almost continually to assist in performing everyday activities.

### How muscles move your trunk

When you twist or rotate your spine, the abdominal and back muscles (collectively known as the muscles of your core) play a key role in the movement. Like most muscles, they work in pairs: when one contracts, its opposite number relaxes. Think of a golfer whose muscles need to create a powerful twisting force to effect a good drive. This force must be balanced by an equal and opposite twisting movement, transmitted along the spine and lower limbs. Over the back muscles lie those of the shoulders and hips. Large, strong muscles support the joints, while smaller, deeper muscles exert a stabilizing force, controlling movement.

### Maintaining healthy muscles

Muscles need a good supply of blood. If a muscle goes into spasm in reaction to pain, or becomes contracted due to poor posture, its blood supply will be reduced. If this lack of supply continues, the muscle may become weak and less elastic.

Muscles need exercise in order to stay strong. If they have been contracted for long periods to maintain a certain posture – when you are sitting at a desk, for example – regular stretching will stop them becoming shorter and weaker. Prolonged pain or even stress can make muscles tense up. Consequently, relaxation is important for maintaining healthy muscles.

Finally, muscles require an intact nerve supply. If an injury or an infection damages a nerve, or its cell unit in the spinal cord, the muscle cannot contract and will waste away.

## SPINAL LIGAMENTS

A network of slightly elastic bands of fibre, or ligaments, helps hold the spinal joints together, keeping the spinal column in one piece and allowing only a limited range of movement in any one direction. Most ligaments contain a large number of nerve endings.

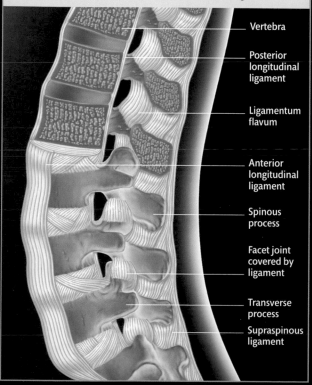

- Vertebra
- Posterior longitudinal ligament
- Ligamentum flavum
- Anterior longitudinal ligament
- Spinous process
- Facet joint covered by ligament
- Transverse process
- Supraspinous ligament

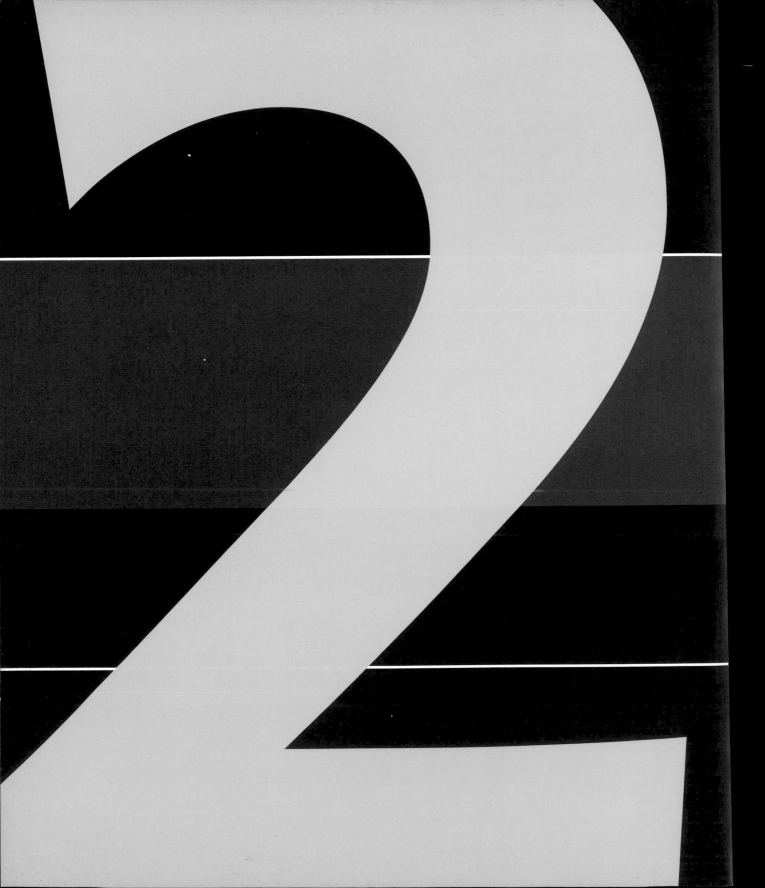

# DIAGNOSIS AND TREATMENT

**Opening with useful symptoms-based diagnostic charts**, this chapter profiles the more common conditions that can affect your back and neck, providing detailed information on symptoms, prognoses, and therapy options, alongside sample timelines for the treatment and rehabilitation of each condition.

# SYMPTOMS CHART: NECK

**This symptoms chart** will help you to determine the potential cause of your neck pain, and cross-refer you to the sections in the book that are relevant to that disorder. These charts are for reference only, however, and you should always ensure you consult your doctor for a firm diagnosis.

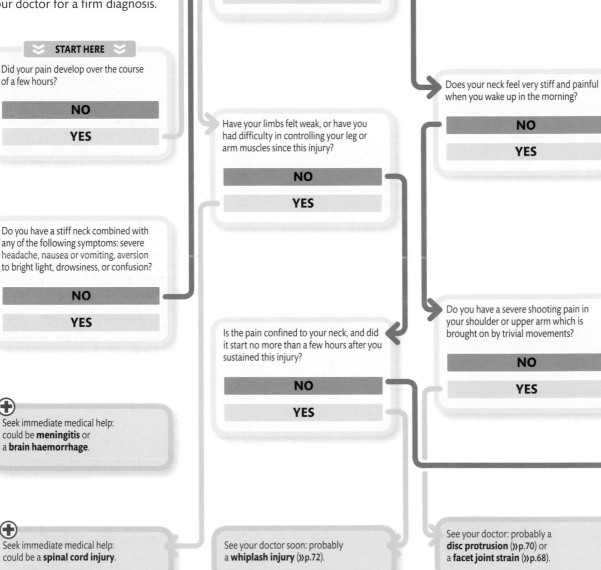

**START HERE**

Did your pain develop over the course of a few hours?

NO

YES

Do you have a stiff neck combined with any of the following symptoms: severe headache, nausea or vomiting, aversion to bright light, drowsiness, or confusion?

NO

YES

Have you had a violent jolt in the last day or two, such as you might receive if you were in a car accident?

NO

YES

Have your limbs felt weak, or have you had difficulty in controlling your leg or arm muscles since this injury?

NO

YES

Is the pain confined to your neck, and did it start no more than a few hours after you sustained this injury?

NO

YES

See your doctor: probably **acute torticollis** (»p.71).

Does your neck feel very stiff and painful when you wake up in the morning?

NO

YES

Do you have a severe shooting pain in your shoulder or upper arm which is brought on by trivial movements?

NO

YES

Seek immediate medical help: could be **meningitis** or a **brain haemorrhage**.

Seek immediate medical help: could be a **spinal cord injury**.

See your doctor soon: probably a **whiplash injury** (»p.72).

See your doctor: probably a **disc protrusion** (»p.70) or a **facet joint strain** (»p.68).

Has the pain or stiffness been developing steadily over a period of several months?

**NO**

**YES**

Did your pain or stiffness follow an episode of acute neck pain?

**NO**

**YES**

See your doctor for diagnosis.

See your doctor: probably **trigger points** (»p.62).

Do you have intermittent numbness or tingling in your hands, or are you over 50 years old?

**NO**

**YES**

Are you under any stress at the moment, or are you experiencing some emotional conflict?

**NO**

**YES**

Does your pain become worse after you remain in one position, such as sitting at a desk, for a long period of time?

**NO**

**YES**

See your doctor: probably **osteoarthritis** (»p.73).

See your doctor: probably **muscular tension** (»p.62).

Do you have pain, numbness, or tingling extending down one arm, possibly to the hand, which is aggravated by certain neck movements?

**NO**

**YES**

See your doctor: probably **postural pain** (»pp.54–55) or **muscular tension** (»p.62).

Do you have pain in your shoulder which is made worse when you breathe in, or do you have a cough or a fever?

**NO**

**YES**

See your doctor soon: could be a **disc protrusion** (»p.70) resulting in arm pain.

(24) See your doctor within 24 hours: could be **pneumonia** or **pleurisy**.

# SYMPTOMS CHART: MID-BACK

**This symptoms chart** will help you to determine the potential cause of pain in your mid-back, and cross-refer you to the sections in the book that are relevant to that disorder. The chart is for reference only, however, and you should always ensure you consult your doctor for a firm diagnosis.

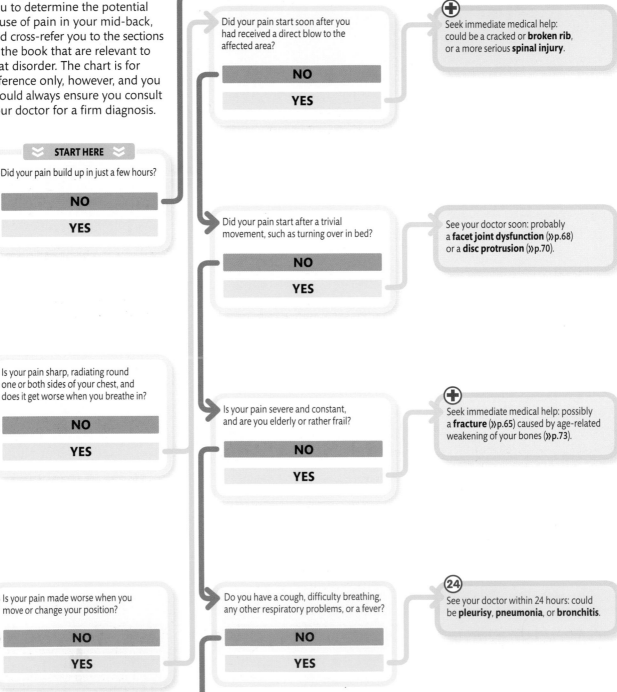

**START HERE**

Did your pain build up in just a few hours?

NO

YES

Did your pain start soon after you had received a direct blow to the affected area?

NO

YES

Seek immediate medical help: could be a cracked or **broken rib**, or a more serious **spinal injury**.

Did your pain start after a trivial movement, such as turning over in bed?

NO

YES

See your doctor soon: probably a **facet joint dysfunction** (»p.68) or a **disc protrusion** (»p.70).

Is your pain sharp, radiating round one or both sides of your chest, and does it get worse when you breathe in?

NO

YES

Is your pain severe and constant, and are you elderly or rather frail?

NO

YES

Seek immediate medical help: possibly a **fracture** (»p.65) caused by age-related weakening of your bones (»p.73).

Is your pain made worse when you move or change your position?

NO

YES

Do you have a cough, difficulty breathing, any other respiratory problems, or a fever?

NO

YES

24
See your doctor within 24 hours: could be **pleurisy**, **pneumonia**, or **bronchitis**.

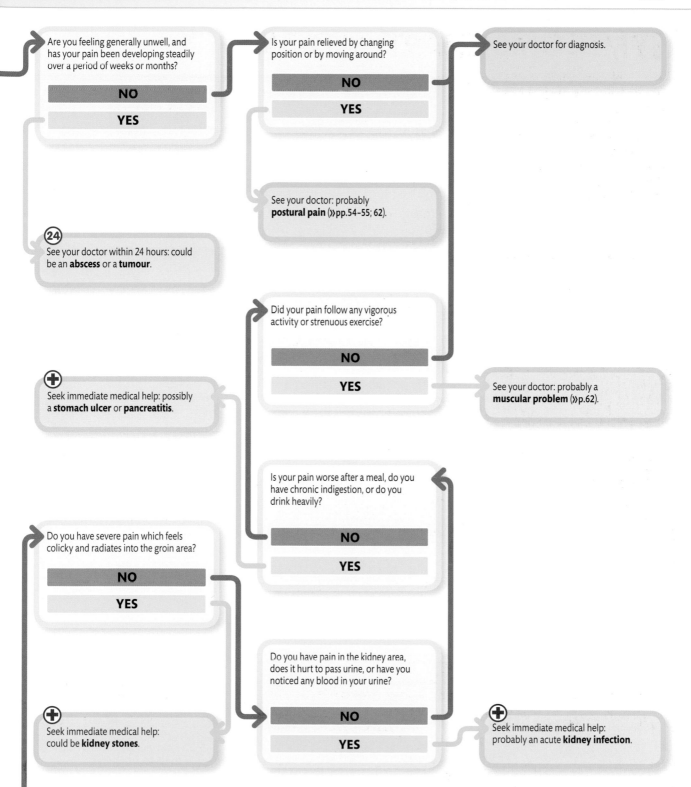

Are you feeling generally unwell, and has your pain been developing steadily over a period of weeks or months?

**NO**

**YES**

Is your pain relieved by changing position or by moving around?

**NO**

**YES**

See your doctor for diagnosis.

See your doctor: probably **postural pain** (》pp.54–55; 62).

(24) See your doctor within 24 hours: could be an **abscess** or a **tumour**.

Did your pain follow any vigorous activity or strenuous exercise?

**NO**

**YES**

See your doctor: probably a **muscular problem** (》p.62).

(+) Seek immediate medical help: possibly a **stomach ulcer** or **pancreatitis**.

Is your pain worse after a meal, do you have chronic indigestion, or do you drink heavily?

**NO**

**YES**

Do you have severe pain which feels colicky and radiates into the groin area?

**NO**

**YES**

Do you have pain in the kidney area, does it hurt to pass urine, or have you noticed any blood in your urine?

**NO**

**YES**

(+) Seek immediate medical help: could be **kidney stones**.

(+) Seek immediate medical help: probably an acute **kidney infection**.

# SYMPTOMS CHART: LOWER BACK AND LEG

**This symptoms chart** will help you to determine the potential cause of pain in your lower back and legs, and cross-refer you to the sections in the book that are relevant to that disorder. These charts are for reference only, however, and you should always consult your doctor for a firm diagnosis.

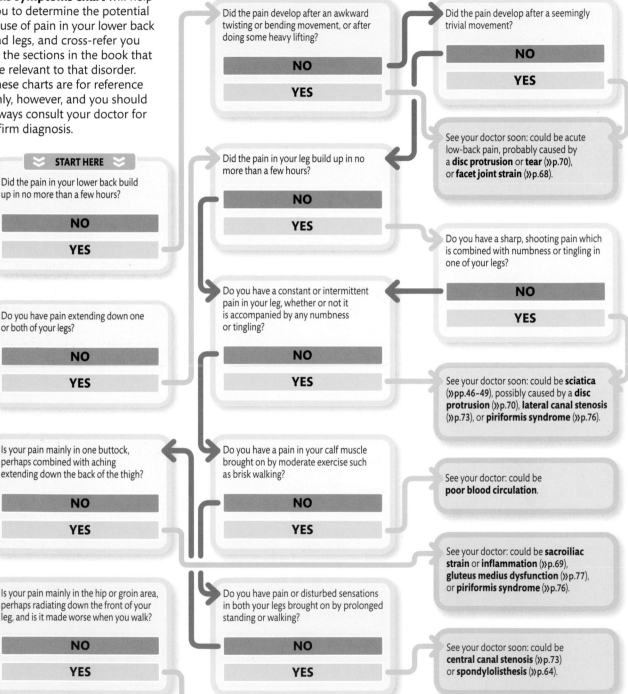

⩔ START HERE ⩔

Did the pain in your lower back build up in no more than a few hours?

**NO**

**YES**

Do you have pain extending down one or both of your legs?

**NO**

**YES**

Is your pain mainly in one buttock, perhaps combined with aching extending down the back of the thigh?

**NO**

**YES**

Is your pain mainly in the hip or groin area, perhaps radiating down the front of your leg, and is it made worse when you walk?

**NO**

**YES**

Did the pain develop after an awkward twisting or bending movement, or after doing some heavy lifting?

**NO**

**YES**

Did the pain in your leg build up in no more than a few hours?

**NO**

**YES**

Do you have a constant or intermittent pain in your leg, whether or not it is accompanied by any numbness or tingling?

**NO**

**YES**

Do you have a pain in your calf muscle brought on by moderate exercise such as brisk walking?

**NO**

**YES**

Do you have pain or disturbed sensations in both your legs brought on by prolonged standing or walking?

**NO**

**YES**

Did the pain develop after a seemingly trivial movement?

**NO**

**YES**

See your doctor soon: could be acute low-back pain, probably caused by a **disc protrusion** or **tear** (》p.70), or **facet joint strain** (》p.68).

Do you have a sharp, shooting pain which is combined with numbness or tingling in one of your legs?

**NO**

**YES**

See your doctor soon: could be **sciatica** (》pp.46–49), possibly caused by a **disc protrusion** (》p.70), **lateral canal stenosis** (》p.73), or **piriformis syndrome** (》p.76).

See your doctor: could be **poor blood circulation**.

See your doctor: could be **sacroiliac strain** or **inflammation** (》p.69), **gluteus medius dysfunction** (》p.77), or **piriformis syndrome** (》p.76).

See your doctor soon: could be **central canal stenosis** (》p.73) or **spondylolisthesis** (》p.64).

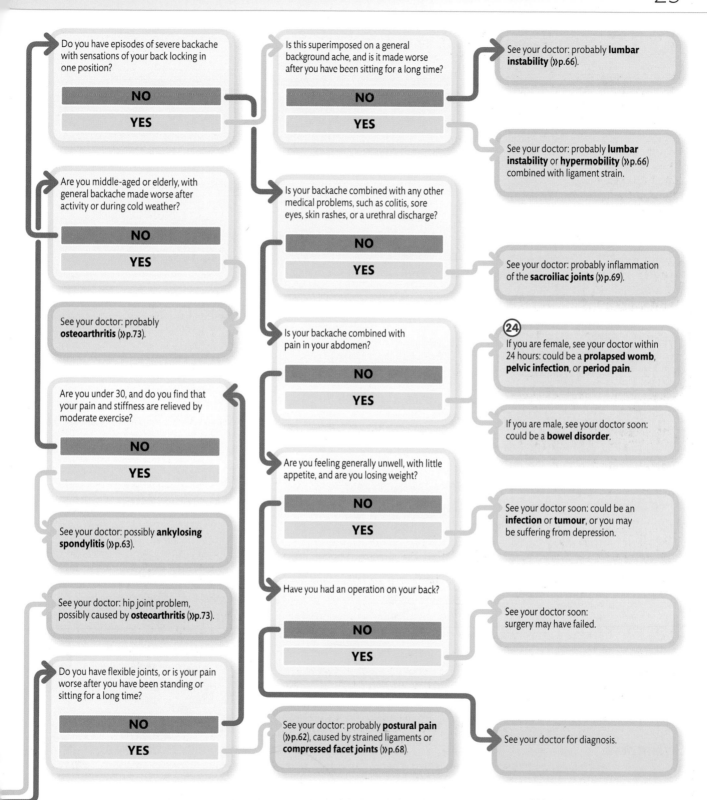

Do you have episodes of severe backache with sensations of your back locking in one position?

**NO**

**YES**

Is this superimposed on a general background ache, and is it made worse after you have been sitting for a long time?

**NO**

**YES**

See your doctor: probably **lumbar instability** (»p.66).

See your doctor: probably **lumbar instability** or **hypermobility** (»p.66) combined with ligament strain.

Are you middle-aged or elderly, with general backache made worse after activity or during cold weather?

**NO**

**YES**

Is your backache combined with any other medical problems, such as colitis, sore eyes, skin rashes, or a urethral discharge?

**NO**

**YES**

See your doctor: probably inflammation of the **sacroiliac joints** (»p.69).

See your doctor: probably **osteoarthritis** (»p.73).

Is your backache combined with pain in your abdomen?

**NO**

**YES**

(24) If you are female, see your doctor within 24 hours: could be a **prolapsed womb**, **pelvic infection**, or **period pain**.

If you are male, see your doctor soon: could be a **bowel disorder**.

Are you under 30, and do you find that your pain and stiffness are relieved by moderate exercise?

**NO**

**YES**

Are you feeling generally unwell, with little appetite, and are you losing weight?

**NO**

**YES**

See your doctor soon: could be an **infection** or **tumour**, or you may be suffering from depression.

See your doctor: possibly **ankylosing spondylitis** (»p.63).

See your doctor: hip joint problem, possibly caused by **osteoarthritis** (»p.73).

Have you had an operation on your back?

**NO**

**YES**

See your doctor soon: surgery may have failed.

Do you have flexible joints, or is your pain worse after you have been standing or sitting for a long time?

**NO**

**YES**

See your doctor: probably **postural pain** (»p.62), caused by strained ligaments or **compressed facet joints** (»p.68).

See your doctor for diagnosis.

# ACUTE NECK AND NERVE-ROOT PAIN

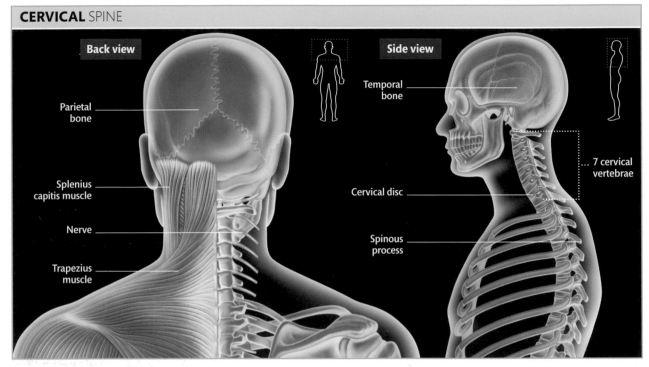

**CERVICAL** SPINE

Back view

Parietal bone

Splenius capitis muscle

Nerve

Trapezius muscle

Side view

Temporal bone

Cervical disc

Spinous process

... 7 cervical vertebrae

**Acute neck and nerve-root pain** describes several conditions that affect the cervical spine region, and can also cause head pain. In the long term, it is rarely as disabling as low-back pain, but the severity of acute nerve-root pain can be just as bad as sciatica (»p.46).

## CAUSES

This pain can be caused by strain of the facet joints (»p.68) and ligaments, and disc herniation (»pp.67; 70). Muscular pain is more of a chronic condition but can flare up (»p.62). Your neck is also vulnerable to external indirect trauma, as in whiplash syndrome (»p.72). When acute neck pain arises spontaneously in young adults or adolescents it is called acute torticollis, or "wry neck" (»p.71). Disc prolapse (»p.70) with nerve-root compression is the cause of the most severe pain.

## SYMPTOMS

You may feel sharp pain, centrally or to one side of the neck, with intense, dull aching that can spread further into the shoulder blade area and half-way down the thoracic spine.

You may have stiffness due to your spine being trapped by a muscle spasm (known as "splinting"), and worse pain on certain movements such as bending forwards, backwards, sideways, or rotating. You may also find it hard to sit in a car or at a computer for long periods. The pain is often troublesome at night and lying down may may make it worse. If a nerve is compressed or irritated, a sharp pain will radiate down your arm as far as your hand, accompanied by sensory disturbance such as pins and needles or numbness. If your motor nerve fibres have been damaged, you may develop weakness in your upper arm and/or forearm.

## RISKS AND COMPLICATIONS

The risk of serious consequences of acute neck pain is extremely small. Most of the time the pain eases over a few weeks without specific treatment. The main risk lies in too much rest, the fear of triggering pain through everyday movements, and the idea that more pain means further harm, as these can lead to loss of confidence and mobility. If you have developed pain after direct trauma such as a blow to the back of the neck, then you should obtain immediate medical advice.

# TREATMENT – CERVICAL DISC HERNIATION

⊕ SEEK IMMEDIATE MEDICAL ATTENTION

## MEDICAL

### IMMEDIATE ▶

■ If you suspect your pain is caused by a cervical disc herniation (》p.67; p.70), you should:
▶ relieve your pain by finding the least painful position – usually semi-recumbent with your legs horizontal, your back elevated, and your neck supported by a firm moulded pillow.
▶ use ice packs for a maximum of 15 minutes every 2 hours for the first day of pain.
▶ take paracetamol or ibuprofen in recommended dosages.
▶ try not to rest for more than 2–3 days.

### SHORT TERM ▶

■ If after 7–10 days you are still feeling pain, you should:
▶ stay as active and mobile as you can, while being careful to avoid extreme movements of your neck.
▶ avoid prolonged reaching or working with your arms extended.
▶ try to avoid driving, and any jolting or jarring movements.
▶ see your doctor for stronger pain-relief medication such as tramadol, codeine, or amitriptyline.

### MEDIUM TERM ▶

■ If after 2–4 weeks you are able to resume normal activities, you should:
▶ talk to your work supervisor or occupational health nurse, if appropriate, about returning to work. Your physiotherapist or doctor may also be able to advise you.
■ If after 2–4 weeks you are not able to resume normal activities, you should:
▶ consult your doctor or physiotherapist for further examination and treatment.
■ If your pain is very severe, your doctor may:
▶ refer you to a specialist for an epidural steroid or nerve-root injection (》pp.86–87).

### LONG TERM

■ If you have regained nearly normal function, you should:
▶ observe good neck posture (》pp.112–14) and rebuild your fitness through a recommended exercise programme (》table below).
■ If after 6–8 weeks you are not recovering as expected, your doctor may:
▶ arrange investigations such as an X-ray, MRI, or bone scans, as well as blood tests (》pp.82–83).
▶ recommend surgery to decompress the nerve or spinal cord (》pp.88–89), although this is very rare.

## PHYSIOTHERAPY

### EARLY STAGE ▶

■ Once your doctor has referred you, your therapist will perform a thorough assessment. Depending on the findings of the assessment, your therapist may:
▶ perform soft-tissue mobilization (》pp.98–99), gentle spinal joint mobilization (》pp.94–95), and manual traction of the involved segment (》pp.94–95).
▶ teach you how to perform active joint-mobilization in a supine position.
■ Your therapist may advise you to:
▶ avoid activities such as bending, lifting, carrying, straining, and prolonged sitting.
▶ use laxatives to avoid straining during bowel movements.
▶ practise breathing from your diaphragm (》pp.148–49) to ease the pressure on your cervical spine.
■ If you have arm or hand pain, or other neurological symptoms, you may be suffering from cervical radiculopathy. You will be advised to:
▶ rest your neck to relieve compression of your spine.

### INTERMEDIATE STAGE ▶

■ After a few days or weeks, depending on your symptoms, your therapist may:
▶ suggest further passive and active mobilizations to increase the range of movement in your neck.
▶ advise you to perform self-positional tractions between treatments.
■ After your symptoms have subsided, you may be ready for more vigorous stretching and strengthening exercises in weight-bearing positions. Your therapist may advise you to:
▶ perform shoulder rotations (》p.161), neck rotations (》p.160), passive and active neck retractions (》p.172), and seated shoulder squeezes (》p.167). Do these several times a day, 10 reps at a time.
■ As your pain diminishes you may:
▶ introduce flexion and extension exercises such as towel neck flexions and towel neck extensions (》p.174), without causing pain.
■ If your pain is not improving or is getting worse, you should:
▶ return to your doctor for review.

### ADVANCED STAGE

■ If your symptoms have decreased in severity and your range of movement is back to normal, you may:
▶ begin isometric strengthening of your neck (》p.163), gradually increasing the amount of resistance applied.
▶ start cardiovascular conditioning and functional activities, using your upper limbs to increase the load.
▶ add sensorimotor training such as kneeling supermans level 2 (》p.191), or standing on a wobble board.
■ If your pain is not improving or is getting worse, you should:
▶ return to your doctor for review.

## TREATMENT – ACUTE TORTICOLLIS

### ✚ SEEK IMMEDIATE MEDICAL ATTENTION

### MEDICAL

| IMMEDIATE ▶ | SHORT TERM ▶ | MEDIUM TERM ▶ | LONG TERM |
|---|---|---|---|
| ■ If you suspect your pain is caused by acute torticollis, you should:<br>▶ find a comfortable position in which to rest your neck such as reclining in a high-backed chair to support your head.<br>▶ use ice packs for a maximum of 15 minutes every 2 hours for the first day of pain.<br>▶ take paracetamol or ibuprofen in recommended dosages.<br>▶ try not to rest for more than 2–3 days, and only use a soft collar (**»p.151**) at night for support. | ■ If after 3 days you can move your neck, you should:<br>▶ consider trying a neck retraction exercise (**»p.172**) and adopting the Alexander Technique posture (**»p.115**).<br>▶ avoid prolonged static positions such as working at a computer or driving, and heavy lifting or carrying.<br>▶ ensure you are performing everyday movements correctly (**»pp.112–14; 124–39**).<br>■ If the pain increases when you are upright, you should:<br>▶ relieve your neck by adopting a semi-recumbent position with your legs horizontal, your back elevated, and your neck supported by a firm pillow. | ■ If after 3–5 days you are able to resume normal activities, you should:<br>▶ talk to your work supervisor or occupational health nurse, if appropriate, about returning to work. A physical therapist or doctor may be able to advise you.<br>■ If after 7–10 days you are not able to resume normal activities, you should:<br>▶ consult your doctor or physical therapist for further examination, advice, or treatment. You may benefit from some manual therapy, manipulation, acupuncture, and more specific guidance on exercises (**»table below**). | ■ If you have regained nearly normal function, you should:<br>▶ observe good neck care (**»pp.112–14**) and rebuild your fitness through a recommended exercise programme (**»table below**).<br>■ If after 6–8 weeks you are not recovering as expected, you should seek further advice. Your doctor may:<br>▶ arrange investigations such as an X-ray, MRI, or bone scan, and blood tests. |

### PHYSIOTHERAPY

| EARLY STAGE ▶ | INTERMEDIATE STAGE ▶ | ADVANCED STAGE |
|---|---|---|
| ■ Once your doctor has referred you, your therapist will perform a thorough assessment. Depending on the findings of the assessment, your therapist may:<br>▶ perform manual therapy, consisting of soft-tissue mobilization (**»pp.98–99**), gentle traction (**»pp.94–95**), passive and active spinal mobilizations (**»pp.94–95**), and muscle-energy techniques (**»p.92**).<br>▶ teach you the correct posture for your daily activities and for sleeping.<br>▶ advise you to avoid lifting, carrying, and pushing.<br>▶ advise you to perform active movements and isometric contractions in the opposite direction to your muscle spasm.<br>■ You may be advised to:<br>▶ perform shoulder shrugs (**»p.166**), shoulder rotations (**»p.161**), neck rotations (**»p.160**), neck side flexions (**»p.160**), and neck extensions and flexions (**»p.161**). | ■ If your neck is now in a more upright position and the pain is significantly less intense, your therapist may:<br>▶ use gentle spinal mobilization.<br>▶ continue with muscle energy techniques.<br>▶ suggest starting passive and active neck retractions (**»p.172**).<br>■ As you continue to recover, you may:<br>▶ perform upper-back stretches (**»p.162**), seated shoulder squeezes (**»p.167**), towel rocks (**»p.173**), and oval shoulder stretches (**»p.175**) as part of your exercise routine.<br>▶ start low-impact cardiovascular training on a cross-trainer or a reclined bike.<br>■ If your pain is not improving or is getting worse, you should:<br>▶ return to your doctor for review. | ■ If you are free of pain and have a full range of movement in your neck, you may:<br>▶ progress to more advanced neck stretching exercises such as levator scapulae stretches (**»p.168**).<br>▶ perform upper-back stretches such as seated back extensions (**»p.170**) and upper-back extensions level 2 (**»p.170**).<br>▶ increase the resistance of your isometric contractions (**»p.163**) or incorporate bands or a Swiss ball into your exercises to increase the difficulty.<br>▶ resume all sports and activities, gradually increasing the load and duration as pain allows.<br>■ You should:<br>▶ maintain good posture (**»pp.112–14**) and take care of your neck to prevent the injury from recurring.<br>■ If your pain is not improving or is getting worse, you should:<br>▶ return to your doctor for review. |

## TREATMENT – WHIPLASH

⊕ SEEK IMMEDIATE MEDICAL ATTENTION

### MEDICAL

**IMMEDIATE**
- If you suspect your pain is caused by whiplash, you should:
  ▶ get your neck assessed at a hospital to exclude more serious bone or nerve injury.
- If only soft tissue is injured, you should:
  ▶ relieve the pain by finding a suitable posture, usually sitting upright in a high-backed chair.
  ▶ use ice packs for a maximum of 15 minutes every 2 hours for the first day of pain.
  ▶ take paracetamol or ibuprofen in recommended dosages.
  ▶ try not to rest for more than 2–3 days, and only use a soft collar (»p.151) at night for support.

**SHORT TERM**
- If after 3 days you are able to move your neck, you should:
  ▶ consider trying a neck retraction exercise (»p.172) and adopting the Alexander Technique posture (»p.115).
  ▶ avoid prolonged static positions such as working at a computer or driving, and heavy lifting or carrying.
  ▶ ensure you are performing everyday movements correctly (»pp.112–14; 124–39).
- If the pain increases when you are upright, you should:
  ▶ relieve your neck by adopting a semi-recumbent posture with head support for short periods.

**MEDIUM TERM**
- If after 7–10 days you are able to resume normal activities, you should:
  ▶ talk to your work supervisor or occupational health nurse, if appropriate, about returning to work. A physiotherapist or doctor may be able to advise you.
- If after 7–10 days you are not able to resume normal activities, you should:
  ▶ consult your doctor or physiotherapist for further examination, advice, or treatment. You may benefit from some manual therapy, manipulation, acupuncture, and more specific guidance on exercises (»table below).

**LONG TERM**
- If you have regained nearly normal function, you should:
  ▶ observe good neck care (»pp.112–15) and rebuild your fitness through a recommended exercise programme (»table below).
- If after 6–8 weeks you are not recovering as expected, your doctor may refer you to a specialist, who may:
  ▶ see if you benefit from facet joint injections (»pp.86–87).
  ▶ suggest an MRI scan (»p.82) if you experience no response to the facet joint injections.
  ▶ refer you to a pain-management programme.

### PHYSIOTHERAPY

**EARLY STAGE**
- If you have suffered a recent trauma to your neck, you should:
  ▶ get thoroughly assessed to eliminate any serious disease. If a serious disease is suspected, you will be referred to the appropriate specialist or department.
- In less serious cases, your therapist may:
  ▶ advise you to rest and apply ice to your swollen and sore tissues.
  ▶ use ibuprofen, if not already prescribed by your doctor.
  ▶ advise you to keep moving within your limits to prevent stiffness.
  ▶ apply strapping to take the strain off the sore tissue in your neck.
- In the period shortly after the injury, your therapist may:
  ▶ perform soft-tissue mobilization (»pp.98–99) and joint mobilization (»pp.94–95).
  ▶ encourage you to actively rotate your neck in both directions (»p.160) within your comfort zone.
  ▶ reassure you that most whiplash injuries heal within 4–5 weeks.

**INTERMEDIATE STAGE**
- If your pain has diminished and the swelling has subsided, your therapist may:
  ▶ use active assisted movements in a supine position to alleviate pain and discomfort.
  ▶ continue soft-tissue mobilization.
- Your therapist may advise you to:
  ▶ begin exercises such as controlled supine neck flexions (»p.169), neck extensions with overpressure (»p.169), and active neck retractions (»p.172).
  ▶ strengthen your upper back by adding seated shoulder squeezes (»p.167), prone shoulder squeezes (»p.167), lat band rows (»p.171), and upper-back band rows (»p.171).
  ▶ stretch your chest with corner chest stretches (»p.176).
  ▶ mobilize your upper back with seated waist stretches (»p.177) and seated waist twists (»p.177).
- If your pain is not improving or is getting worse, you should:
  ▶ return to your doctor for review.

**ADVANCED STAGE**
- If you are free of pain and have a full range of neck movement and good control, your therapist will:
  ▶ monitor your progress, but encourage you to continue your exercises at home.
- Your therapist may:
  ▶ design an aerobic programme for you and suggest sensorimotor exercises (»p.93) to establish better control of your muscles in day-to-day activities.
- You should:
  ▶ remain as active as possible and gradually resume all sports and other activities.
  ▶ consider an occupational assessment if your work is sedentary and involves computers, in order to maintain good posture during your working hours.
  ▶ consider an occupational assessment if your work involves lifting and carrying heavy objects, and implement any changes in order to prevent further injuries.
- If your pain is not improving or is getting worse, you should:
  ▶ return to your doctor for review.

# CHRONIC NECK AND NERVE-ROOT PAIN

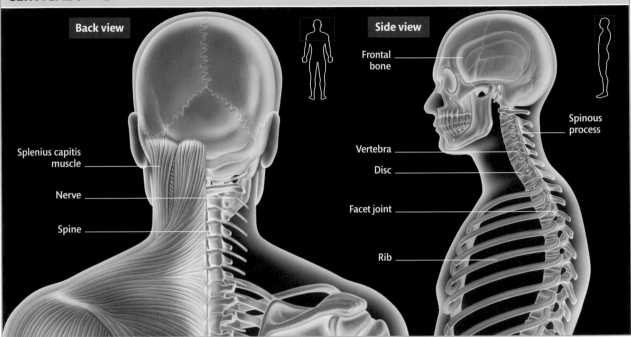

**CERVICAL** SPINE

**Back view**

Splenius capitis muscle

Nerve

Spine

**Side view**

Frontal bone

Spinous process

Vertebra

Disc

Facet joint

Rib

**If you have suffered** from a neck problem for three months or more, your pain will be described as "chronic". The pain may be severe or mild, constant or intermittent; these factors will determine the degree to which it affects your life.

## CAUSES
Precise causes of chronic neck pain are often difficult to determine. In more than 50 per cent of sufferers, it stems from the facet joints as a result of osteoarthritis, spondylosis (**»p.64**), or a previous trauma such as a whiplash injury (**»p.72**). If you have nerve-root pain, the most probable cause is a prolapsed disc (**»p.70**). Less common causes of chronic neck pain include myofascial pain and, very rarely, cancer.

## SYMPTOMS
The symptoms of chronic neck pain are similar to those of acute neck pain (**»p.26**). Older people with degenerative changes in their neck may experience grinding or grating when moving, causing stiffness and aching. Recurrent episodes of more disabling pain can be triggered by trivial movements

such as rotating your neck suddenly, jolting or jarring, and extending your neck or bending forwards for sustained periods of time. Numbness, pins and needles, and weakness in your hands may be a sign of cervical myelopathy – when the spinal cord in the neck is squeezed by degenerative changes in the bones and discs, leading to impairment of the nerves, affecting the arms and sometimes the legs – or spinal cord compression (**»p.65**). Advanced cervical myelopathy may affect walking and gait. Chronic nerve-root pain may cause neuropathic features – when a nerve or nerves are damaged over a long period, leading to abnormal processing of pain – such as burning sensations. Mood and sleep patterns may become disturbed; the impact of the pain on your life can cause frustration and sometimes depression.

## RISKS AND COMPLICATIONS
The physical risks of chronic neck pain are associated with the more serious conditions of major disc prolapse or cervical myelopathy leading to spinal cord compression. In rheumatoid disease, the neck can become unstable due to ligament damage. Other significant complications of chronic pain relate to its effect on your life, work, relationships, mood, and fitness.

## TREATMENT – FACET JOINT PAIN

### MEDICAL

#### IMMEDIATE

■ If your pain has been diagnosed as being caused by a facet joint problem, you should:
► stay as active as you can.
► take paracetamol or ibuprofen in recommended dosages.
► learn what relieves your pain, and what increases it.
► try to retain a normal range of movement in your neck.
► consult your physical therapist or doctor for advice on manual manipulation (>>pp.94–95), exercises (>>table below), postural training (>>pp.112–15), and acupuncture (>>pp.100–01).

#### SHORT TERM

■ If your pain is moderate or severe, and you have not improved with physical therapy, your doctor may refer you to a specialist. The specialist may:
► perform further imaging investigations and diagnostic blocks (>>pp.86–87) of the facet joints in your neck. This process may lead to significant improvement in your condition.
► perform radiofrequency thermal denervation of the joints (>>pp.86–87).

#### MEDIUM TERM

■ If your specialist decides that injections and diagnostic blocks are not appropriate or are not working, he may:
► suggest a functional rehabilitation programme to improve your control of movement, posture, strength, and flexibility, as well as general fitness (>>table below).
► offer a pain-management programme, which includes psychological help on learning to live with pain.
► suggest an operation. Two vertebrae may be fused together to strengthen your spine, or your injured disc may be replaced altogether (>>pp.88–89).

#### LONG TERM

■ If a more specific diagnosis leading to effective treatment has not been made, and if further treatment has been ruled out, pain-management experts will help you to learn how to:
► pace yourself.
► relax your muscles.
► use medication wisely and appropriately.
► cope with your disability.
► live with minimum disruption to your daily routine.

### PHYSIOTHERAPY

#### EARLY STAGE

■ Once your doctor has referred you, your therapist will perform a thorough assessment. Depending on the findings of the assessment, your therapist may:
► perform manual therapy consisting of soft-tissue mobilization (>>pp.94–95; 98–99), gentle traction, passive and active spinal mobilization, and muscle-energy techniques (>>p.92).
► educate you about posture (>>pp.112–115), ergonomics, and relaxation techniques (>>pp.148–49).
► advise you to pace yourself, staying as active as your pain allows.
■ You may be advised to perform:
► mobilizing exercises such as neck rotations (>>p.160), neck extensions and flexions (>>p.161), shoulder rotations (>>p.161), upper-back stretches (>>p.162), and active neck retractions (>>p.172).
► strengthening exercises such as supine neck flexions (>>p.169) and neck extensions with overpressure (>>p.169).

#### INTERMEDIATE STAGE

■ If your pain has diminished and you have an improved range of movement, you may:
► continue with self-mobilizations, adding isometric strengthening exercises such as manual isometrics (>>p.163), and more advanced stretching such as levator scapulae stretches (>>p.168) and passive neck retractions (>>p.172).
■ Your therapist will:
► monitor your progress.
■ You may be advised to perform:
► seated back extensions (>>p.170), corner chest stretches (>>p.176), and seated waist stretches (>>p.177), particularly if you work on a computer a lot.
► arm movements while maintaining the correct posture of your neck and upper back such as doorway chest stretches (>>p.168), wall sit presses (>>p.181), and kneeling supermans level 1 (>>p.191).
► low-load aerobic exercises and fast walking on a treadmill or outdoors.
■ If your pain is not improving or is getting worse, you should:
► return to your doctor for review.

#### ADVANCED STAGE

■ If you are now almost free of symptoms, you may:
► start more advanced conditioning exercises such as swimming, aqua-aerobics, jogging on soft ground, or training on a cross-trainer; gradually increase speed and duration, as pain allows.
■ For preventative purposes, you should:
► continue to follow the postural advice given in the early stage.
► stretch daily.
■ You may be advised to:
► alter your technique for any sports you play. Your therapist may be able to help you with this.
► invest in a chair that places less strain on your back.
► have your eyesight checked regularly, as there is a strong connection between eye strain and neck pain.
■ If your pain is not improving or is getting worse, you should:
► return to your doctor for review.

# TREATMENT – MYOFASCIAL PAIN SYNDROME

## MEDICAL

| IMMEDIATE ▶ | SHORT TERM ▶ | MEDIUM TERM ▶ | LONG TERM |
|---|---|---|---|
| ■ If your pain is diagnosed as being caused by a myofascial problem (muscle and fascia dysfunction), you should:<br>▶ adopt the most comfortable body position for your neck.<br>▶ stay as active as you can.<br>▶ take paracetamol or ibuprofen in recommended dosages.<br>▶ avoid worrying about minor symptoms, as this will only tighten your muscles more.<br>▶ consult your physical therapist or doctor for advice on manual manipulation, exercise, postural training, and acupuncture (**≫table below**). | ■ If your pain is moderate or severe and it has not improved with physical therapy, you should:<br>▶ if appropriate, request a workstation assessment if your work is desk-based.<br>▶ consider some sessions with an Alexander Technique therapist (**≫p.115**). | ■ If you are still in pain, your doctor may refer you to a specialist, who may:<br>▶ consider giving you a low dose of an antidepressant called amitriptyline to relax your muscles and improve sleep quality (**≫pp.84–85**).<br>▶ identify trigger points. If these are found, he may use trigger-point injections (**≫pp.86–87**) and, in some cases, botulinus toxin to relax these for up to 3 months, allowing your muscles to return to normal.<br>▶ advise against prolonged or regular use of analgesics to control headaches caused by muscle tension. | ■ If after several months you are still in pain, your specialist may:<br>▶ give you a functional rehabilitation programme to improve your movement, posture, strength, and flexibility, as well as general fitness (**≫table below**).<br>■ It is likely that your pain will be treatable and manageable, but if you wish, you may consult a pain-management expert who will help you to:<br>▶ maintain good posture.<br>▶ relax your muscles.<br>▶ use medication wisely and appropriately.<br>▶ cope with your disability.<br>▶ continue working. |

## PHYSIOTHERAPY

| EARLY STAGE ▶ | INTERMEDIATE STAGE ▶ | ADVANCED STAGE |
|---|---|---|
| ■ Once your doctor has referred you, you will be thoroughly assessed for muscle imbalances and joint dysfunction. Depending on the findings of the assessment, your therapist may:<br>▶ suggest deactivation of your trigger points using deep massage, myofascial manipulations, acupressure, muscle-energy techniques (**≫p.92**), ultrasound, dry needling, or massage with ice cubes or cooling spray, combined with stretching.<br>▶ suggest stretching and strengthening techniques such as Proprioceptive Neuromuscular Facilitation (**≫p.92**).<br>▶ suggest relaxation such as autogenic training (**≫pp.148–49**) or Jacobson's technique.<br>▶ recommend progressive stretching exercises such as levator scapulae stretches (**≫p.168**), upper-back extensions (**≫p.170**), upper-back stretches (**≫p.162**), and roll-down stretches (**≫p.176**), depending on the location of the trigger points.<br>▶ teach you how to release the trigger points responsible for your pain. | ■ After identifying the causes of your muscle tightening and consequently the origin of your trigger points, your therapist may:<br>▶ suggest altering postures and habits to alleviate further tightening. It is essential that you comply with the instructions and carry on with home exercises.<br>■ You may be advised to:<br>▶ use heat rub cream, take hot baths or showers, and perform relaxation exercises combined with deep breathing from your diaphragm (**≫pp.148–49**).<br>▶ treat your trigger points by using a foam roller (**≫p.185**) or two tennis balls joined together in a sock.<br>▶ start low-impact cardiovascular training.<br>■ If your pain is not improving or is getting worse, you should:<br>▶ return to your specialist for review. | ■ If you are now in control of your symptoms and gently stretching regularly, your pain should diminish significantly. You may:<br>▶ continue cardiovascular training, increasing speed and duration, as pain allows.<br>▶ attend the gym, but do not overexert yourself by using loads that are too heavy. Use low-weight loads and perform a greater number of reps. This way you will increase your strength and endurance without making your condition worse.<br>■ If your pain is not improving or is getting worse, you should:<br>▶ return to your specialist for review. |

## TREATMENT – DISC-RELATED PAIN

✚ SEEK IMMEDIATE MEDICAL ATTENTION

### MEDICAL

| IMMEDIATE ▶ | SHORT TERM ▶ | MEDIUM TERM ▶ | LONG TERM |
|---|---|---|---|
| ■ If your pain has been diagnosed as disc-related, you should:<br>▸ stay as active as you can.<br>▸ take paracetamol or ibuprofen in recommended dosages, sparingly, on a regular schedule.<br>▸ pay attention to your body and be aware of any discomfort.<br>▸ try to keep your movement as normal as possible.<br>▸ consult your physical therapist or doctor for advice on manual manipulation, exercise, postural training, and acupuncture (»table below). | ■ If your pain is moderate or severe and it has not improved with physical therapy, then you should consult a specialist. He may:<br>▸ perform further imaging investigations, diagnostic blocks (»pp.86–87), and discography to ascertain possible causes of pain in your neck.<br>▸ offer further treatment, such as prolotherapy (»p.86), to reduce excessive motion and strain on the disc.<br>■ If your spine has degenerated or the disc is badly damaged, your specialist may:<br>▸ suggest surgery to fuse the spine, or replace the disc (»pp.88–89). | ■ If your specialist feels that treatment is not working, he may suggest:<br>▸ a functional rehabilitation programme to improve your control of movement, posture, strength, and flexibility, as well as general fitness (»table below).<br>▸ a pain-management programme that includes physical and psychological help.<br>▸ suggest surgery to fuse the spine, or replace the disc (»pp.88–89). | ■ If treatment has improved your symptoms, you should:<br>▸ continue to practise good neck care (»pp.112–14).<br>■ If after several months a more specific diagnosis leading to effective treatment has not been made, and if further treatment has been ruled out, pain-management experts will help you to learn how to:<br>▸ pace yourself.<br>▸ relax your muscles.<br>▸ use medication wisely and appropriately.<br>▸ cope with your disability.<br>▸ continue working. |

### PHYSIOTHERAPY

| EARLY STAGE ▶ | INTERMEDIATE STAGE ▶ | ADVANCED STAGE |
|---|---|---|
| ■ Once your doctor has referred you, your therapist will perform a thorough assessment. Depending on the findings of the assessment, your therapist may:<br>▸ perform manual therapy consisting of soft-tissue mobilizations (»pp.94–95; 98–99), gentle traction, passive and active spinal mobilizations (»p.91), muscle-energy techniques (»p.92), and postural strapping (»p.93).<br>▸ educate you about posture (»pp.112–14), ergonomics, and relaxation techniques (»pp.148–49).<br>■ Your therapist may:<br>▸ perform mobilizing exercises such as passive neck retractions (»p.172), neck rotations (»p.160), neck side flexions (»p.160), neck extensions and flexions (»p.161), shoulder shrugs (»p.166), and shoulder rotations (»p.161).<br>▸ suggest upper-back stretches (»p.162), seated shoulder squeezes (»p.167), seated waist stretches (»p.177), trunk rotations (»p.163), towel rocks (»p.173), and towel neck extensions and flexions (»p.174). | ■ If you now have fewer symptoms, you may begin:<br>▸ a strengthening programme for your neck and upper back by adding exercises such as active neck retractions (»p.172), supine neck flexions (»p.169), neck extensions with overpressure (»p.169), manual isometrics (»p.163), lat band rows (»p.171), and upper-back band rows (»p.171).<br>▸ a mobilizing programme for your back, adding cat stretches (»p.165), alligators (»p.184), lying waist twists (»p.184), and cat and camels (»p.187).<br>▸ sensorimotor training (static and dynamic phase) such as balancing, standing on one leg, and moving your upper limbs in various directions.<br>▸ low-impact cardiovascular training on a cross-trainer, or walking on a treadmill or outdoors, gradually increasing your speed and duration, as pain allows.<br>■ If your pain is not improving or is getting worse, you should:<br>▸ return to your specialist for review. | ■ You should now experience minimum pain and possess a good range of movement. You may be advised to:<br>▸ start a more advanced upper-body strengthening programme, maintaining core stability with exercises such as kneeling supermans (»p.191), Swiss ball roll-outs (»p.212), and planks (»p.188).<br>▸ progress to the functional phase of sensorimotor training by introducing wobble boards or an air cushion.<br>▸ increase the impact of your cardiovascular training by introducing jogging or aqua aerobics. You could also consider starting t'ai chi classes.<br>▸ increase your activities and begin or resume sports.<br>■ If your pain is not improving or is getting worse, you should:<br>▸ return to your specialist for review. |

# THORACIC PAIN

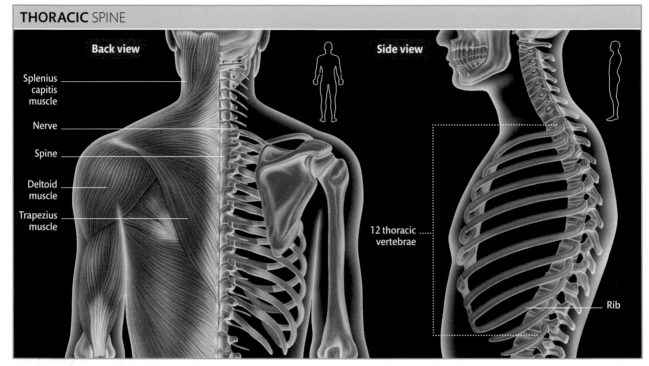

Back view

Splenius capitis muscle

Nerve

Spine

Deltoid muscle

Trapezius muscle

Side view

12 thoracic vertebrae

Rib

**Pain in the mid-back** or thoracic spine (also known as the dorsal spine) usually arises in similar ways to pain in the lower back or neck, except that disc protrusions are less common and nerves are less likely to be trapped. Thoracic pain should always be investigated by a doctor.

## CAUSES

Acute attacks may be caused by a fall or stumble, repeated heavy lifting, an awkward bend, a violent twist or wrench, a cough or sneeze, or a trivial uncoordinated movement, such as turning over in bed or getting up from a chair. The actual physical causes are probably due to mechanical dysfunction: a facet or rib joint strain ("locking"), a muscle strain, or, more rarely, a disc strain or protrusion. More long-standing pain that develops gradually may be related to scoliosis (»p.74).

## SYMPTOMS

The thorax houses important organs, such as the heart and lungs, which can refer pain to the front, side, or back of the chest. Symptoms include central or one-sided

thoracic pain: it may hurt more when coughing, sneezing, or breathing deeply, and it invariably hurts to rotate the trunk in one direction more than the other. Central, severe pain that is made worse by bending forwards or backwards and radiates through to the front directly is more suggestive of a disc problem. In an older person who is coughing violently, a stress fracture of a rib is a possibility. Similarly, a young athlete may develop a stress fracture through repetitive strain, or may pull or tear one of the large muscles of the back in a violent movement. Pain that is constant, unaffected by movement or position, and worse at night may signify an underlying illness or disease. Pain may be referred to the abdomen or as low as the groin in any of the above conditions.

## RISKS AND COMPLICATIONS

It is important that you rule out any potentially serious causes of thoracic pain, as it may be linked to diseases of the heart, aorta, lungs, pancreas, or kidneys. Infection in a disc or vertebra involves the thoracic spine more than any other area of the back. Very rarely, the cause of pain is secondary cancer.

# TREATMENT – MECHANICAL

⊕ SEEK IMMEDIATE MEDICAL ATTENTION

## MEDICAL

### IMMEDIATE
- If you have acute thoracic pain of mechanical origin, you should:
  ▸ consult your doctor.
  ▸ relieve your back by finding the least painful position – usually sitting with full back support, or semi-recumbent.
  ▸ use ice packs for a maximum of 15 minutes every 2 hours for the first day of pain.
  ▸ take paracetamol or ibuprofen in recommended dosages for the first few days of pain.
  ▸ try not to rest for more than 2–3 days.

### SHORT TERM
- If after 3 days you are able to move around, you should:
  ▸ consider trying a simple trunk rotation or McKenzie extension (»pp.163; 192).
  ▸ avoid bending, prolonged inactivity, and static postures brought on by activities such as driving.
  ▸ try holding onto an overhead bar or beam and stretching your back by allowing your full body weight to hang. Do this several times a day for as long as you can.
- If your condition is slow to improve, you should:
  ▸ consult a physical therapist for treatment.

### MEDIUM TERM
- If after 7–14 days you are able to resume normal activities, you should:
  ▸ talk to your work supervisor or occupational health nurse to discuss ways of making it easier to return to work. A physiotherapist or doctor may be able to advise you.
- If after 14–21 days you are not able to resume normal activities, you should:
  ▸ consult your doctor or physical therapist for further examination, advice, or treatment. You may benefit from some manual therapy, manipulation, acupuncture, and more specific guidance on exercises (»table below).

### LONG TERM
- If you have regained nearly normal function, you should:
  ▸ observe good back care (»pp.112–15) and rebuild your fitness through a recommended exercise programme (»table below).
- If, after 6–8 weeks, you are not recovering as expected, you should:
  ▸ seek further advice from your doctor, who may consider arranging investigations such as an X-ray, MRI or bone scan, as well as blood tests (»pp.82–83).

## PHYSIOTHERAPY

### EARLY STAGE
- Once your doctor has referred you, your therapist will perform a thorough assessment. Depending on the findings of the assessment, your therapist may:
  ▸ perform spinal mobilization and manipulation and trigger-point therapy (»pp.90–93).
  ▸ suggest acupuncture (»pp.100–01).
  ▸ use strapping.
  ▸ teach you about posture (»pp.112–15), ergonomics, and breathing techniques.
- Your therapist may advise you to:
  ▸ stretch your thoracic spine with seated back extensions (»p.170), upper-back stretches (»p.162), roll-down stretches (»p.176), seated twist stretches (»p.177), seated waist stretches (»p.177), and corner chest stretches (»p.176).
  ▸ strengthen your deep spinal stabilizers with single arm and leg raises (»p.182), dead bugs (»p.182), kneeling supermans (»p.191), and prone arm and leg lifts (»p.210).
  ▸ strengthen your abs with four-point supine knee lifts (»p.204) and Swiss ball roll-outs (»p.212).

### INTERMEDIATE STAGE
- If you are experiencing less pain and are able to perform specific stabilizing exercises for your thoracic spine, your therapist may advise you to:
  ▸ perform doorway chest stretches (»p.168) progressing to wall sit presses (»p.181).
  ▸ increase the load on your upper limbs by adding weights to kneeling supermans level 1, progressing to levels 2 and 3 (»p.191).
  ▸ use a foam roller to release trigger points with exercises such as thoracic foam rollers (»p.185) and lat foam rollers (»p.185).
  ▸ add lat band rows (»p.171), upper-back band rows (»p.171), and prone shoulder squeezes (»p.167).
  ▸ increase your level of endurance by increasing the number of reps and number of sets, as pain allows.
- If your pain is not improving or is getting worse, you should:
  ▸ return to your doctor for review.

### ADVANCED STAGE
- If you are free of pain and able to maintain good stability within your thoracic spine, your therapist may advise you to:
  ▸ progress to functional exercises and sensorimotor training such as single-leg stands (»p.199).
  ▸ include cardiovascular training such as aqua aerobics, using a cross-trainer, and running (on a treadmill or outdoors) in your exercise programme.
  ▸ consider t'ai chi or Pilates classes to ensure further strengthening and prevent any recurrence of your injury.
- If your pain is not improving or is getting worse, you should:
  ▸ return to your doctor for review.

# ACUTE LOW-BACK PAIN

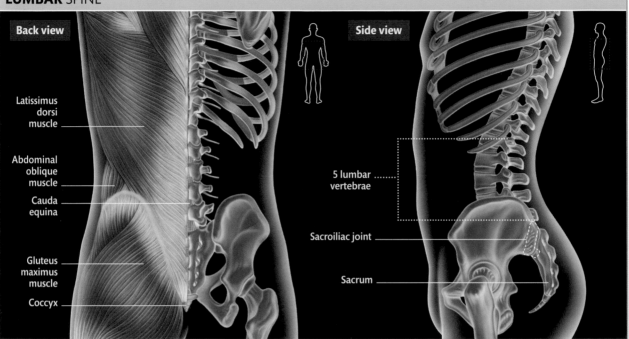

**LUMBAR** SPINE

**Back view**

Latissimus dorsi muscle

Abdominal oblique muscle

Cauda equina

Gluteus maximus muscle

Coccyx

**Side view**

5 lumbar vertebrae

Sacroiliac joint

Sacrum

**Acute attacks of low-back pain** commonly afflict young and middle-aged adults. They can occur with little warning, or can develop slowly over a number of days. In about half of these cases, no obvious trigger for the pain can be identified. The pain can be severe and temporarily disabling, and last for 10–14 days on average.

## CAUSES

The causes of acute low-back pain may include a fall or stumble, repeated heavy lifting, an awkward bend, prolonged bending and stooping, or a cough or sneeze. Occasionally it may occur suddenly, without any obvious cause, such as waking in the morning and finding it impossible to get out of bed. The actual physical causes of the pain are probably one of the following: acute dysfunction of a segment of the lumbar spine, lumbar disc internal disruption or herniation (**»p.70**), irritation of a sciatic nerve (**»p.70**), a sacroiliac strain (**»p.69**), ligament strain or, very occasionally, a muscle strain. Accompanying muscle "spasm" is a common result of these strains, but is not the cause in itself.

## SYMPTOMS

The symptoms of acute low-back pain are sharp pain, either centrally or to one side of your lower back, with an intense dull aching which can spread further into your buttocks, groin, and even thighs. Muscle spasm can grip your spine – known as "splinting" – causing immobility and stiffness; the pain may be worse with one or two particular movements such as bending forwards, backwards, or sideways, and you may find it hard to sustain some positions, such as sitting, for long.

## RISKS AND COMPLICATIONS

Normally, episodes of acute low-back pain will resolve within a few weeks without the need for specific treatment, and the threat of any serious complications as a result of them is very small. The main risks are associated with resting for too long, which can cause stiffness. You may become fearful of any movement because of the memory of the initial pain or the idea that any pain caused by moving means further harm. Rarely, a disc strain can develop into cauda equina syndrome, when the disc prolapses or herniates (**»p.70**) fully into the spinal canal and damages the nerves that run into the legs, bladder, and bowels.

# TREATMENT – ACUTE LUMBAR DYSFUNCTION

➕ SEEK IMMEDIATE MEDICAL ATTENTION

## MEDICAL

### IMMEDIATE ▶

- If you suspect your pain is caused by acute lumbar dysfunction, you should:
  ▸ find the most comfortable position – this will usually involve lying down, possibly with your knees bent.
  ▸ use ice packs for a maximum of 15 minutes every 2 hours for the first day of pain.
  ▸ take paracetamol or ibuprofen in recommended dosages for the first few days of pain.
  ▸ try not to rest for more than 2–3 days.

### SHORT TERM ▶

- If after 3 days you are able to move, you should:
  ▸ consider trying a basic pelvic tilt exercise (**》pp.200-01**) or a McKenzie extension (**》p.192**).
  ▸ avoid prolonged sitting (especially in sofas and deep armchairs), driving, and bending.
  ▸ ensure you are following the correct advice for performing basic movements (**》pp.150-57**).
- If the pain increases when you are upright, you should:
  ▸ relieve your back by lying flat for short periods.
- If, after 3 days, you are still unable to move, you should:
  ▸ seek medical attention.

### MEDIUM TERM ▶

- If after 7–10 days you are able to resume normal activities, you should:
  ▸ talk to your work supervisor or occupational health nurse about returning to work, if appropriate. Your physical therapist or doctor may be able to advise you on this.
- If after 7–10 days you are not able to resume normal activities, you should:
  ▸ consult your doctor or physical therapist for further examination and treatment. You may benefit from manual therapy, acupuncture, and further guidance on exercise (**》table below**).

### LONG TERM

- If you have regained nearly normal function, you should:
  ▸ observe good back care (**》pp.112-15**) and rebuild your fitness through an exercise programme (**》table below**).
- If after 6–8 weeks you are not recovering as expected, your doctor may:
  ▸ arrange investigations such as an X-ray, MRI, or bone scans, as well as blood tests (**》pp.82–83**).

## PHYSIOTHERAPY

### EARLY STAGE ▶

- Once your doctor has referred you, your therapist will perform a thorough assessment. Depending on the findings of the assessment, your therapist may:
  ▸ perform manual techniques such as spinal mobilizations and spinal manipulations (**》pp.90–95**), soft-tissue mobilization (**》pp.98–99**), muscle-energy techniques (**》p.92**), and relaxation techniques (**》pp.148–49**).
  ▸ perform acupuncture for pain relief (**》pp.100–01**).
  ▸ explain basic ergonomics, and advise you on good posture (**》pp.112–15**) and how to restore your range of functional movements.
- You therapist may advise you to:
  ▸ perform cat and camels (**》p.187**), back rotations (**》p.203**), McKenzie extensions (**》p.192**), neural glides (**》p.162**), and knees-to-chest stretches (**》p.202**).

### INTERMEDIATE STAGE ▶

- If you are now able to perform daily activities with a reduced level of discomfort, your therapist may:
  ▸ check for muscle imbalances and shortening of your muscles.
  ▸ recommend that you perform stretches for your hamstrings (**》p.196**), hip flexors (**》p.209**), quadriceps (**》p.196**), calves (**》p.198**), adductors (**》p.197**), and latissimus dorsi (**》p.196**).
  ▸ recommend a strengthening programme.
- You may begin:
  ▸ low-intensity, core-stability exercises such as four-point supine knee lifts (**》p.204**), clams (**》p.181**), bridges (**》p.195**), and curl-ups (**》p.186**).
  ▸ non-impact cardiovascular exercises such as fast walking and using a cross-trainer. Start with 5 minutes and gradually increase the duration.
- If your pain is not improving or is getting worse, you should:
  ▸ return to your doctor for review.

### ADVANCED STAGE

- If you are now pain-free, or nearly pain-free, and your range of spinal movement has returned to normal, you may:
  ▸ begin exercises such as kneeling supermans (**》p.191**), prone arm and leg lifts (**》p.210**), bridges (**》p.195**), curl-ups (**》p.186**), curl-ups on the Swiss ball (**》p.186**), Swiss ball side crunches (**》p.190**), Swiss ball back extensions (**》p.170**), and Swiss ball roll-outs (**》p.212**). Gradually increase the number of reps and sets, as pain allows.
  ▸ go back to sports or activities, gradually increasing effort and duration.
- If your pain is not improving or is getting worse, you should:
  ▸ return to your doctor for review.

## TREATMENT – DISC HERNIATION AND SCIATICA

➕ SEEK IMMEDIATE MEDICAL ATTENTION

### MEDICAL

| IMMEDIATE ▶ | SHORT TERM ▶ | MEDIUM TERM ▶ | LONG TERM |
|---|---|---|---|
| ■ If you suspect your pain is caused by sciatica, you should:<br>▶ consult your doctor for examination, diagnosis, and prescription of strong painkillers.<br>▶ find a comfortable position, either lying in the Fowler position (»p.150) or sitting.<br>▶ be prepared to be unable to perform normal activities for 7–10 days. Mild cases usually resolve within 4–6 weeks without further treatment. | ■ If after 3 days you are able to move, you should:<br>▶ try a supine pelvic tilt (»p.200) or McKenzie extension (»p.192).<br>▶ avoid prolonged sitting, driving, and bending.<br>▶ follow the correct advice for basic movement (»pp.150–57).<br>■ If the pain increases when you are upright, you should:<br>▶ lie flat for short periods.<br>▶ seek advice from a physical therapist on exercise, back care, and posture (»table below).<br>■ If your sciatica is caused by piriformis syndrome (»p. 76), you should:<br>▶ try massage, stretching, and acupuncture. | ■ If after 7–10 days you are able to resume normal activities, you should:<br>▶ talk to your work supervisor or occupational health nurse about returning to work, if appropriate. Your doctor or physical therapist may be able to advise you on this.<br>■ If after 7–10 days you are unable to resume normal activities, consult your doctor or physical therapist, who may:<br>▶ give you further advice on exercise (»table below).<br>▶ refer you for an epidural steroid injection (»pp.86–87) or a nerve-root block (»pp.86–87). This should happen within 2–12 weeks. | ■ If after 6–8 weeks you have regained nearly normal function, you should:<br>▶ observe good back care and rebuild your fitness through a recommended exercise programme (»table below).<br>■ If after 6–8 weeks you are not recovering as expected, you should:<br>▶ seek further advice from your doctor, who may arrange an MRI (»pp.82–83).<br>■ If you have not responded to therapy within 3 months, then:<br>▶ your doctor may refer you to a spinal surgeon to consider removing disc protrusions that may be causing pain (»pp.88–89). |

### PHYSIOTHERAPY

| EARLY STAGE ▶ | INTERMEDIATE STAGE ▶ | ADVANCED STAGE |
|---|---|---|
| ■ Once your doctor has referred you, your therapist will perform a thorough assessment. Depending on the findings of the assessment, your therapist may:<br>▶ perform soft-tissue mobilization and spinal-joint mobilization (»pp.90–95), and acupuncture (»pp.100–01), to relieve pain.<br>▶ apply tape to your leg and buttock to reduce neuro-muscular tension.<br>■ If you have a lateral shift in your spine, your therapist may:<br>▶ teach you the procedure for self-correction (»pp.90–93).<br>▶ advise you to perform side glides (»p.206) to centralize your pain. If your pain increases or moves to your legs, stop.<br>■ Once your pain has centralized, or if you have no lateral shift, your therapist may:<br>▶ suggest performing McKenzie extensions (»p.192; 202) as a form of self-mobilization several times a day, 10 reps each time.<br>■ You should:<br>▶ avoid slouching, and use a lumbar support when you sit.<br>▶ use a raised toilet seat and laxatives to ease pressure during defecation. | ■ If your condition has improved, and you are able to perform daily activities with less discomfort, your therapist will:<br>▶ select passive joint-mobilization techniques (»pp.90–95) to restore mobility in your lower back.<br>■ You may begin:<br>▶ cat and camels (»p.187), Lancelot stretches (»p.197), quad stretches (»p.196), hamstring stretches (»p.196), and hip flexor stretches (»p.209).<br>▶ low-intensity core exercises such as kneeling supermans (»p.191), bridges (»p.195), four-point supine knee lifts (»p.204), and dead bugs (»p.182).<br>▶ hamstring stretches, levels 1–2 (»p.196), and simple leg kicks, if the pain is in the front of your thigh.<br>▶ exercising on a cross-trainer.<br>■ If your pain is not improving or is getting worse, you should:<br>▶ return to your doctor for review. | ■ If you have a full range of movement, good postural muscle strength, and little or no pain during daily activities, you may begin:<br>▶ low-intensity running, swimming, and aqua aerobics.<br>▶ a training programme, gradually increasing the number of reps and the duration, as pain allows.<br>▶ exercises such as stationary lunges (»p.207), psoas lunges (»p.209), reverse lunges with knee lifts (»p.208), weight-based strengthening exercises for your flexor, abductor, and extensor muscles, Swiss ball roll-outs (»p.212), curl-ups on a Swiss ball (»p.186), Swiss ball side crunches (»p.190), and Swiss ball side crunches with twists (»p.190).<br>■ If your pain is not improving or is getting worse, you should:<br>▶ return to your doctor for review. |

# TREATMENT – SACROILIAC STRAIN

## MEDICAL

| IMMEDIATE ▶ | SHORT TERM ▶ | MEDIUM TERM ▶ | LONG TERM |
|---|---|---|---|
| ■ If you suspect your pain is caused by a sacroiliac strain, you should:<br>▶ adopt a position or movement of comfort such as sitting, gentle walking, or exercises (**》table below**).<br>▶ use ice packs for a maximum of 15 minutes every 2 hours for the first day of pain.<br>▶ take paracetamol or ibuprofen in recommended dosages for the first few days of pain.<br>▶ try not to rest for more than 2–3 days. | ■ If, after 3 days, the pain has settled, you should:<br>▶ seek advice from a registered physical therapist if it recurs.<br>▶ ensure you are following the correct advice for performing exercises (**》table below**).<br>■ If, after 3 days, the pain has not settled, you should:<br>▶ consult your doctor or physical therapist for examination, manipulation, and an exercise programme (**》table below**). | ■ If, after several weeks, you are progressing as expected, you should:<br>▶ continue to perform your exercise programme (**》table below**).<br>■ If, after several weeks, you are still unable to resume normal activities, you should:<br>▶ consult your doctor or physical therapist for further examination, advice, or treatment.<br>▶ seek further manual therapy, manipulation, and more specific guidance on exercise (**》table below**). | ■ If, after 6–8 weeks, you have recovered nearly normal function, you should:<br>▶ observe good back care and rebuild your fitness through an exercise programme (**》table below**).<br>■ If, after 6–8 months, you still have recurring pain, you should:<br>▶ seek further advice from a musculoskeletal physician, who may give you diagnostic blocks to the joint or prolotherapy injections (**》pp.86–87**) to strengthen the ligaments and stabilize the joint. |

## PHYSIOTHERAPY

| EARLY STAGE ▶ | INTERMEDIATE STAGE ▶ | ADVANCED STAGE |
|---|---|---|
| ■ Once your doctor has referred you, your therapist will perform a thorough assessment. Depending on the findings of the assessment, your therapist may:<br>▶ perform soft-tissue mobilization (**》pp.98–99**) and gentle joint-mobilization techniques (**》pp.90–95**).<br>▶ apply ultrasound (**》p.92**).<br>▶ strap your back for comfort and support (**》p.93**).<br>▶ advise you to apply ice and rest frequently, lying on your side with the painful side uppermost and a pillow between your knees.<br>▶ suggest using a supportive sacroiliac belt, especially if your sacroiliac joint is painful (this may be pre-childbirth, post-childbirth, or post-trauma). Wear the belt during activities, and take it off when sitting or lying down.<br>▶ advise you to minimize weight-bearing activities such as walking, standing, and sitting. | ■ If you are feeling less pain, your therapist will:<br>▶ perform active and passive mobilization techniques (**》pp.90–95**) to restore your joint mobility, and ensure optimal alignment and motor control of your pelvic girdle.<br>▶ advise you to work on the strength and endurance of your quadratus lumborum, gluteus medius, and gluteus maximus muscles.<br>▶ recommend you perform prone arm and leg lifts (**》p.210**), kneeling supermans (**》p.191**), Swiss ball twists (**》p.187**), lying waist twists (**》p.184**), isometric hip flexions (**》p.184**), side planks from knees (**》p.188**), clams (**》p.181**), isometric hip abductions lying sideways (**》p.194**), side-lying leg raises (**》p.192**), hip-hitchers (**》p.180**), kneeling hip flexors (**》p.194**), and single-leg bridges (**》p.195**). Increase the number of reps and sets as your fitness and strength improve, as pain allows.<br>■ If your pain is not improving or is getting worse, you should:<br>▶ return to your specialist for review. | ■ If you are nearly pain-free, you may:<br>▶ stabilize your lower back by performing stationary lunges (**》p.207**), forward lunges (**》p.207**), and reverse lunges with knee lifts (**》p.208**).<br>▶ try chair squats (**》p.213**) and regular squats (**》p.179**).<br>▶ begin sensorimotor training such as single-leg stands (**》p.199**).<br>▶ gradually increase the number of reps and sets when performing these exercises in order to build muscle endurance.<br>▶ introduce aerobic exercises such as jogging, hopping, and jumping.<br>■ If your pain is not improving or is getting worse, you should:<br>▶ return to your specialist for review. |

# CHRONIC LOW-BACK PAIN

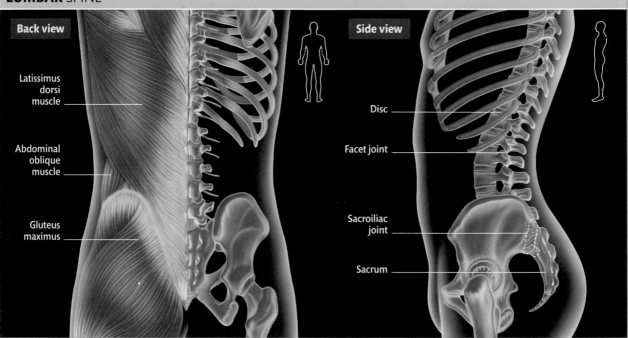

**LUMBAR** SPINE

**Back view**

Latissimus dorsi muscle

Abdominal oblique muscle

Gluteus maximus

**Side view**

Disc

Facet joint

Sacroiliac joint

Sacrum

**Chronic low-back pain** is pain in the lumbar region of your spine that has lasted for more than three months. It may be constant or intermittent, mild or severe, and is often caused by certain postures or activities. Pain may consist of acute episodes with little pain in between, or constant pain with occasional flare-ups. Its impact on your life will be dictated by these factors.

## CAUSES

In 70 per cent of cases of chronic low-back pain, the cause is one of the following: a lumbar disc internal strain or disruption (**》p.67**), a facet joint problem (**》p.68**), or a strain of the sacroiliac joint and/or ligaments (**》p.69**). These causes can sometimes be determined by diagnostic blocks (**》p.87**). Occasionally, the pain is caused by a combination of spinal segment changes that lead to an "instability" syndrome (**》p.66**). There are many other physical and environmental factors that can cause low-back pain, and most of these can be addressed. Serious conditions, such as cancer or fracture, account for less than one per cent of low-back pain.

Sometimes, however, there will be no identifiable cause of your pain – this is commonly known as non-specific low-back pain.

## SYMPTOMS

Facet joint pain tends to occur in older people and is usually worse with upright activity. Recurrent episodes of more severe pain can be triggered by trivial factors such as twisting, stooping, sneezing, lifting, or prolonged sitting. Your back may feel weak and unstable (known as "lumbar instability"). Chronic sacroiliac pain can cause this symptom, but the pain will be in your buttock, rather than your lumbar area. At times pain may shoot or move down one of your legs, like sciatica – this is often the result of a disc injury. The pain can develop more nerve-related features, such as burning sensations.

## RISKS AND COMPLICATIONS

If serious causes of disease and pathology such as infection or tumour have been ruled out, the risks of chronic low-back pain are both psychological and physical: your mood and sleep patterns may become disturbed and the effect on your life may cause frustration and even depression.

# TREATMENT – DISC-RELATED PAIN

## MEDICAL

| IMMEDIATE ▶ | SHORT TERM ▶ | MEDIUM TERM ▶ | LONG TERM |
|---|---|---|---|
| ■ If your pain has been diagnosed as coming from a disc, you should: <br> ▶ stay as active as you can. <br> ▶ take paracetamol or ibuprofen in recommended dosages, sparingly, on a regular schedule, rather than only when the pain becomes unbearable. <br> ▶ consult your doctor or physical therapist for advice on how to reduce disc pressure and strain (**»table below**). | ■ If the pain is moderate or severe and you have not improved with physical therapy, your doctor will refer you to a specialist who may: <br> ▶ suggest a rehabilitation programme to improve your control of movement, posture, strength, flexibility, and general fitness (**»table below**). | ■ If further treatment does not help, your specialist may: <br> ▶ give you further imaging investigations, psychological assessment, and/or diagnostic blocks of specific structures in your spine (**»pp.86–87**). <br> ▶ recommend a trial of intradiscal therapy of the disc (**»pp.86–87**). <br> ▶ consider prolotherapy (**»pp.86–87**) to control segmental strain on the disc <br> ▶ recommend an operation, to fuse two vertebrae together to strengthen the spine, or to replace the damaged disc altogether (**»pp.88–89**). | ■ If you continue to experience pain and no further treatment is available, you should seek advice from a specialist who may: <br> ▶ provide a pain-management programme that includes physical and psychological help (**»table below**). <br> ▶ help you to moderate your expectation of what you can do. <br> ▶ advise you on how to use medication sensibly and appropriately. <br> ▶ advise you on how to cope with your disability and live with minimum disruption to your daily routine. |

## PHYSIOTHERAPY

| EARLY STAGE ▶ | INTERMEDIATE STAGE ▶ | ADVANCED STAGE |
|---|---|---|
| ■ Once your doctor has referred you, your therapist will perform a thorough assessment. Depending on the findings of the assessment, your therapist may: <br> ▶ perform manual techniques to increase soft-tissue pliability, if you have myofascial tension. <br> ▶ perform acupuncture for pain relief (**»p.100–01**). <br> ▶ apply a tape to decrease neuromuscular tension, if you have buttock or leg pain. <br> ▶ suggest spinal extension exercises, such as McKenzie extensions (**»p.192**) or neural glides (**»p.162**). <br> ▶ teach you the best practice for sitting, working at a desk, driving, lifting, carrying, and sleeping (**»pp.124–57**). | ■ Depending on your progress, your therapist may: <br> ▶ suggest muscle-energy techniques (**»p.92**), and active dynamic rehabilitation to stabilize your lumbar spine. <br> ▶ assess your muscles for any imbalances and suggest an exercise programme to rectify any problems. <br> ■ You may begin: <br> ▶ low-level core exercises such as kneeling supermans level 1 (progressing in later stages to level 2) (**»p.191**), bridges (**»p.195**), four-point supine knee lifts (**»p.204**), and dead bugs (**»p.182**). <br> ▶ mobilizing exercises such as cat and camels (**»p.187**), back rotations (**»p.203**), lying waist twists (**»p.184**), and single-leg elongations (**»p.205**). <br> ■ If your pain is not improving or is getting worse, you should: <br> ▶ return to your doctor for review. | ■ If you have recovered a full range of movement in your lumbar region, and you are able to perform daily activities with less pain and discomfort, you may: <br> ▶ perform moderate- to high-level core exercises such as planks from knees (**»p.188**), side planks levels 1–2 (**»p.189**), and single-leg bridges (**»p.195**). <br> ■ Your therapist may: <br> ▶ suggest that you start cardiovascular training to build endurance, preventing fatigue of the muscles that stabilize your spine. Aqua aerobics and using cross-trainers are best for this. <br> ▶ perform a functional kinetic chain exercise programme to restore balance in your body. <br> ■ If your pain is not improving or is getting worse, you should: <br> ▶ return to your doctor for review. |

## TREATMENT – FACET JOINT PAIN

### MEDICAL

| IMMEDIATE ▶ | SHORT TERM ▶ | MEDIUM TERM ▶ | LONG TERM |
|---|---|---|---|
| ■ If your pain has been diagnosed as the result of facet joint problems, you should:<br>▶ stay as active as you can.<br>▶ take paracetamol or ibuprofen in recommended dosages, sparingly, on a regular schedule.<br>▶ learn what relieves pain and what increases it.<br>▶ remember that pain doesn't mean harm or more injury.<br>▶ consult your doctor or physical therapist (**»table below**). | ■ If the pain is moderate or severe and has not improved with treatment and physical therapy, you should seek more specialist help. Your specialist may:<br>▶ give you further imaging investigations (**»pp.82–83**), psychological assessment, and/or diagnostic blocks of the facet joint blocks in your spine (**»pp.86–87**).<br>▶ perform radiofrequency denervation (**»pp.86–87**) to bring lasting relief from pain. | ■ If further treatment does not help, your specialist may:<br>▶ suggest a rehabilitation programme to improve your control of movement, posture, strength, flexibility, and general fitness (**»table below**).<br>▶ recommend an operation to fuse two vertebrae together to strengthen your spine (**»pp.88–89**). | ■ If you continue to feel pain, and no further treatment is available, you should seek advice from a specialist on how to:<br>▶ moderate your expectation of what you can do.<br>▶ use medication sensibly and appropriately.<br>▶ cope with your disability.<br>▶ live with minimum disruption to your daily routine. |

### PHYSIOTHERAPY

| EARLY STAGE ▶ | INTERMEDIATE STAGE ▶ | ADVANCED STAGE |
|---|---|---|
| ■ Once your doctor has referred you, your therapist will perform a thorough assessment. Depending on the findings of the assessment, your therapist may:<br>▶ perform gentle manual rhythmic traction on your legs (**»pp.94–95**), passive rotational joint mobilizations (**»pp.90–91**), specific and non-specific rotational manipulations (**»p.94**), and acupuncture for pain relief (**»pp.100–01**).<br>■ Your therapist may:<br>▶ recommend relaxation techniques such as autogenic training and progressive relaxation therapy (**»pp.102–03**).<br>▶ suggest gentle stretching and self-mobilizing techniques such as single-leg elongations (**»p.205**), hip-hitchers (**»p.180**), side glides (**»p.206**), supine pelvic tilts (**»p.200**), seated pelvic tilts (**»p.201**), alligators (**»p.184**), knees-to-chest stretches (**»p.202**), back rotations (**»p.203**), child's poses (**»p.212**), and cat and camels (**»p.187**). | ■ If you have an almost full range of movement in your lumbar region and are experiencing slightly less pain, you may:<br>▶ begin a functional rehabilitation programme including gentle core-stability exercises such as kneeling supermans (**»p.191**), prone arm and leg lifts (**»p.210**), four-point supine knee lifts (**»p.204**), bridges (**»p.195**), and dead bugs (**»p.182**).<br>▶ continue stretching, adding modified self-traction press-ups (**»p.180**) and isometric hip flexions (**»p.205**) to your exercise programme.<br>■ Your therapist may:<br>▶ advise you on aerobic training, such as using a cross-trainer and taking up aqua aerobics.<br>■ If your pain is not improving or is getting worse, you should:<br>▶ return to your doctor for review. | ■ If you have a full range of movement in your lumbar region and are pain-free, you may:<br>▶ begin more intense stabilizing exercises such as planks from knees (**»p.188**), progressing to prone planks (**»p.188**), Swiss ball roll-outs (**»p.212**), Swiss ball twists (**»p.187**), planks levels 1–2 (**»p.188**), and single-leg bridges (**»p.195**).<br>▶ perform sensorimotor training such as single-leg stands (**»p.199**).<br>▶ extend your cardiovascular training to running on the treadmill or outdoors, preferably on soft ground.<br>▶ attend yoga or Pilates classes.<br>▶ resume other sports by gradually increasing effort and duration, as pain allows.<br>■ If your pain is not improving or is getting worse, you should:<br>▶ return to your doctor for review. |

## TREATMENT – SPONDYLOLYSIS AND SPONDYLOLISTHESIS

### MEDICAL

| IMMEDIATE ▶ | SHORT TERM ▶ | MEDIUM TERM ▶ | LONG TERM |
|---|---|---|---|
| ■ If your pain has been diagnosed as the result of spondylolysis or spondylolisthesis, you should:<br>▶ follow the advice given by your physical therapist or specialist.<br>▶ perform any exercises you have been prescribed by your therapist.<br>▶ be patient. | ■ If treatment and exercise do not help, your doctor may:<br>▶ send you for an X-ray (»p.82).<br>■ If the X-rays show evidence of spondylolysis or spondylolisthesis, your doctor may:<br>▶ send you for further investigations with a specialist including an MRI, bone, or CT scan (»pp.82–83). | ■ Depending on the results of further testing, your specialist may:<br>▶ attempt to control your symptoms by suggesting you modify your activities, that is, maintaining fitness while avoiding competitive sport and continuing your rehabilitation programme (»table below). This may last for 3–6 months.<br>▶ recommend an operation to fuse two vertebrae together to strengthen your spine (»pp.88–89). | ■ If you continue to feel pain, and no further treatment is available, you should seek advice from a specialist on how to:<br>▶ moderate your expectation of what you can do.<br>▶ use medication sensibly and appropriately.<br>▶ cope with your disability.<br>▶ live with minimum disruption to your daily routine. |

### PHYSIOTHERAPY

| EARLY STAGE ▶ | INTERMEDIATE STAGE ▶ | ADVANCED STAGE |
|---|---|---|
| ■ Once your doctor has referred you, your therapist will perform a thorough assessment. Depending on the findings of the assessment, your therapist may:<br>▶ perform manual passive joint mobilization (»pp.90–95), non-specific passive rotational manipulations (»pp.90–95), neuro-mobilization techniques (»p.92), segmental spinal movements (»pp.94–95), and acupuncture (»pp.100–01) to relieve pain.<br>▶ advise you to sit in a flexed position, and lie on your back with a pillow under your knees or in a crook position (»pp.150–51).<br>▶ teach you relaxation techniques such as autogenic or Jacobson training (»pp.102–03), and isometric hip flexions (»p.205) to increase the strength of your deep stabilizing muscles.<br>■ You may:<br>▶ perform supine pelvic tilts (»p.200), kneeling pelvic tilts (»p.200), seated pelvic tilts (»p.201), knees-to-chest stretches (»p.202), and neural glides (»p.162). | ■ If you are experiencing slightly less pain, your therapist may:<br>▶ assess any imbalances around your pelvic area and lower limbs.<br>▶ advise you to stretch any tight muscles, and strengthen your weak ones.<br>■ You may now:<br>▶ progress to low-level core-stabilizing exercises such as four-point supine knee lifts (»p.204), oblique crunches (»p.211), curl-ups levels 1–3 (»p.186), clams (»p.181), and dead bugs (»p.182).<br>▶ begin sensorimotor training (»p.93), gradually increasing in difficulty, using special equipment such as a wobble board and air cushion.<br>▶ begin cardiovascular work in the form of aqua aerobics or exercise on a cross-trainer, gradually increasing in speed and duration, as pain allows.<br>■ If your pain is not improving or is getting worse, you should:<br>▶ return to your doctor for review. | ■ If you are experiencing significantly less pain, you may begin:<br>▶ more advanced core-stabilizing exercises such as kneeling supermans (»p.191), planks from knees (»p.188), side planks level 1 (»p.189), Swiss ball roll-outs (»p.212), and curl-ups (»p.186).<br>▶ increasing your leg strength by practising sit-to-stand and stand-to-sit chair squats (»p.213), stationary lunges (»p.207), forward lunges (»p.207), and reverse lunges with knee lifts (»p.208).<br>▶ resuming sports, gradually increasing the load and duration, bearing in mind that you may have to modify your technique to accommodate pain. Sports involving spinal extension, such as gymnastics, dance, cricket, and tennis, are the most hazardous activities for these conditions, and should be approached with caution.<br>■ If your pain is not improving or is getting worse, you should:<br>▶ return to your doctor for review. |

# TREATMENT – INSTABILITY SYNDROME AND SACROILIAC STRAIN

## MEDICAL

### IMMEDIATE ▶

■ If your pain has been diagnosed as the result of an instability syndrome, you should:
▶ stay as active as you can.
▶ take paracetamol or ibuprofen in recommended dosages when pain flares up.
▶ try to manage the phases in between flare-ups by building up your exercise programme (»**table below**).
▶ learn what triggers acute episodes, and find ways to avoid these activities or movements.

### SHORT TERM ▶

■ You doctor may refer you to a specialist who understands the nature of your problem. Your specialist may:
▶ recommend manual treatment to reduce the length of instability episodes.
▶ suggest specific stabilizing exercises and general exercise to help your back feel more stable and provide partial protection (»**table below**).

### MEDIUM TERM ▶

■ Your specialist may recommend that you:
▶ try a 3–6 month period of functional rehabilitation, including stabilizing exercises and/or Pilates-like exercises (»**table below**).
▶ undergo a course of prolotherapy to the ligaments of the involved segments of the spine or sacroiliac joints (»**pp.86–87**).
▶ assess whether it will be beneficial to surgically fuse two vertebrae, or replace the disc altogether (»**pp.88–89**).

### LONG TERM

■ If your specialist has exhausted all treatment options and you are still experiencing pain, you should:
▶ request a pain-management programme to help minimize the physical and psychological impact of pain on your life.

## PHYSIOTHERAPY

### EARLY STAGE ▶

■ Once your doctor has referred you, your therapist will perform a thorough assessment. Depending on the findings of the assessment, your therapist may:
▶ suggest manual passive mobilizations of hypomobile joints (often accompanying hypermobile segments).
▶ perform soft-tissue mobilization.
▶ apply strapping to stabilize hypermobile segments, or suggest you use an sacroiliac joint belt.
▶ advise you to change your daily routine and to practise crouching within pain-free limits.
▶ advise you to avoid sitting with your legs crossed, bending forwards and twisting, and stretching the joint.
■ You may:
▶ start isometric lumbar and sacroiliac joint stabilizing exercises such as bracing your abdomen and back muscles.
▶ try dynamic exercises such as kneeling supermans (»**p.191**), four-point supine knee lifts (»**p.204**), and prone arm and leg lifts (»**p.210**).

### INTERMEDIATE STAGE ▶

■ If you are experiencing less pain due to improved stability, you may:
▶ stretch tight muscles such as your hip adductors with adductor stretches (2) (»**p.197**), piriformis stretches (»**p.198**), and lying waist twists (»**p.184**).
▶ strengthen weak muscles such as your gluteus maximus and gluteus medius with side-lying leg raises (»**p.193**), reverse leg raises (»**p.193**), and clams (»**p.181**).
▶ progress to more advanced stabilizing exercises such as planks from knees (»**p.188**), side planks level 1(»**p.189**), bridges (»**p.195**), and prone arm and leg lifts (»**p.210**), gradually increasing the length of time holding the contraction and the number of reps in the set, as pain allows. To improve your endurance, gradually increase the number of sets.
▶ start walking on the treadmill or outdoors, gradually increasing the speed and distance. During these activities you should brace your core muscles at 30 per cent of your maximum.

### ADVANCED STAGE

■ If you are free of pain with good stability in your lumbar region and sacroiliac joint, you may:
▶ begin sensorimotor training such as single-leg stands (»**p.199**).
▶ introduce squats and lunges, beginning with stationary lunges (»**p.207**), forward lunges (»**p.207**), and reverse lunges with knee lifts (»**p.208**).
▶ begin working your rectus abdominis, obliques, and quadratus lumborum muscles by performing curl-ups (»**p.186**), planks (»**p.188**), and side planks, level 2 (»**p.189**), before progressing to Swiss ball side crunches (»**p.190**), and Swiss ball side crunches with twists (»**p.190**).
▶ develop your cardiorespiratory workout by using a cross-trainer and running on a treadmill, gradually increasing the duration.

## TREATMENT – NON-SPECIFIC/LUMBAR DYSFUNCTION

### MEDICAL

| IMMEDIATE ▶ | SHORT TERM ▶ | MEDIUM TERM ▶ | LONG TERM |
|---|---|---|---|
| ■ If your pain has been diagnosed as the result of a lumbar dysfunction, and a solution cannot be found, you should:<br>▶ stay as active as you can (**》table below**).<br>▶ take paracetamol or ibuprofen in recommended dosages, sparingly, on a regular schedule, rather than only when the pain becomes unbearable.<br>▶ learn what your back can and cannot cope with.<br>▶ remember that pain does not necessarily indicate harm or further injury. | ■ If the pain is moderate or severe, and physiotherapy has not improved your condition, your doctor may refer you to a specialist. Your specialist may:<br>▶ decide whether to perform further imaging investigations, psychological assessment, and/or diagnostic blocks (**》p.87**) of specific structures in your spine. | ■ If your condition is not improving, your specialist may:<br>▶ suggest a functional rehabilitation programme to improve your strength, flexibility, control of movement and posture, and general fitness (**》table below**).<br>▶ suggest a pain-management programme, which includes psychological assistance to help you minimize the impact of living with pain. | ■ After a year or two, if you continue to feel pain, and no further treatment is available, you should seek advice from your specialist on how to:<br>▶ moderate your expectation of what you can do.<br>▶ use medication sensibly and appropriately.<br>▶ cope with your disability.<br>▶ live with minimum disruption to your daily routine.<br>▶ get in touch with patient self-help organizations and other people suffering from the same condition. |

### PHYSIOTHERAPY

| EARLY STAGE ▶ | INTERMEDIATE STAGE ▶ | ADVANCED STAGE |
|---|---|---|
| ■ Once your doctor has referred you, your therapist will perform a thorough assessment. Depending on the findings of the assessment, your therapist may:<br>▶ perform soft tissue and joint mobilization and manipulation.<br>▶ teach you posture (**》pp.112–15**) and relaxation techniques (**》pp.102–03**).<br>▶ recommend acupuncture (**》pp.100–01**).<br>▶ suggest specific exercises that address your pain.<br>▶ apply strapping to immobilize hypermobile segments, or use special tape to facilitate more functional movement of specific segments (**》p.93**).<br>▶ suggest incorporating McKenzie extensions (**》p.192**) and standing back extensions (**》p.202**), or neuro-mobilization exercises such as neural glides (**》p.162**), into your exercise programme.<br>▶ teach you about the physiology of pain to help you deal with it more successfully. | ■ If your pain has diminished and you are able to perform daily activities more easily, you should:<br>▶ pace yourself to prevent flare-ups of your condition.<br>■ Your therapist may:<br>▶ address any muscle shortening or imbalance, and design an exercise programme for you.<br>■ Your therapist may advise you to begin:<br>▶ low-level core stability exercises, such as kneeling supermans (**》p.191**), four-point supine knee lifts (**》p.204**), and bridges (**》p.195**).<br>▶ more advanced mobilizing exercises such as Swiss ball back extensions (**》p.170**), supine pelvic tilts (**》p.200**), single-leg elongations (**》p.205**), and back rotations (**》pp.173; 203**).<br>▶ neural mobility exercises such as prone knee bends (**》p.206**), one-leg circles (**》p.183**), and neural glides (**》p.162**)<br>▶ non-impact conditioning exercises such as reclined cycling, cross-trainer workouts, and walking on a treadmill or outdoors.<br>■ If your pain is not improving or is getting worse, you should:<br>▶ return to your doctor for review. | ■ If you are able to perform daily activities without pain, you may begin:<br>▶ moderate-level core exercises such as curl-ups (**》p.186**), Swiss ball twists (**》p.187**), side crunches (**》p.211**), prone arm and leg lifts (**》p.210**), planks from knees (**》p.188**), planks (**》p.188**), single-leg bridges (**》p.195**), and side planks (**》p.189**); progressing to higher levels.<br>▶ functional training such as squats (**》p.179**), stationary lunges (**》p.207**), forward lunges (**》p.207**), reverse lunges with knee lifts (**》p.208**), and walking lunges (**》p.179**).<br>▶ sensorimotor training such as single-leg stands (**》p.199**).<br>▶ running on a treadmill or on soft ground outdoors.<br>■ If you do not enjoy sports, you should:<br>▶ keep doing the exercises listed in the intermediate stage (**》left**), but increase the number of repetitions and sets. This will help you build up your muscle strength and endurance, which in the long term will prevent the pain from recurring.<br>■ If your pain is not improving or is getting worse, you should:<br>▶ return to your doctor for review. |

# CHRONIC SCIATICA

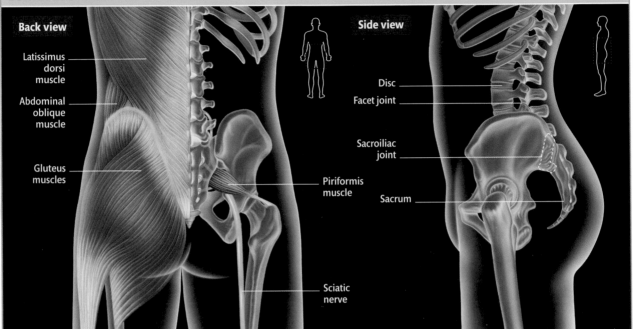

**LUMBAR SPINE** AND UPPER LEG

Back view
- Latissimus dorsi muscle
- Abdominal oblique muscle
- Gluteus muscles

Side view
- Disc
- Facet joint
- Sacroiliac joint
- Piriformis muscle
- Sacrum
- Sciatic nerve

**When a disc** in your lower back presses on the sciatic nerve, you will feel pain running down one leg, possibly accompanied by numbness or tingling in the nerve root. Pain in this area is known as sciatica. Normally, this pain subsides within 3–6 months: if it persists for longer it is described as chronic.

## CAUSES

Chronic sciatica may be the result of stenosis (》**p.73**) of the central or lateral canals of the spine, or of irritation of the nerve by the piriformis muscle (》**p.76**). The former is diagnosed by an MRI or CT scan, while the latter is diagnosed by physical examination or how your piriformis muscle responds to an anaesthetic block (》**pp.86–87**).

## SYMPTOMS

Chronic nerve-root pain can be just like acute nerve-root pain, though not as severe. You may feel a shooting pain in your affected leg, accompanied by a tingling electrical sensation. Changes in your spinal cord and brain – the central nervous system – can lead to nerve-related ("neuropathic") symptoms such as a burning sensation. You may feel pressure deep in your leg, which may also "squeeze" or pulsate. You may have numbness in your leg, and a tingling feeling, similar to pins and needles. You may experience hypersensitivity to light touch or pressure, and normal movement may cause you pain. Your skin may discolour, sweat, or appear to swell and be sensitive to temperature change. All these neuropathic symptoms indicate structural changes in your affected nerve, its cells, and the wiring in your spinal cord and brain.

## RISKS AND COMPLICATIONS

There is no real risk of physical complications from chronic sciatic pain. However, the consequences of living with pain over a prolonged period of time can lead to practical complications, including difficulty staying active and continuing to work, and the psychological challenge related to remaining optimistic about your prospect of continuing to lead a full life.

## TREATMENT – NON-SPECIFIC NERVE-ROOT PAIN

**MEDICAL**

| IMMEDIATE ▶ | SHORT TERM ▶ | MEDIUM TERM ▶ | LONG TERM |
|---|---|---|---|
| ■ If the cause of your pain is non-specific chronic nerve-root pain, you should:<br>▶ discuss with your specialist whether all testing and treatment options have been considered.<br>■ Your specialist may:<br>▶ suggest further imaging investigations to find a cause (**»pp.82–83**).<br>▶ advise on options such as injections (epidural or nerve block with steroids) (**»pp.86–87**), if they have not already been tried.<br>▶ consider surgery to relieve pressure on the damaged nerve. | ■ If treatment does not help to relieve your pain, you should:<br>▶ ask your doctor about medication such as amitryptyline. Gabapentin or pregabalin can also help reduce neuropathic pain.<br>▶ ask your doctor about a trial of TENS (transcutaneous electrical nerve stimulation) (**»p.104**), in which the nerves are stimulated by an electric current. | ■ If you are still feeling pain after specialist treatment and advice, you should:<br>▶ moderate your expectation of what you can do.<br>▶ use painkillers sparingly but on a regular schedule.<br>▶ follow a home exercise programme (**»table below**).<br>▶ practise self-help techniques such as relaxation, mindfulness, or meditation (**»pp.102–03**).<br>▶ request a pain-management programme to help you cope with the pain. | ■ For many people, the pain from chronic sciatica does improve very slowly over time. If you continue to feel pain, you should:<br>▶ not exert yourself too heavily until you have learned to pace your activities and listen to your body.<br>▶ be realistic about what you can achieve.<br>▶ continue to follow a home exercise programme (**»table below**). |

**PHYSIOTHERAPY**

| EARLY STAGE ▶ | INTERMEDIATE STAGE ▶ | ADVANCED STAGE |
|---|---|---|
| ■ Once your doctor has referred you, your therapist will perform a thorough assessment. Depending on the findings of the assessment, your therapist may:<br>▶ suggest manual therapies such as spinal mobilization and manipulation (**»pp.90–95**), soft-tissue mobilization (**»pp.98–99**), neuromobilization (**»p.92**), and muscle-energy techniques (**»p.92**).<br>▶ teach you about posture (**»pp.112–15**), basic ergonomics (**»pp.124–27**), and relaxation techniques (**»pp.102–03**).<br>▶ recommend acupuncture (**»pp.100–01**).<br>▶ advise you on an appropriate rehabilitation programme.<br>■ You may begin:<br>▶ neural glides (**»p.162**) and side glides (**»p.206**). Start gently, with a few reps each time; gradually increase the reps but never hold these positions for longer than 2 seconds.<br>▶ perform self-traction techniques, such as modified press-ups (**»p.180**) and single-leg elongations (**»p.205**). | ■ If your symptoms have subsided, you may:<br>▶ begin mobilizing exercises such as supine pelvic tilts (**»p.200**), kneeling pelvic tilts (**»p.200**), knees-to-chest stretches (**»p.202**), and back rotations (**»pp.173; 203**).<br>▶ perform strengthening exercises such as kneeling supermans (**»p.191**), curl-ups (**»p.186**), oblique crunches (**»p.211**), side planks level 1 (**»p.189**), reverse leg raises (**»p.193**), and bridges (**»p.195**).<br>▶ begin sensorimotor training such as single-leg stands (**»p.199**), walking on the treadmill or outside, and aqua aerobics.<br>■ If you have shortened muscles, your therapist may:<br>▶ advise you to incorporate leg raises (**»p.192**), adductor lifts (**»p.194**), hamstring stretches (**»p.196**), Lancelot stretches (**»p.197**), and hip flexor stretches (**»pp.209–10**) into your exercise programme.<br>■ If your pain is not improving or is getting worse, you should:<br>▶ return to your doctor for review. | ■ If you can perform most daily activities without pain and demonstrate an increased range of movement, you may:<br>▶ start cardiovascular advanced training using a cross-trainer, running on a treadmill or outside on soft ground.<br>▶ consider participating in less strenuous activities such as yoga, Pilates, or t'ai chi.<br>■ If your pain is not improving or is getting worse, you should:<br>▶ return to your doctor for review. |

## TREATMENT – SPINAL STENOSIS

### MEDICAL

| IMMEDIATE ▶ | SHORT TERM ▶ | MEDIUM TERM ▶ | LONG TERM |
|---|---|---|---|
| ■ If your pain is caused by spinal stenosis, you should:<br>▶ learn how to stand and even walk with your spine slightly flexed (**》pp.112–14**).<br>▶ plan short trips within your limits, so that if the symptoms come on severely you can rest if you need to.<br>▶ carry a "shooting stick" (a stick with a seat attached) to prop yourself on.<br>▶ use a buggy or a walking frame to lean on. | ■ In order to treat your condition, your specialist will:<br>▶ order a scan to ascertain the severity of the problem and the number of spinal levels involved.<br>■ If your pain is not too disabling, you should:<br>▶ perform self-help measures to stay mobile. A physiotherapist can help you to adjust your posture to keep your spinal canal as wide as possible (**》table below**).<br>■ If your condition is getting worse, your specialist may:<br>▶ perform an epidural steroid injection. This can provide pain relief for 3–6 months or more. | ■ If your mobility is very limited or nerve damage is occurring, your specialist may:<br>▶ recommend surgery.<br>■ If one lumbar level is affected, a surgeon may:<br>▶ insert a spacer called an "X-stop" between your spinous processes to hold the canal open.<br>■ If two or more levels are affected, a surgeon may:<br>▶ remove a "window" of bone from the vertebral arch (lamina) of each level. This is known as "decompression". | ■ If your condition is stable, your specialist may:<br>▶ prescribe a course of 2–3 epidural injections (**》pp.86–87**) per year, for an indefinite period of time.<br>■ If your condition cannot be improved with surgery, or surgery is not appropriate, you should:<br>▶ help your condition by cycling longer distances rather than walking. |

### PHYSIOTHERAPY

| EARLY STAGE ▶ | INTERMEDIATE STAGE ▶ | ADVANCED STAGE |
|---|---|---|
| ■ Once your doctor has referred you, your therapist will perform a thorough assessment. Depending on the findings of the assessment, your therapist may:<br>▶ perform manual therapy such as spinal mobilizations and manipulations (**》pp.90–95**), soft tissue manipulations (**》p.91**), and neuro-mobilization (**》p.92**) to restore segmental mobility and improve neuro-muscular function.<br>▶ educate you in pain management (**》pp.142–47**), ergonomics (**》pp.124–27**), and relaxation techniques (**》pp.102–03**).<br>▶ recommend a functional training programme and a graded walking programme, if your pain level increases with walking.<br>■ You may be advised to:<br>▶ perform stretching exercises such as knees-to-chest stretches (**》p.202**), supine pelvic tilts (**》p.200**), child's poses (**》p.212**), and neural glides (**》p.162**).<br>▶ adopt forward flexing positions and avoid bending backwards. | ■ If you are now able to avoid painful positions and pace yourself, your therapist will:<br>▶ monitor your progress and continue to perform manual therapy if appropriate.<br>■ You may be advised to:<br>▶ perform low-level, core-strengthening exercises such as four-point supine knee lifts (**》p.204**), dead bugs (**》p.182**), and curl-ups levels 1–4 (**》p.186**).<br>▶ perform active and passive stretches of your hip flexors such as hip flexor stretches (**》p.209**), psoas lunges (**》p.209**), and kneeling hip flexors (**》p.210**).<br>▶ strengthen your hip abductors and extensors by performing bridges (**》p.195**), single-leg bridges (**》p.195**), clams (**》p.181**), side-lying leg raises (**》p.193**), and sensorimotor training such as single-leg stands (**》p.199**).<br>▶ gradually increase the number of repetitions, add ankle weights, and increase the number of sets for these exercises.<br>■ If your pain is not improving or is getting worse, you should:<br>▶ return to your doctor for review. | ■ If you are nearly pain-free, you may:<br>▶ perform more advanced core-stability exercises such as oblique crunches (**》p.211**), progressing to side crunches (**》p.211**) and Swiss ball twists (**》p.187**).<br>▶ try more advanced functional training exercises such as stationary lunges (**》p.207**), one-leg circles (**》p.183**), forward lunges (**》p.207**), reverse lunges with knee lifts (**》p.208**), walking lunges (**》p.179**), and squats (**》p.179**).<br>▶ increase the level of difficulty of your sensorimotor training by adding arm and leg movements; for example, throwing and catching a ball, and using a wobble board, an air cushion, or airex foam.<br>▶ add general conditioning exercises to your cardiovascular training. Aqua aerobics, cycling, and inclined treadmill walking are the most suitable for this condition.<br>■ If your pain is not improving or is getting worse, you should:<br>▶ return to your doctor for review. |

# TREATMENT – PIRIFORMIS SYNDROME

## MEDICAL

### IMMEDIATE ▶

- If you have a chronic pain in your buttock that travels down your leg, you should:
  ▶ seek a diagnosis from a registered physical therapist or musculoskeletal specialist.
  ▶ be aware that there are many possible causes of sciatic pain, and piriformis syndrome tends to be over-diagnosed. It is rarely possible to be certain that this condition is a primary cause of this kind of pain.
- Your specialist may:
  ▶ recommend a programme of stretching exercises to relieve pain (**》table below**).

### SHORT TERM ▶

- If you are able to move around normally, you should:
  ▶ avoid prolonged sitting on hard chairs or sitting with objects (such as a wallet) in your back pocket.
  ▶ perform the prescribed stretching exercises regularly.

### MEDIUM TERM ▶

- If your condition is not settling down, you should:
  ▶ consult a musculoskeletal specialist for further examination and a more specific diagnosis.
- If your specialist has ruled out other causes of pain, such as sacroiliitis or disc or dural irritation, he may:
  ▶ offer you an image-guided injection of the muscle with anaesthetic and steroid (**》pp.86–87**). If successful this may be followed with a botulinum injection.
  ▶ order further investigation with imaging studies to rule out more serious causes (**》pp.82–83**).

### LONG TERM

- If you have recovered well enough to regain most of your usual functions, you should:
  ▶ observe good back care (**》pp.112–15**) and rebuild your fitness through a recommended exercise programme (**》table below**).
  ▶ continue to perform your specific stretching exercises for 6 months.
  ▶ remember that it is rare for this condition to persist indefinitely or require surgery.

## PHYSIOTHERAPY

### EARLY STAGE ▶

- Once your doctor has referred you, your therapist will perform a thorough assessment. Depending on the findings of the assessment, and after other causes of your pain are eliminated, your therapist may:
  ▶ perform manual therapies such as soft tissue mobilization and muscle-energy techniques (**》p.92**).
  ▶ suggest passive and active stretching to the piriformis muscle.
  ▶ use electrotherapy treatment in order to relax the piriformis muscle and enhance the healing process.
  ▶ advise you on an appropriate rehabilitation programme.
  ▶ recommend acupuncture.
- You may be advised to perform:
  ▶ stretching exercises such as adductor stretches (**》p.197**), piriformis stretches (**》p.198**), and lying waist twists (**》p.184**).
  ▶ strengthening exercises such as clams (**》p.181**), side-lying leg raises (**》p.193**), reverse leg raises (**》p.193**), and bridges (**》p.195**).

### INTERMEDIATE STAGE ▶

- If you have less pain in your buttock and leg, your therapist may:
  ▶ screen your legs and pelvis area for any muscle imbalances, and prescribe specific stretching and strengthening exercises to balance your body.
- You may now:
  ▶ progress to more advanced strengthening exercises such as single-leg bridges (**》p.195**), squats (**》p.179**), and stationary lunges (**》p.207**).
  ▶ start low cardiovascular training on a bike, cross-trainer, or in water.
- If your pain is not improving or is getting worse, you should:
  ▶ return to your doctor for review.

### ADVANCED STAGE

- If you are now free of pain, your therapist may advise you to resume all physical activities. You may:
  ▶ start running, gradually increasing your speed and duration.
  ▶ continue with your stretching and strengthening programme in order to prevent further injuries.
  ▶ advance to a high-level, core-stability programme, incorporating exercises such as Swiss ball roll-outs (**》p.212**), Swiss ball side crunches (**》p.190**), Swiss ball side crunches with twists (**》p.190**), and side-lying leg raises and reverse leg raises (**》p.193**) with a gradual increase to ankle weights.
- If your pain is not improving or is getting worse, you should:
  ▶ return to your doctor for review.

# BUTTOCK AND COCCYX PAIN

## BUTTOCK AND COCCYX

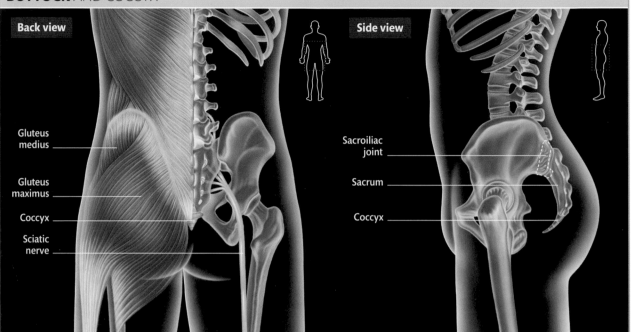

**Back view**

Gluteus medius

Gluteus maximus

Coccyx

Sciatic nerve

**Side view**

Sacroiliac joint

Sacrum

Coccyx

**Pain in the buttocks** commonly emanates from the spine, but can also stem from the sacroiliac joints and ligaments, and the muscles and bursae – fluid-filled cushioning sacs – of the hip. Most pain in the tail bone area originates in the coccyx.

## CAUSES

Lumbar and lower-thoracic sources such as facet joints, discs, nerves, and even muscles can produce pain in this area. Injuries to the lower-thoracic vertebrae such as compression fractures (**»p.65**) also create pain lower down the back. The sacroiliac joints (**»p.69**) and ligaments of the pelvis can cause pain more locally – deep into the buttock, sometimes to the side of the hip and groin, and occasionally down the leg. Muscles in the buttock may develop tension, trigger points, and tears, and can rub the bursae between layers, leading to bursitis – inflammation of the bursa – in the side of the hip. The gluteus medius muscle can tighten and cause hip and buttock pain. The tail bone or coccyx can be painful long after a fall or blow (**»p.75**), while the hip joint and associated structures such as the labrum (cartilaginous rim) can cause buttock pain.

## SYMPTOMS

Lumbar spine nerve-root irritation can radiate to your buttock, and may cause piriformis syndrome (**»p.76**). Sacroiliac pain can cause spontaneous, severe pain in inflammatory conditions (sacroiliitis and ankylosing spondylitis (**»p.63**)). Mechanical pain from the joint and ligaments is common and may arise from a fall, or more progressively from ligament laxity during pregnancy or after childbirth. It causes aching pain with sharp stabs, locking sensations, and a sense of instability, and may interfere with walking – see hypermobility (**»p.66**). Muscle dysfunction may also arise, due to overload from sport, or from asymmetrical back, hips, or legs, causing a dull ache that worsens with exercise. If the hip is the source, walking or running will cause aching, stiffness, and pain at night. Bursitis in the hip causes pain from pressure – lying, walking, and sitting; coccydynia is painful mainly when sitting.

## RISKS AND COMPLICATIONS

The main risk here is incorrect diagnosis: treatments for inflammatory and mechanical conditions are quite different. Cancer from the pelvic organs can spread to the bony structure, so ruling out more serious problems is vital.

## TREATMENT – COCCYDYNIA

### MEDICAL

| IMMEDIATE | SHORT TERM | MEDIUM TERM | LONG TERM |
|---|---|---|---|
| ■ If you suspect you have coccydynia as the result of a blow or fall, you should:<br>▶ avoid sitting directly on your coccyx by using a coccyx cushion, which has an area removed to avoid pressure on the coccyx.<br>▶ avoid becoming constipated. | ■ If after 2–3 weeks you are still in pain, you should consult your doctor. He may:<br>▶ assess the painful area to decide whether an X-ray is required to rule out a fracture.<br>▶ prescribe pain-relief medication, if necessary.<br>▶ offer you a local injection to relieve pain. | ■ If an injection has not worked, or has only relieved pain temporarily, your doctor may:<br>▶ refer you to a specialist for further examination, and more specific diagnosis.<br>■ If causes such as sacroiliac problems or referred pain from the lumbar spine or pelvis have been ruled out, your specialist may:<br>▶ assess your mobility with an X-ray. You will be scanned sitting and standing.<br>▶ recommend manual therapy such as coccygeal manipulation via the rectum, and specific exercises (》table below). | ■ If you have almost regained normal function, you should:<br>▶ continue to use a coccyx cushion for 6 months.<br>■ If, after a trial of conservative treatment, you are not recovering as expected, your specialist may:<br>▶ recommend surgery. This is rarely necessary, unless your pain is caused by a sharp bony projection from the tip of the coccyx (a painful hypermobile segment which has not responded to a course of prolotherapy), or if you have a rigid, non-mobile coccyx which is projecting slightly backwards rather than flexing forwards. |

### PHYSIOTHERAPY

| EARLY STAGE | INTERMEDIATE STAGE | ADVANCED STAGE |
|---|---|---|
| ■ Once your doctor has referred you, your therapist will perform a thorough assessment. Depending on the findings of the assessment, your therapist may:<br>▶ perform manual therapy such as manipulation of the coccyx, massage, and stretching of the ligaments attached to the coccyx.<br>▶ perform electrotherapy or acupuncture.<br>■ Your therapist may advise you to:<br>▶ sit only for short periods of time and use a coccyx cushion (》table above) to take the pressure off your tail bone. If you do not have a cushion, you can roll up a towel or fold a pillow.<br>▶ apply ice packs for the first few days after the pain starts.<br>▶ apply heat packs after the first few days, several times a day.<br>▶ take stool-softening medication and increase fibre and water intake in order to reduce the pressure on your coccyx during bowel movements. | ■ Once your pain has reduced, you may:<br>▶ start a rehabilitation programme.<br>■ You therapist may advise you to:<br>▶ perform sit-to-stand and stand-to-sit chair squats (》p.213), squats (》p.179), clams (》p.181), McKenzie extensions (》p.192), leg raises (》p.192), side-lying leg raises (》p.193), one-leg circles (》p.183), and supine and kneeling pelvic tilts (》p.200).<br>■ You may:<br>▶ start low-impact cardiovascular training on the cross-trainer or in the water in the form of aqua aerobics.<br>▶ perform deep breathing and relaxation exercises.<br>■ If your pain is not improving or is getting worse, you should:<br>▶ return to your doctor for review. | ■ Once you are nearly pain-free, you may:<br>▶ increase the impact of cardiovascular training such as jogging or running on the treadmill, cycling, and aerobics.<br>▶ continue strengthening your hip with leg raises (》p.192), side-lying leg raises (》p.193), and adductor lifts (》p.194) by gradually adding weights to your legs (such as ankle weights).<br>▶ continue stretching your back, hip flexors, and extensors with knees-to-chest stretches (》p.202), McKenzie extensions (》p.192), kneeling hip flexors (》p.210), and hamstring stretches (》p.196).<br>▶ resume sports, gradually increasing the load and duration.<br>■ If your pain is not improving or is getting worse, you should:<br>▶ return to your doctor for review. |

# TREATMENT - SACROILIITIS

## MEDICAL

### IMMEDIATE ▶

- If you have acute pain in the buttock, the most likely source is your lumbar spine. You should:
  ▶ rest your back by finding the least painful position – usually lying flat on your back or with your knees bent.
  ▶ use ice packs for a maximum of 15 minutes every 2 hours for the first day of pain.
  ▶ take paracetamol or ibuprofen in recommended dosages for the first few days of pain.
  ▶ try not to rest for more than 2–3 days.

### SHORT TERM ▶

- If the pain does not settle after a few days, you should consult your doctor. He will:
  ▶ analyze your symptoms.
  ▶ refer you to a rheumatologist, if he suspects you have sacroiliitis.
  ▶ prescribe anti-inflammatory medication, which may help to control your symptoms.
  ▶ send you for an X-ray.

### MEDIUM TERM ▶

- Your specialist will:
  ▶ perform further examinations and blood tests, including an MRI to rule out other causes of pain such as sacral insufficiency fracture or a serious problem with your pelvis.
- If you are diagnosed with sacroiliitis, your specialist may:
  ▶ give you a steroid injection, or a more powerful anti-inflammatory agent to treat your condition.

### LONG TERM

- Your specialist will:
  ▶ confirm the diagnosis by a period of observation over the long term.
  ▶ keep you under review on a regular basis to ensure there is no escalation of inflammatory joint problems elsewhere in your body.
- One the acute inflammation is under control, your specialist may:
  ▶ recommend physiotherapy to counteract any muscle weakness and imbalance resulting from the condition (**》table below**).

## PHYSIOTHERAPY

### EARLY STAGE ▶

- Once your doctor has referred you, your therapist will perform a thorough assessment. Depending on the findings of the assessment, your therapist may:
  ▶ teach you about posture (**》pp.112–15**), ergonomics (**》pp.124–27**), and how to modify or avoid the type of activities that aggravate your pain.
  ▶ recommend stretching exercises to maintain joint flexibility.
  ▶ suggest strengthening exercises to build stability.
  ▶ advise you to start functional training.
  ▶ perform manual therapy such as soft-tissue massage.
- If only one joint is affected, your therapist may advise you to:
  ▶ fold a small towel and place it under your buttock on your good side while sitting. This may alleviate the pain.
- You may:
  ▶ perform knees-to-chest stretches (**》p.202**), clams (**》p.181**), adductor stretches (**》p.197**), and kneeling hip flexors (**》p.210**).

### INTERMEDIATE STAGE ▶

- If you are feeling less pain, you may:
  ▶ continue with your previous exercises, and begin psoas lunges (**》p.209**), hamstring stretches (**》p.196**), and crouching as low as your pain allows to practise sit-to-stand and stand-to-sit chair squats (**》p.213**).
  ▶ gradually add more advanced core-stability exercises such as plank from knees (**》p.188**), side planks levels 1–2 (**》p.189**), leg raises (**》p.192**), side-lying leg raises (**》p.193**), and reverse leg raises (**》p.193**).
- Your therapist may advise you to:
  ▶ move as much as your pain allows and to sit as little as possible.
- If your pain is not improving or is getting worse, you should:
  ▶ return to your doctor for review.

### ADVANCED STAGE

- If you are continuing to improve, you may:
  ▶ begin functional training by practising patterns in movements and positions that you can adopt in daily routines.
  ▶ add stationary lunges (**》p.207**), forward lunges (**》p.207**), and reverse lunges with knee lifts (**》p.208**) to your routine.
  ▶ begin sensorimotor training, gradually increasing the difficulty level by using special equipment such as a wobble board or air cushion.
- Your therapist may advise you to:
  ▶ begin cardiovascular training, either on the cross-trainer or with aqua aerobics.
- If your pain is not improving or is getting worse, you should:
  ▶ return to your doctor for review.

## TREATMENT – GLUTEUS MEDIUS DYSFUNCTION

⊕ SEEK IMMEDIATE MEDICAL ATTENTION

### MEDICAL

**IMMEDIATE** ▶

■ If you have chronic pain in your buttock, the most likely source is a problem in your lumbar spine. It this has been ruled out, your doctor will:
▶ perform palpation and muscle testing to ascertain if the source of pain is your gluteus medius muscle.
▶ examine your hip and sacroiliac joints to identify the primary cause of your dysfunction.

**SHORT TERM** ▶

■ Your doctor will:
▶ refer you to a physiotherapist specializing in sports medicine (》table below).
■ Your therapist will:
▶ teach you how to retrain the muscle and restore your balance with the action of surrounding muscles.
▶ manage causes such as overuse, referred pain from the lumbar area, an inflamed bursa, and hip joint problems such as osteoarthritis.
▶ suggest an exercise programme (》table below).

**MEDIUM TERM** ▶

■ If after 6–10 sessions your condition has improved, your specialist will:
▶ provide a maintenance exercise programme for you to follow (》table below).
■ If your condition has not improved, and you do not need hip surgery, you doctor will refer you to a sports therapist or musculoskeletal specialist, who may:
▶ reassess your case and consider investigations such as a diagnostic ultrasound or an MRI to rule out a tear of the tendon.
▶ suggest local injection therapy or deep acupuncture (》p.92) to normalize muscle function.

**LONG TERM**

■ If you have recovered nearly normal function, you should:
▶ maintain a recommended exercise programme for 3 months; this should include some stretching and strengthening exercises (》table below).
■ If your problem is the result of a hip joint dysfunction or osteoarthritis, you should:
▶ consult a specialist who will advise you on treating these conditions.

### PHYSIOTHERAPY

**EARLY STAGE** ▶

■ Once your doctor has referred you, your therapist will perform a thorough assessment. Depending on the findings of the assessment, your therapist may:
▶ perform manual therapy such as the hold-relax technique if you are experiencing pain, or the contract-relax technique if you are not.
▶ perform trigger-point therapy (》pp.86–87), ultrasound (》p.92), or acupuncture (》pp.100–01).
▶ suggest an exercise programme to balance your body and gradually enhance motor control, endurance, and strength.
■ You may:
▶ begin side-lying leg raises (》p.193), clams (》p.181), adductor stretches levels 1–2 (》p.197), and single-leg stands (》p.199).
▶ begin gentle stretching such as lying waist twists (》p.184).

**INTERMEDIATE STAGE** ▶

■ If you are able to hold your pelvis level during a single-leg stand for 30 seconds, your therapist may advise you to:
▶ progress to weight-bearing exercises and stability training using functional patterns. You may be asked to perform these exercises while moving your centre of gravity horizontally by stepping forwards and backwards, reducing the width of the base of support, and to practise them on unstable surfaces.
■ You may:
▶ perform stationary lunges (》p.207), forward lunges (》p.207), reverse lunges with knee lifts (》p.208), walking lunges (》p.179), and sensorimotor training such as single-leg stands (》p.199).
▶ increase the height of your centre of gravity by elevating your arms or by holding weights.
■ If your pain is not improving or is getting worse, you should:
▶ return to your doctor for review.

**ADVANCED STAGE**

■ If you have good strength in your hip abductors, and good lower-limb stability, you may:
▶ progress to functional training for sport-specific movement patterns.
▶ start running on the treadmill, cycling, and swimming in order to train your cardiovascular system.
■ If your pain is not improving or is getting worse, you should.
▶ return to your doctor for review.

# WHOLE SPINE CONDITIONS

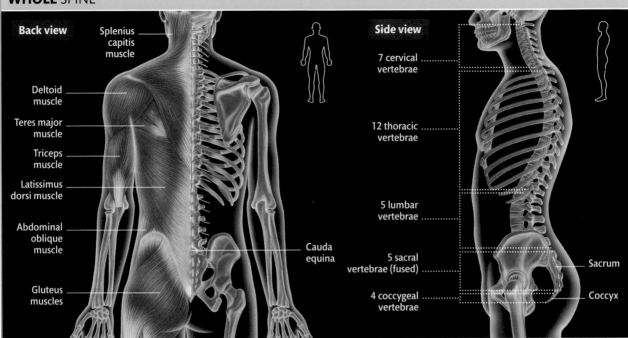

**WHOLE** SPINE

**Back view**
Splenius capitis muscle
Deltoid muscle
Teres major muscle
Triceps muscle
Latissimus dorsi muscle
Abdominal oblique muscle
Gluteus muscles
Cauda equina

**Side view**
7 cervical vertebrae
12 thoracic vertebrae
5 lumbar vertebrae
5 sacral vertebrae (fused)
4 coccygeal vertebrae
Sacrum
Coccyx

**Some diseases involve** the whole spine (inflammatory conditions such as ankylosing spondylitis, for instance) or develop suddenly in a specific area, for example, as a result of an osteoporotic compression fracture (**»p.65**). Other conditions develop gradually and cause symptoms in several areas, such as postural pain and muscle tension, scoliosis, and hypermobility syndrome.

## CAUSES

The causes of a problem that affects the whole spine depend on the specific condition. The spine is a single functioning unit with 25 mobile segments, controlled by muscles that can span nearly its whole length: as a result, a condition that starts at the bottom can spread upwards, involving new areas of the spine by a chain reaction or "knock-on" effect. Furthermore, the joints of the spine are made of the same lining tissues as other joints in the body, so an inflammatory disease (inflammation of the joints by a rheumatic process) can involve several joints. In addition, bones lose mineral content with age and progressively weaken as a result.

## SYMPTOMS

Symptoms of postural disorders or advanced scoliosis (**»pp.58; 74**) that affects the whole spine will vary from pain and aching due to sustained contraction of muscles, fascia, and ligaments being stretched or strained. In inflammatory disorders, aching is symmetrical and is usually worse in the morning or after a period of inactivity (**»p.55**). In osteoporosis, there are no symptoms apart from a gradual change in posture until a trivial fall or knock causes a vertebra to collapse – a vertebral compression fracture (**»p.65**) – producing intense pain. Hypermobile joints will seem to keep "catching" and clicking, and will feel unstable (**»p.56; 66**).

## RISKS AND COMPLICATIONS

The risks are related to the condition that is causing your symptoms. Some spinal pains are part of a chronic pain condition called fibromyalgia, which involves other regions of the body. A diagnosis of fibromyalgia will prevent you from receiving unnecessary and excessive localized treatment. Some metabolic conditions, such as vitamin D deficiency, may cause widespread aching, and this requires careful medical screening.

# TREATMENT – INFLAMMATORY DISEASE

## MEDICAL

### IMMEDIATE

- It is important that you seek medical attention if you exhibit the symptoms of inflammatory disease of the spine. Your doctor will:
  ▶ order appropriate blood tests and may take X-rays of your pelvis and spine (**》pp.80–81**).
  ▶ refer you to a rheumatologist who specializes in these disorders.
  ▶ prescribe anti-inflammatory medication such as ibuprofen or diclofenac.

### SHORT TERM

- Your specialist may:
  ▶ establish a diagnosis based on your symptoms and the tests organized by your doctor.
  ▶ order some additional tests. (X-rays of your sacroiliac joints may not show changes for the first 5 years, but an MRI scan will reveal the characteristic changes sooner.)
- If you have ankylosing spondylitis, your specialist will:
  ▶ continue to prescribe anti-inflammatory medication.
  ▶ refer you to a physiotherapist who specializes in treatment of the disease (**》table below**).

### MEDIUM TERM

- If you have a more aggressive form of inflammatory disease, your specialist will:
  ▶ consider giving you sulphasalazine, or a biological agent.
  ▶ monitor the inflammatory markers in your blood tests.
  ▶ monitor the side-effects of any strong medication.

### LONG TERM

- Once your condition has been diagnosed, you should:
  ▶ perform the daily exercises recommended by your physiotherapist (**》table below**).
  ▶ remain under regular review by your specialist.
  ▶ maintain your lifestyle as much as possible.

## PHYSIOTHERAPY

### EARLY STAGE

- Once your doctor has referred you, your therapist will perform a thorough assessment. Depending on the findings of the assessment, your therapist may:
  ▶ perform manual therapy such as soft-tissue manipulation (**》p.91**).
  ▶ teach you about posture (**》pp.112–15**), ergonomics (**》pp.124–27**), and relaxation techniques (**》pp.102–03**).
  ▶ recommend deep-breathing exercises (**》pp.148–49**).
- You may be advised to:
  ▶ begin exercising in water. The buoyancy of water supports your weight and takes the load off your joints, which can result in decreased joint pain and help you to relax.
  ▶ start mobility exercises such as cat and camels (**》p.187**), bridges (**》p.195**), alligators (**》p.184**), lying waist twists (**》p.184**), Lancelot stretches (**》p.197**), seated and lying trunk rotations (**》pp.163; 164**), and neck rotations (**》p.160**).

### INTERMEDIATE STAGE

- If you are now feeling less pain, you may:
  ▶ begin stretching exercises such as upper-back extensions (**》p.170**), Swiss ball back stretches (**》p.170**), corner chest stretches (**》p.176**), seated waist stretches (**》p.177**), hamstring stretches (**》p.196**), kneeling hip flexors (**》p.210**), prone knee bends (**》p.206**), and oval shoulder stretches (**》p.175**).
  ▶ begin strengthening exercises such as prone arm and leg lifts (**》p.210**), kneeling supermans (**》p.191**), single-leg bridges (**》p.195**), cat stretches (**》p.165**), prone breaststroke (**》p.166**), and prone shoulder squeezes (**》p.167**).
  ▶ begin postural exercises such as doorway chest stretches (**》p.168**) and wall sit presses (**》p.181**).
  ▶ begin sensorimotor training (**》p.93**).
- If your pain is not improving or is getting worse, you should:
  ▶ return to your doctor for review.

### ADVANCED STAGE

- If your symptoms have improved significantly, you may:
  ▶ begin low-impact cardiovascular training such as aqua aerobics, swimming, fast walking on a treadmill or outdoors, and cross-training.
  ▶ perform a physical activity such as t'ai chi.
  ▶ avoid contact sports such as rugby and wrestling. (High-impact sports such as netball, basketball, tennis, and step aerobics may also worsen your symptoms.)
- If your pain is not improving or is getting worse, you should:
  ▶ return to your doctor for review.

# TREATMENT – HYPERMOBILITY SYNDROME

## MEDICAL

### IMMEDIATE ▶

■ If you have aching, "clicking" joints, poor coordination, balance, and movement control, and feelings of instability in areas such as the pelvis, shoulders, neck, and back, you should:
▶ consult your doctor.
■ If your doctor suspects benign hypermobility syndrome, he will:
▶ refer you to a rheumatologist or a specialist physiotherapist to confirm the diagnosis.
■ Your specialist will:
▶ look for more serious or extreme forms of the condition, and screen for evidence of it throughout your body.

### SHORT TERM ▶

■ Once a diagnosis has been confirmed, you condition will become more manageable. Start a programme of recommended exercises. You should aim to:
▶ build up muscle tone and strength in the core muscles of your spine and pelvis (**»table below**).
▶ practise the correct movement patterns for the normal use of your spine and limb joints.
▶ work on your balance, posture, and position sense – in particular, consider the Alexander Technique (**»p.115**).

### MEDIUM TERM ▶

■ In the medium term, a pain specialist may be the most appropriate person to help you find the right balance of medication. You should:
▶ use medication for the alleviation of pain sensibly and sparingly.
▶ enquire about the availability of prolotherapy (**»pp.86–87**) for specific regions in your body such as the pelvis, lumbar, and thoracic spinal joints. (These injections have a beneficial and stabilizing influence when used as part of a package of overall management.)

### LONG TERM

■ With chronic pain, it is important to address any psychological, social, or occupational issues you may have. You should:
▶ deal with negative thinking patterns such as fear of pain and movement.
▶ pace yourself.
▶ learn to relax your muscles voluntarily through regular or daily practice of mindfulness and meditation (**»pp.102–03**).
▶ seek help if you suffer from depressed feelings and mood swings (**»pp.146–47**).

## PHYSIOTHERAPY

### EARLY STAGE ▶

■ Once your doctor has referred you, your therapist will look at your feet, knees, and posture, analyze the way you walk and the way you stand on one foot, and test the length and strength of your muscles. Depending on the findings of the assessment, your therapist may:
▶ perform manual therapy.
▶ teach you about posture (**»pp.112–15**) and ergonomics (**»pp.124–27**).
▶ provide a rehabilitation programme for the whole musculoskeletal system.
▶ recommend orthotics if your feet are over-pronating (**»p.113**).
■ Your therapist may advise you to:
▶ begin a regular strengthening programme, including kneeling supermans (**»p.191**), prone arm and leg lifts (**»p.210**), bridges (**»p.195**), curl-ups (**»p.186**), oblique crunches (**»p.211**), cat stretches (**»p.165**), and clams (**»p.181**).
▶ begin stretching using calf stretches (**»p.198**), hamstring stretches (**»p.196**), and adductor stretches (**»p.197**), starting gently and increasing the intensity as your strength improves.

### INTERMEDIATE STAGE ▶

■ If your therapist is happy with your progress, you may:
▶ perform more advanced strengthening exercises such as single-leg bridges (**»p.195**), side planks levels 1–2 (**»p.189**), planks from knees (**»p.188**), prone planks (**»p.188**), leg raises (**»p.192**), side-lying leg raises (**»p.193**), reverse leg raises (**»p.193**), adductor lifts (**»p.194**), upper-back band rows (**»p.171**), lat band rows (**»p.171**), and prone breaststroke (**»p.166**). Progress gradually, increasing the intensity before adding weights to develop strength.
■ Your therapist may advise you to:
▶ start sensorimotor training such as single-leg stands (**»p.199**).
■ If you have over-pronating feet, you may be advised to:
▶ begin calf raises (**»p.198**) and wall-supported foot lifts (**»p.199**).
■ If your pain is not improving or is getting worse, you should:
▶ return to your doctor for review.

### ADVANCED STAGE

■ If your therapist continues to be happy with your progress, you may:
▶ develop your strengthening programme by performing high-load, core-stability exercises such as Swiss ball side crunches (**»p.190**) and Swiss ball side crunches with twists (**»p.190**).
▶ progress to weight-bearing exercises and stability training using functional patterns. You may be asked to perform these exercises shifting your centre of gravity horizontally by stepping forwards and backwards, reducing the width of the base of support, and performing the exercises on unstable surfaces.
▶ perform stationary lunges (**»p.207**) and squats (**»p.179**) using hand weights and bands.
▶ resume sports, gradually increasing the intensity and duration.
■ If your pain is not improving or is getting worse, you should:
▶ return to your doctor for review.

# TREATMENT – POSTURAL PAIN

## MEDICAL

| IMMEDIATE ▶ | SHORT TERM ▶ | MEDIUM TERM ▶ | LONG TERM |
|---|---|---|---|
| ■ If you are suffering from postural pain (pain arising from the overload of muscles and/or joints due to posture), you should:<br>▶ take paracetamol or ibuprofen in recommended dosages sparingly on a regular schedule, rather than only when the pain becomes unbearable.<br>▶ stay as active as you can.<br>▶ listen to your body and respond to any signals of discomfort.<br>▶ try not to worry about minor symptoms, as this will only further tighten your muscles.<br>▶ consult your doctor or physical therapist if pain persists. | ■ If the pain is moderate or severe, and physiotherapy has not improved your condition, seek further medical help. Your doctor may:<br>▶ order blood tests to rule out muscle disease or inflammation.<br>▶ suggest assays of nutrients such as vitamin D.<br>▶ order hormone tests such as thyroid function, or other biochemical tests.<br>▶ prescribe low-dose tricyclic antidepressants to relax your muscles and improve sleep.<br>▶ consider trigger-point injections (**》pp.86–87**) (and, in severe cases, botulinum toxin), to relax the trigger point for up to 3 months and normalize muscle behaviour. | ■ If you have not received a specific diagnosis or truly effective treatment, or if you have been diagnosed with fibromyalgia or chronic fatigue syndrome, your specialist may offer:<br>▶ a functional rehabilitation programme to improve your strength, flexibility, control of movement and posture, and general fitness (**》table below**).<br>▶ a pain-management programme (including psychological help).<br>▶ appropriate medication such as antidepressants, gabapentin, or pregabalin (**》pp.84–85**). | ■ Most of these pains are treatable or mild enough to be manageable. However, if your condition is severe and disabling, and further treatment has been ruled out, pain management experts will teach you how to adapt. You should:<br>▶ pace yourself.<br>▶ maintain good posture.<br>▶ use medication wisely and appropriately.<br>▶ relax your muscles.<br>▶ cope with the disability.<br>▶ keep working.<br>▶ get in touch with patient self-help organizations (**》pp.216–17**) and other people suffering from the same condition. |

## PHYSIOTHERAPY

| EARLY STAGE ▶ | INTERMEDIATE STAGE ▶ | ADVANCED STAGE |
|---|---|---|
| ■ Once your doctor has referred you, your therapist will perform a thorough assessment. Depending on the findings of the assessment, your therapist may:<br>▶ perform soft-tissue massage, passive mobilizations, and postural taping (**》p.93**).<br>▶ teach you about posture (**》pp.112–15**) and ergonomics (**》pp.124–27**).<br>▶ recommend biomechanical correction (insoles in your shoes for arch support).<br>▶ begin functional re-training.<br>■ You may begin:<br>▶ mobilizing exercises such as McKenzie extensions (**》p.192**), seated and lying trunk rotations (**》pp.163; 164**), and cat and camels (**》p.187**).<br>▶ strengthening exercises such as four-point supine knee lifts (**》p.204**), kneeling supermans (**》p.191**), and clams (**》p.181**).<br>▶ stretching exercises such as knees-to-chest stretches (**》p.202**), side glides (**》p.206**), levator scapulae stretches (**》p.168**), seated back extensions (**》p.170**), seated waist stretches (**》p.177**), and seated twist stretches (**》p.177**). | ■ If you have a lot more mobility and less pain, and have modified your daily activities to prevent postural strain, your therapist may advise you to:<br>▶ move from moderate core-strengthening exercises to high-level exercises such as curl-ups (**》p.186**), Swiss ball twists (**》p.187**), side crunches (**》p.211**), prone arm and leg lifts (**》p.210**), planks from knees (**》p.188**), single-leg bridges (**》p.195**), and side planks (**》p.189**).<br>▶ begin functional training such as squats (**》p.179**), stationary lunges (**》p.207**), forward lunges (**》p.207**), reverse lunges with knee lifts (**》p.208**), and walking lunges (**》p.179**).<br>▶ begin sensorimotor training such as single-leg stands (**》p.199**).<br>▶ begin cardiovascular training by using a cross-trainer, or running on the treadmill or outdoors.<br>■ If your pain is not improving or is getting worse, you should:<br>▶ return to your doctor for review. | ■ If you now have no pain and a full range of movement in your back, your therapist may advise you to:<br>▶ begin more intense strengthening exercises such as prone breaststroke (**》p.166**), Swiss ball side crunches (**》p.190**), Swiss ball side crunches with twists (**》p.190**), and Swiss ball back stretches (**》p.170**).<br>▶ begin swimming, t'ai chi, or Pilates.<br>■ If your pain is not improving or is getting worse, you should:<br>▶ return to your doctor for review. |

# TREATMENT – SCOLIOSIS

## MEDICAL

| IMMEDIATE ▷ | SHORT TERM ▷ | MEDIUM TERM ▷ | LONG TERM |
|---|---|---|---|
| ■ If you are concerned about your spinal shape, consult your doctor. He will:<br>▶ assess the shape of your spine when you are standing, ask you to bend forwards and backwards, and inspect your profile.<br>■ Depending on the outcome of the assessment, your doctor may:<br>▶ refer you to a specialist in scoliosis (**》p.74**). | ■ The scoliosis specialist will also assess you, and may:<br>▶ refer you for X-rays of your whole spine.<br>▶ measure the angles of curvature.<br>▶ decide on the appropriate management of your condition.<br>▶ refer you to a physiotherapist for a programme of exercise (**》table below**). | ■ If you have been diagnosed with a structural scoliosis, you should follow the medical advice given to you. This may involve:<br>▶ attending regular follow-up appointments.<br>▶ performing any exercises you have been prescribed (**》table below**).<br>▶ wearing a brace. | ■ There is no medical treatment available for this problem, but if you are suffering from age-related scoliotic degeneration of your lumbar region, your specialist may:<br>▶ recommend pain-relief injections.<br>■ If the angles between the curve get close to or exceed 45 degrees, your specialist may:<br>▶ suggest corrective surgery. This operation is major and will involve months of recovery time, but the long-term results may make it worthwhile. |

## PHYSIOTHERAPY

| EARLY STAGE ▷ | INTERMEDIATE STAGE ▷ | ADVANCED STAGE |
|---|---|---|
| ■ Once your doctor has referred you, your therapist will perform a thorough assessment. Depending on the findings of your assessment, your therapist may:<br>▶ educate you on your condition, best posture (**》pp.112–15**), and diaphragmatic breathing in corrective positions to enhance lung function (**》p.103**).<br>▶ recommend a programme of exercise to minimize asymmetric posture.<br>▶ recommend that you wear a spinal brace.<br>▶ recommend that you perform deep-breathing exercises.<br>▶ perform manual therapy, including myofascial release, Proprioceptive Neuromuscular Facilitation, and trigger-point therapy, if you are experiencing pain (**》pp.90–93**). | ■ At this stage, your therapist will treat you using the Schroth method (**》p.91**). This will help you to:<br>▶ correct your posture.<br>▶ elongate your trunk.<br>▶ perform deep breathing from your diaphragm (**》p.103**).<br>▶ stretch any tight, overactive muscles.<br>▶ strengthen weak, underactive muscles.<br>■ Your therapist will recommend an exercise programme appropriate to the type of scoliosis you have. You may:<br>▶ perform safe stretches such as upper-back extensions (**》p.170**), wall sit presses (**》p.181**), corner chest stretches (**》p.176**), upper band rows (**》p.171**), child's poses (**》p.212**), prone breast strokes (**》p.166**), and prone shoulder squeezes (**》p.167**).<br>■ If your pain is not improving or is getting worse, you should:<br>▶ return to your doctor for review. | ■ If you have been exercising 4–6 times per week, you should now be able to:<br>▶ maintain a better posture in everyday activities.<br>■ You may:<br>▶ consider taking up swimming or joining a special aqua aerobic class.<br>■ If your pain is not improving or is getting worse, you should:<br>▶ return to your doctor for review. |

# TREATMENT – ACUTE VERTEBRAL COMPRESSION FRACTURE

✚ SEEK IMMEDIATE MEDICAL ATTENTION

## MEDICAL

| IMMEDIATE ▶ | SHORT TERM ▶ | MEDIUM TERM ▶ | LONG TERM |
|---|---|---|---|
| ■ If your doctor suspects an acute vertebral compression fracture, he will:<br>▶ arrange for an X-ray of your thoracic and/or lumbar spine. If this shows more than one area of collapse or compression, he may want to do blood tests to rule out other causes. | ■ Your doctor may:<br>▶ prescribe potent painkillers such as tramadol, or a combination of codeine and paracetamol.<br>▶ explain the prognosis.<br>▶ advise modified activities and rest.<br>▶ recommend that you sleep in a chair or in a semi-recumbent position, especially if the compression is in your thoracic spine. | ■ Your doctor will review any other medication you may be taking, such as steroids or proton pump inhibitors (for indigestion), and consider whether you need to make any changes, as these medicines may cause osteoporosis. He will:<br>▶ recommend further imaging, such as a bone scan or MRI, if the radiologist reporting on the X-ray is uncertain about the cause.<br>▶ advise further investigation such as blood tests.<br>▶ review your pain medication after the first week to ensure you are receiving adequate relief. | ■ If you have recovered fully, your doctor may:<br>▶ order a DEXA scan or bone densitometry, to ascertain the degree of mineral loss in your bones. If the score is too low below, you will be prescribed supplements to delay the progressive loss of bone mineral content. This is a long-term treatment and will be reviewed every 2 years or so.<br>▶ refer you for a programme of rehabilitation (»table below).<br>■ If you have not recovered fully, or are still in severe pain after 6 weeks, your doctor may:<br>▶ refer you to a pain specialist or radiologist to consider vertebroplasty. |

## PHYSIOTHERAPY

| EARLY STAGE ▶ | INTERMEDIATE STAGE ▶ | ADVANCED STAGE |
|---|---|---|
| ■ Once your doctor has referred you, your therapist will perform a thorough assessment. Depending on the findings of the assessment, your therapist may:<br>▶ recommend you rest from activities that aggravate the injured vertebra.<br>▶ apply a postural brace and educate you on good posture (»pp.112–15), relaxation (»pp.148–49), and modifying your daily activities.<br>■ Your therapist may advise you to:<br>▶ perform exercises to stabilize your spine and improve posture, strength, and mobility.<br>▶ stay active during the 6–8 weeks it usually takes to recover. | ■ If you have been wearing a brace and it has been removed, you may:<br>▶ perform mobilizing exercises such as back rotations (»p.203), supine pelvic tilts (»p.200), cat and camels (»p.187), and alligators (»p.184).<br>▶ perform strengthening exercises such as clams (»p.181), lat band rows (»p.171), and upper-back band rows (»p.171).<br>▶ begin functional training such as sit-to-stand and stand-to-sit chair squats (»p.213).<br>▶ begin cardiovascular training on the treadmill or outdoors<br>▶ begin gentle exercises in water.<br>■ Your therapist will:<br>▶ monitor your progress and, if necessary, use massage to relieve pain.<br>■ If your pain is not improving or is getting worse, you should:<br>▶ return to your doctor for review. | ■ If you are feeling a lot less pain, and your range of movement has improved, you may:<br>▶ begin moderate-level core exercises to develop more stability around your spine and develop the strength of other muscles supporting your back.<br>▶ increase the intensity of your cardiovascular training by increasing your walking speed or by incline walking.<br>■ Your therapist may advise you to:<br>▶ perform kneeling supermans levels 1–2 (»p.191), four-point supine knee lifts (»p.204), prone arm and leg lifts (»p.210), leg raises (»p.192), side-lying leg raises (»p.193), reverse leg raises (»p.193), adductor lifts (»p.194), and bridges (»p.195).<br>■ If your pain is not improving or is getting worse, you should:<br>▶ return to your doctor for review. |

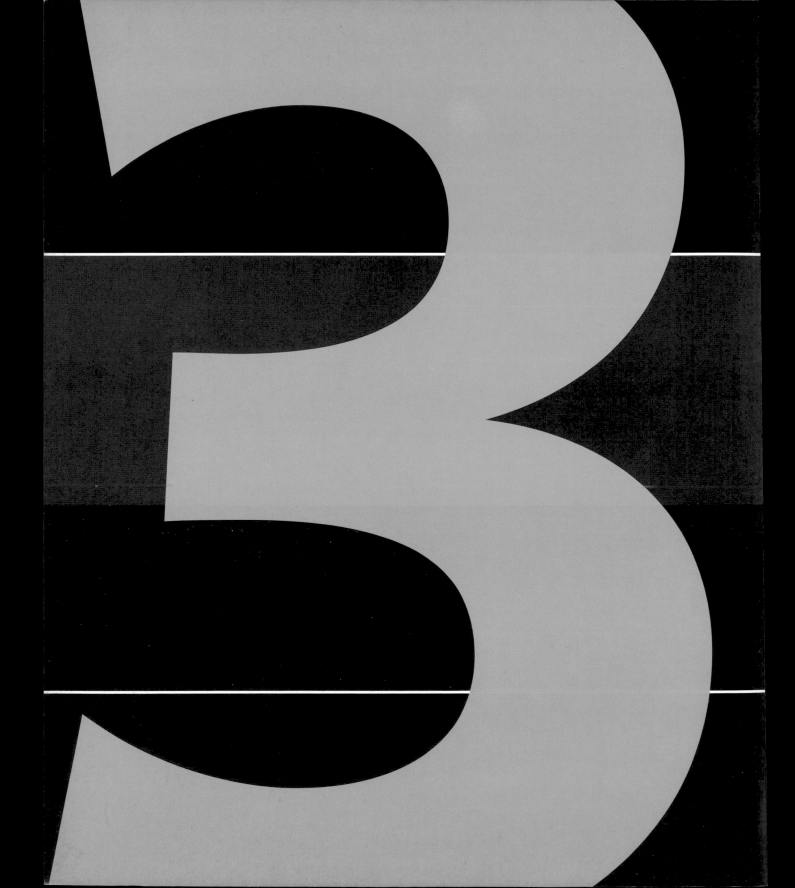

# CAUSES OF BACK AND NECK PAIN

**This chapter provides additional information** on a range of specific causes of back and neck conditions, with fully annotated anatomical diagrams. Entries describe the typical symptoms of each cause, along with details of common methods of diagnosis, the potential medium- to long-term risks, and average recovery periods.

# MUSCULAR TENSION

## MUSCULAR TENSION

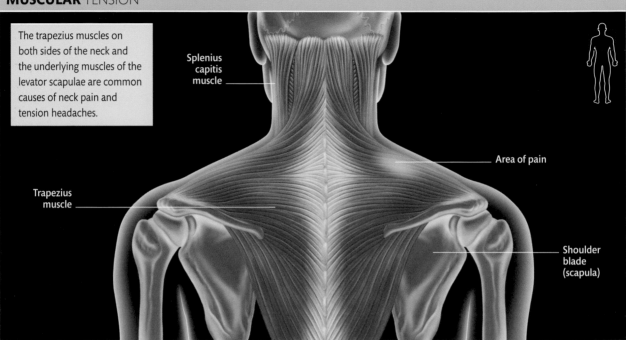

The trapezius muscles on both sides of the neck and the underlying muscles of the levator scapulae are common causes of neck pain and tension headaches.

Splenius capitis muscle

Trapezius muscle

Area of pain

Shoulder blade (scapula)

**Tensing your muscles** is a normal response to stress and heightened emotions, such as anger, nerves, or frustration. You may also get into the habit of holding certain sets of muscles in a tense, fixed position when performing basic everyday actions, such as moving around or sitting at your desk. This tension, however, is a major cause of neck and back pain.

### CAUSES

Poor posture, injury, overexertion, differences in leg length, and conditions such as scoliosis (»p.74) can all cause you to tense specific sets of muscles, as the muscles compensate for any difficulties these problems create. Stress and emotional pressures are the main triggers for over-tense muscles, but difficulty sleeping or poor nutrition can also cause an increase in muscular tension. Holding your muscles for any length of time in a tense, contracted position limits blood flow to your muscles and restricts the supplies of nutrients and oxygen that they need to work properly. Poor blood flow also allows toxins to build up in your muscle tissues.

All this can lead to pain and muscle spasms, which in turn put strain on the joints and ligaments so that they too become tender and sore.

### SYMPTOMS AND DIAGNOSIS

Pain from excess muscle tension may start with a dull ache, but can become extremely painful. Muscles that are regularly held in a contracted and tense position for extended periods of time may also develop "knots", or trigger points. These are particularly tender areas that are easily irritated, sending waves of pain out to other, often distant, parts of your body. Your doctor or physical therapist will make a diagnosis by performing a physical examination.

### RISKS AND RECOVERY

Trying to lead a calmer, less stressful life is the ultimate cure for this condition; incorporating relaxation techniques into your routine will help (»pp.102-03; 148-49). You should always check that the pain is due solely to chronic muscular tension, rather than any illness or physical problem. If you hold your muscles in a tight, tense state for a very long time, they can become permanently shortened and stop functioning properly.

# ANKYLOSING SPONDYLITIS

**Ankylosing spondylitis (AS)** tends to occur in young adults, and usually affects men more severely than women. A form of spinal arthritis, it leads to inflammation and a calcification, or hardening, of the ligaments in the sacroiliac joints and in the intervertebral joints that link the vertebrae together. It is also known as Marie-Strümpell or Bechterev's disease.

## CAUSES

Generally, sufferers of ankylosing spondylitis are genetically predisposed towards the disease. Little is known about what causes it, although it is known to be an autoimmune disease, which means that the body's immune system not only fights invading infections but also attacks the body's own cells. It is thought that AS may start when an immune response to bacteria or a virus continues once the infection has gone.

## SYMPTOMS AND DIAGNOSIS

The onset of the disease usually occurs between the mid-teens and mid-30s. It affects the sacroiliac joint first, and will cause pain and stiffness in your lower back and buttocks that is worse on waking. You may find it difficult to bend forwards and your hip joints will be stiff. It advances gradually over several years into the thoracic and cervical spine, causing pain and stiffness in the rest of your back and neck. Extreme stiffness can result in you hunching forwards, flattening your chest and curving your spine. In some people, the inflammation and calcification may eventually affect the joints between the ribs and the mid-spine so that movement of the ribcage is limited, impairing breathing. Your doctor will make a diagnosis by considering your symptoms and performing tests, including blood tests, X-rays, an MRI scan, and an ultrasound (**»pp.82–83**).

## RISKS AND RECOVERY

It is important to identify and treat the condition as early as possible to prevent irreversible deterioration in posture and mobility. Treatment includes physiotherapy, exercise, and medication. People with ankylosing spondylitis have an increased risk of osteoporosis in the spine and of heart and circulatory problems, such as stroke. In rare cases, the nerves at the base of the spine compress, leading to numbness in the lower back and buttocks, and sometimes incontinence.

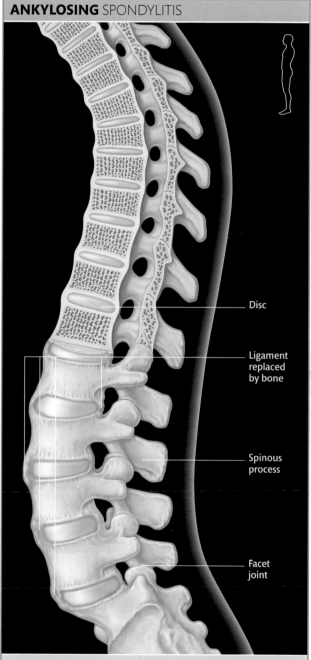

**ANKYLOSING SPONDYLITIS**

Disc

Ligament replaced by bone

Spinous process

Facet joint

Ankylosing spondylitis causes the discs and ligaments of the spine to harden and become bonelike over time. The resulting stiffness decreases flexibility, resulting in a hunched posture with a flat chest and curved spine.

# SPONDYLOLYSIS AND SPONDYLOLISTHESIS

**These linked conditions** generally affect your lower back but may occur in any part of your spine. Spondylolysis occurs when a defect or weakness in a vertebra develops into a fracture. The vertebra is then at risk of slipping out of line with the vertebrae adjacent to it, leading to spondylolisthesis, which can be debilitating and painful, or may be painless and go unnoticed.

## CAUSES

Spondylolysis may start with a minor crack across the narrow arch of bone in a vertebra, known as the neural arch. In some cases, this crack is present at birth, but usually it is the result of a fall or due to strain and overuse. Some sports, such as cricket and football, repeatedly put stress on the arches of the vertebrae, which can lead to minor cracks or breaks. Spondylolisthesis generally develops from spondylolysis, with the crack widening to a complete break due to further stresses and strains. This break allows the damaged vertebra to slip out of line, which can irritate the linked facet joints and ligaments and possibly trap a nerve.

## SYMPTOMS AND DIAGNOSIS

The pain from a displaced vertebra due to spondylolisthesis depends on the degree of slippage. A slight slip may cause little or no pain, while a greater degree of slippage can lead to more intense pain because of the irritation to the spinal joints and ligaments. If your nerve is trapped, there may be some pain, numbness, or "pins and needles" in one or both of your legs. Your doctor will make a diagnosis through a physical examination and testing including an X-ray, MRI scan, and myelogram (**»pp.82–83**).

## RISKS AND RECOVERY

Back-strengthening exercises can help stabilize your posture, but where vertebrae have severely slipped, nerve entrapment can develop that may require surgery (**»pp.88–89**). Young people diagnosed with spondylolisthesis should avoid contact sports and activities with a high risk of back injury. A young person who is still growing should be monitored every six months, using X-rays to detect further movements and shifts in the spinal column. Once growth stops, the vertebrae are unlikely to slip any further.

### SPONDYLOLYSIS

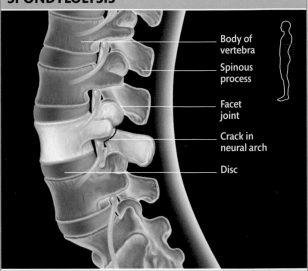

Body of vertebra
Spinous process
Facet joint
Crack in neural arch
Disc

Spondylolysis begins as a minor crack across the neural arch, which spans the spinous and inferior articular processes, and the transverse and superior articular processes (**»p.12**).

### SPONDYLOLISTHESIS

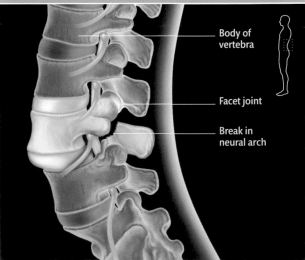

Body of vertebra
Facet joint
Break in neural arch

Spondylolisthesis is the widening of a crack in the neural arch into a fully-fledged break. As a consequence of this, the vertebra slips out of line. This may lead to nerve pain.

# VERTEBRAL COMPRESSION FRACTURE

**Weakening of the bones** is fairly common in old age and may also occur in younger people who are in poor health. When this loss of structural strength affects the vertebrae of the spinal column, even a slight increase in pressure on them – perhaps due to a fall or sudden vigorous activity – can cause cracks and fractures, especially in the mid- and lower back.

## CAUSES

Osteoporosis is the most common cause of bones (including the vertebrae) becoming weaker and more susceptible to injury. The condition causes loss of minerals from the bones, making them less dense and more fragile. It mainly affects women after the menopause, due to hormonal changes, but men also develop osteoporosis to some degree as they age. If you are a heavy smoker, alcoholic, do little exercise, or have suffered from an eating disorder (such as anorexia) and are still underweight and very thin, you have a high risk of developing osteoporosis. In a few cases, taking steroids (**»pp.84–85**) for a particular medical condition may weaken your bones, as can certain forms of cancer.

## SYMPTOMS AND DIAGNOSIS

If you fracture a vertebra, you will feel a sudden, severe pain in the area of your back where the injury has occurred. Damaged vertebrae in your lower back may also cause pain around your pelvis and, if any nerves are irritated, numbness and tingling in your legs. In the upper part of your back, the pain may radiate around your chest and make breathing difficult. You may find it hard to move around, and even lying down can cause pain; coughing or sneezing may hurt too. This pain and lack of mobility is likely to take several weeks to subside. Your doctor may arrange for a CT or an MRI scan (**»pp.82–83**) to assess the extent of the fracture.

## RISKS AND RECOVERY

Although compression fractures in the spine usually heal within a matter of weeks without any special treatment, the shape of your spine and your posture may be permanently affected. While the pain lasts you are likely to find it difficult to perform everyday activities.

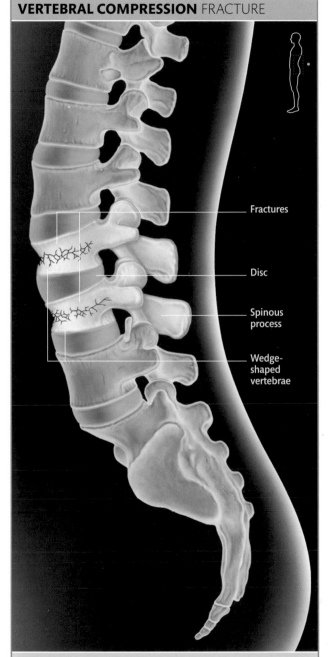

**VERTEBRAL COMPRESSION** FRACTURE

Fractures

Disc

Spinous process

Wedge-shaped vertebrae

In vertebral compression fractures, it is usually the front of the vertebra that collapses. This can create a wedge-shaped vertebra, which causes a "hump" in the spine.

# HYPERMOBILITY AND INSTABILITY

**A common cause** of lower back and neck pain, hypermobility of the spine occurs as a result of ligament laxity (loose ligaments) and/or disc degeneration. It may affect the whole spine, just one joint or segment of the spine, or be part of a generalized syndrome affecting many or all joints and soft tissues of the body. If laxity is limited to one or two segments and is accompanied by degeneration, this is known as instability syndrome.

### CAUSES

Commonly known as being "double-jointed", hypermobility usually runs in families. It is caused by an inherited deficiency in the production of collagen, which results in the ligaments that support the joints being weaker than normal. Slackening of the ligaments may also occur with ageing – as the discs between spinal vertebrae become thinner they gradually move closer together, which leads to looser ligaments and spinal segments. The joints become more susceptible to injury from stresses and strains, which can loosen them further. In addition, the surrounding muscles may have to work harder to stabilize the affected area. This overworking of the muscles can lead to tension.

### SYMPTOMS AND DIAGNOSIS

Minor strains and changes of position, such as bending over, can cause a feeling of your back "going" or locking, resulting in a sharp pain followed by aching and stiffness. If your ligaments are weak, long periods of sitting or inactivity can bring on pain, particularly in your neck and lower back. You may experience a dull ache first thing in the morning, but this usually wears off with movement. Your doctor will make a diagnosis through physical examination, and may carry out X-rays and blood tests (**»pp.82–83**) to rule out conditions such as arthritis.

### RISKS AND RECOVERY

Contact sports or trauma can cause further injury but exercise that builds up muscle tone and stamina will help. Your doctor or a physiotherapist may prescribe an exercise regime to strengthen your muscles and improve the stability of your spine. Prolotherapy (**»pp.86–87**) is a useful treatment if you have only one or two spinal segments that are unstable.

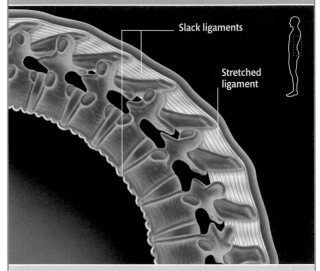

**HYPERMOBILITY** OF THE SPINE

Slack ligaments

Stretched ligament

Hypermobility causes the ligaments of the spine to be much looser. As a result, there is increased flexibility, leading to an ability to bend further forwards or backwards.

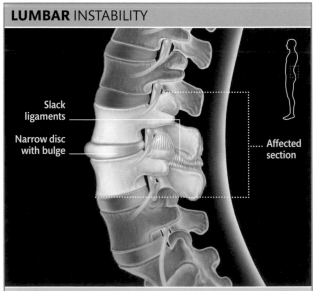

**LUMBAR** INSTABILITY

Slack ligaments

Narrow disc with bulge

Affected section

Lumbar instability is caused by narrowing and tears in the disc, which leads to slackening of the ligaments. These loose ligaments weaken the affected section of the spine.

# DISCOGENIC PAIN

**DAMAGED** DISC

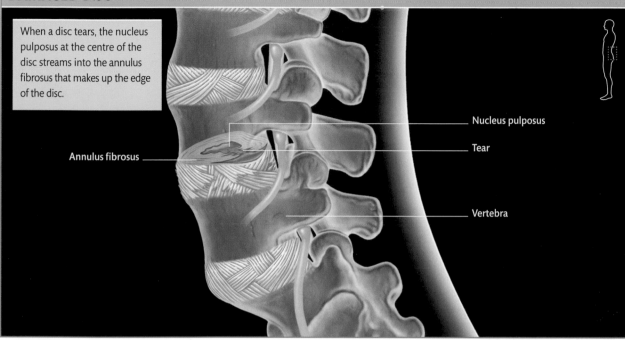

When a disc tears, the nucleus pulposus at the centre of the disc streams into the annulus fibrosus that makes up the edge of the disc.

Nucleus pulposus

Tear

Annulus fibrosus

Vertebra

**Degeneration of the discs** in your neck and lower back commonly occurs with age. To some extent, this degeneration explains the frequency of back problems in adult populations. The result of disc degeneration varies, from no symptoms at all to significant pain and disability.

## CAUSES

As your discs age, they are more susceptible to damage, such as tears and cracks. This can cause chemicals from the soft, pulpy interior of the disc (the nucleus pulposus) to leak into the fibrous outer band of the disc (the annulus fibrosus), which will irritate any nerves that are located nearby. Some people are genetically predisposed to having weak discs, and it is also thought that heavy lifting and lack of regular exercise may exacerbate the problem. Smoking is also believed to be a contributing factor. Acute disc tears can occur as a result of trauma, such as an injury incurred from a sporting activity, or as a result of a combination of degeneration and trauma.

## SYMPTOMS AND DIAGNOSIS

Back or neck pain, either constant or intermittent, may be triggered by simple everyday activities that put pressure or strain on any weakened spinal discs, such as sitting still for a long time, bending over, or even coughing and sneezing. This may be accompanied by referred pain in your leg. Your specialist will perform an MRI scan (**»pp.82–83**) first, to assess the state of the discs. He may then recommend a provocation discography (**»pp.88–89**) to reproduce your pain and assess the internal structure of the disc.

## RISKS AND RECOVERY

The risks of chronic discogenic pain are reduced ability to carry out everyday activities, depression, abuse of painkillers such as opioids (**»pp.84–85**), and side effects from other pain medication. Currently, there are no known methods of prevention, and few effective treatments exist. Less severe cases can respond to prolotherapy (**»pp.86–87**), while more serious cases may be treated with spinal fusion or disc replacement (**»pp.88–89**).

# FACET JOINT STRAIN

**Pain often occurs** when one of the facet joints that link the vertebrae in your spinal column is suddenly twisted or jerked. A joint that is damaged in this way may stick or "lock", making movement difficult as well as painful. Facet joint strain can occur throughout your spine.

## CAUSES

Awkward twisting or bending of your neck or back can injure the ligaments, muscles, or the capsule of a facet joint. Whiplash (»p.72) from a car accident is a good example of this type of injury, but it can also result from failure to warm up before exercising or playing sport, or from lifting heavy objects. Even simply turning over in bed or sleeping awkwardly can have the same effect. Your muscles may then go into an uncontrollable spasm, making the joint stiff and immobile. Facet joints are more vulnerable to strains from middle age onwards, when osteoarthritis may flare up, the discs in your spine have degenerated significantly, and the ligaments that are supporting the joints become more slack.

## SYMPTOMS AND DIAGNOSIS

In the early stages, disabling pain in your neck or back is often accompanied by restricted movement. Pain from facet joint strain in your lower back may also radiate into your buttocks, hips, lower abdomen, and thighs. Movement may be limited for only a few weeks; however, it can last for months, and in some cases years, unless you receive appropriate treatment, which usually involves manipulation or, in chronic cases, an injection (»pp.86–87). Facet joint strain in your neck may extend down to your shoulders, making it difficult to bend your neck or turn your head. Your doctor or therapist will make a diagnosis by giving you a physical examination.

## RISKS AND RECOVERY

There is no serious risk from facet joint strain, but failure to relieve pain or inflammation can lead to permanently stiff joints. Joint strain in the middle of your back, although the least common, may cause pain to radiate around your chest, making it painful and difficult to breathe, especially if the joints between the ribs and thoracic vertebrae become "locked".

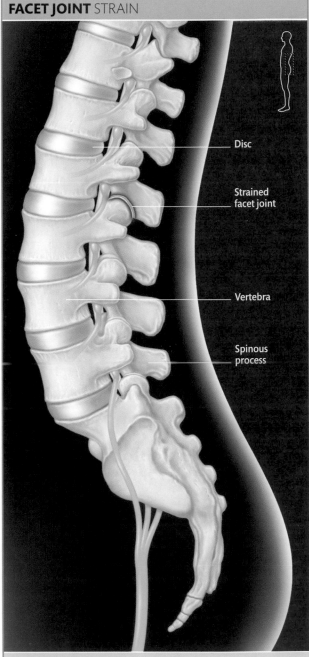

**FACET JOINT** STRAIN

Disc

Strained facet joint

Vertebra

Spinous process

Twisting or jerking your spine may lead to a strained facet joint. If the strain is maintained by a local muscle spasm, this is known as a facet joint dysfunction.

# SACROILIAC STRAIN

**Located on either side** of your spine at the very bottom of the back, the sacroiliac joints link your sacrum (the fused bones at the base of your spine) to your hip bones, forming the rear part of your pelvic girdle. They assist the twisting movements of your legs when you walk or run. Problems arise when they either become "locked", restricting movement, or too mobile.

## CAUSES

Sacroiliac strain is usually the result of a sudden impact, such as a heavy blow or fall, which damages the ligaments supporting the joint. Sudden, unexpected twisting or bending movements, where your muscles are unprepared to take the strain and the pressure is absorbed by the ligaments, can have the same effect. Mechanical changes in these joints may also occur over a period of time due to an imbalanced use of the surrounding muscles, abnormalities (such as a slight difference in leg length), or osteoarthritis. Strained ligaments lead to loosening of the joints, making them more mobile. It is also common for pregnant women to suffer from hypermobile sacroiliac joints, because of hormonal changes that soften and slacken the ligaments of the pelvis in preparation for giving birth.

## SYMPTOMS AND DIAGNOSIS

You will feel a sharp pain in the upper inner part of your buttock when you put your foot down, making walking or running very uncomfortable. There will also be dull pain radiating deep into your lower buttock; sometimes you will also experience referred pain in your legs. Movement of your legs may be restricted, which will also make walking difficult. Your specialist may use an MRI scan or X-ray (**»pp.82–83**) to identify any inflammatory cause of your symptoms. If inflammation is present, you may be given a blood test to check if this is being caused by an infection.

## RISKS AND RECOVERY

If you sit still or lie down for a long time, you may feel stiffness and immobility. Ligaments take longer to heal than fractured bone, and may fail to heal completely. Prolotherapy injections (**»pp.86–87**) may help regenerate and strengthen any weak ligaments.

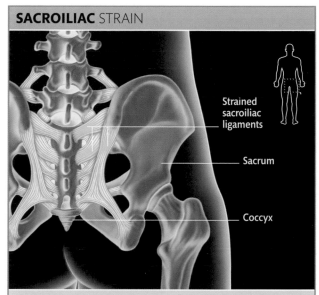

**SACROILIAC** STRAIN

Strained sacroiliac ligaments

Sacrum

Coccyx

A heavy fall or a blow to the bottom of the back – usually as a result of a sports injury – can cause the ligaments that surround the sacroiliac joints to become strained.

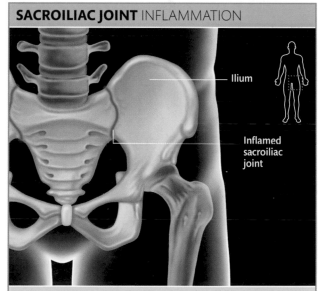

**SACROILIAC JOINT** INFLAMMATION

Ilium

Inflamed sacroiliac joint

The sacroiliac joints are located on either side of the spine, and connect the sacrum (the fused bones at the base of the spine) with the two ilia (the largest pelvic bones). These weight-bearing joints support the spine.

# DISC HERNIATION

**Sandwiched between each** of the vertebrae in your spinal column is a disc of cartilage that acts as a shock-absorbing pad. These discs have a soft, jelly-like centre and a tough, fibrous outer layer. A tear in this outer layer will allow some of the soft centre to bulge out. This bulge may press on the nerve roots emerging from the spine in the region of the damaged disc.

## CAUSES

Any activity that puts increased pressure on the discs of your spine can lead to a disc herniation. This can occur in the cervical spine (**»p.27**), or, more commonly, the lower back (**»p.38**). The general wear and tear that comes with age can also contribute, making middle-aged people susceptible to herniation if they bend suddenly or lift an awkward weight.

## SYMPTOMS AND DIAGNOSIS

Depending on the location of the herniated disc, symptoms can vary, but there is usually severe pain and restriction of movement. In the lower back, the pain tends to be a deep unrelenting ache, which may radiate out to your hips, groin, buttocks, and legs. You may also develop sciatica – a sharp pain, radiating down one leg, accompanied by numbness or tingling (**»pp.46–49**). Herniated discs can also occur in the neck, causing severe pain that may spread into your shoulders, arms, and hands, making it difficult to turn your head or move it backwards or forwards. You will usually feel pain in only one side of your body. Your doctor will make a diagnosis by performing a physical examination; if your symptoms persist, he may order further tests, such as an MRI or CT scan (**»pp.82–83**).

## RISKS AND RECOVERY

Recovery from a slipped disc usually takes 4–6 weeks, and the risk of further serious developments occurring are few. However, if a disc herniation protrudes fully into the spinal canal, it can compress the cauda equina (**»p.14**) and damage the nerves leading to your legs, bladder, and bowels. This may result in weakness and numbness in both legs and the lower part of your body, loss of bladder and bowel control, and even impotence. Although this rarely happens, it is an emergency and you should seek immediate medical help.

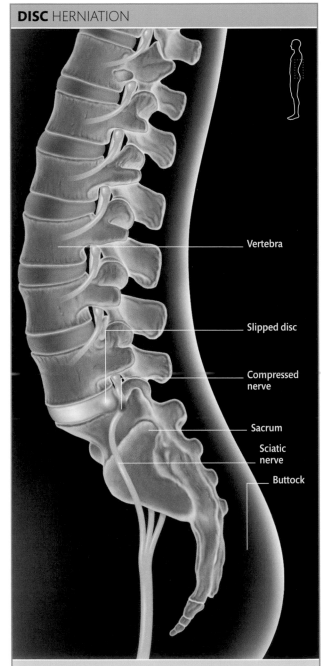

**DISC** HERNIATION

Vertebra

Slipped disc

Compressed nerve

Sacrum

Sciatic nerve

Buttock

The discs of the spine are located between the vertebrae. Herniation causes the soft centre of the disc to bulge, leading to irritation of the nerve nearest the disc.

# ACUTE TORTICOLLIS

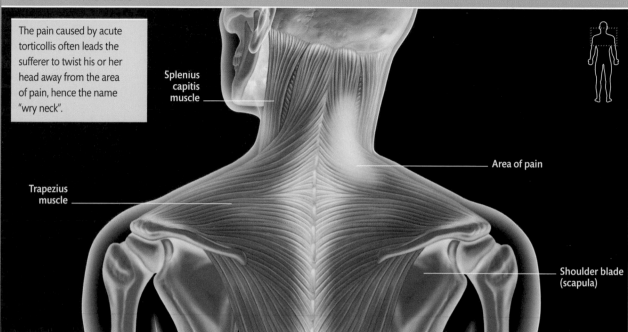

**ACUTE** TORTICOLLIS

The pain caused by acute torticollis often leads the sufferer to twist his or her head away from the area of pain, hence the name "wry neck".

Splenius capitis muscle

Area of pain

Trapezius muscle

Shoulder blade (scapula)

**Sometimes called wry neck**, this is the most common form of torticollis – literally "twisted neck". The condition often seems to appear from nowhere, such as when you wake after a long night's sleep. It is more likely to occur in children, adolescents, and young adults, although babies and infants can also sometimes show signs of torticollis.

## CAUSES

The cause of acute torticollis usually depends on the age of the sufferer. In infants it can be caused by instability of the upper cervical joint, which is often the result of birth trauma or inherited problems. In older children, the condition is often an indirect effect of irritation of the pharyngeal muscles – muscles that sit directly behind the mouth and nasal cavity – from a throat or ear infection. In young adults, the most likely cause of acute torticollis is dysfunction of a localized section of the cervical spine: this usually occurs as the result of lying down or sleeping in an awkward position for a sustained period of time.

## SYMPTOMS AND DIAGNOSIS

Sometimes described as an acute stiff and painful neck, torticollis generally makes turning your head extremely painful and difficult. Often, it is also just as hard to move your head backwards and forwards. The pain is usually sharp and will either run along the middle of your neck or along one side of it. You may also feel an intense dull background ache that can spread down as far as your shoulder blades. Your doctor will make a diagnosis by performing a physical examination.

## RISKS AND RECOVERY

Acute torticollis is not a serious problem, and you should recover in around 7–10 days without any form of treatment. Massage and manipulation (**»pp.96–99**) can help speed up recovery, but need to be carried out with great care so as not to further aggravate your condition. If symptoms persist for more than two weeks, you should consult your doctor because torticollis can be an early indicator of acute disc herniation (**»p.70**) or, rarely, something more serious.

# WHIPLASH

**A form of neck strain**, whiplash arises from the head being jolted violently back and forth, usually as a result of a sudden blow or impact. The most common situation in which this occurs is a car accident, but a fall or an assault can have the same effect. You also have an increased risk of whiplash when you take part in certain contact sports, such as rugby and boxing.

### CAUSES
If your head is suddenly forced violently backwards and forwards, or sideways, causing it to move beyond its normal range, this can strain the soft tissues – the muscles, tendons, and ligaments – in your neck. An unexpected blow or collision tends to increase the severity of the damage, as the muscles have no time to prepare for the impact.

### SYMPTOMS AND DIAGNOSIS
Initially you may feel little pain, but over the next day or so both the front and back of your neck and shoulders will become stiff and painful, and possibly swollen. You may also experience muscle spasms, limited neck movement, nausea, headaches, blurring of vision, and "ringing" in your ears, along with a general feeling of tiredness and, sometimes, difficulty thinking. A pain or tingling in your shoulder that runs down your arm and possibly into your hand may indicate nerve-root irritation from a disc injury. In severe cases, your doctor may request an X-ray or advanced imaging (**»pp.82–83**), but in most cases this is not necessary, and a physical examination will reassure your doctor that it is only a soft-tissue injury.

### RISKS AND RECOVERY
You should always seek immediate treatment for any direct trauma to the neck, as it has the potential to cause paralysis and even death. However, the risk of any serious problems arising from an indirect whiplash injury is very low. Most of the symptoms will disappear within a few weeks without any specific treatment other than rest and taking extra care in your daily routine. Too much rest and inactivity, however, can delay healing, and, as whiplash can lead to long-term problems, such as restricted movement and difficulties with sleeping and concentration, a thorough medical examination is important.

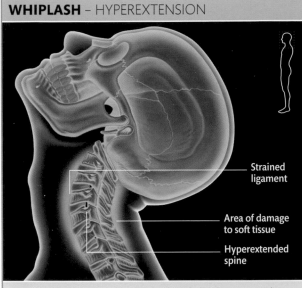

**WHIPLASH** – HYPEREXTENSION

Strained ligament

Area of damage to soft tissue

Hyperextended spine

A car accident, in which the car is hit from behind, can cause the head to be jerked violently backwards and forwards without any warning, resulting in overstretched and/or torn ligaments. The discs, muscles, and facet joints in the neck may also be damaged.

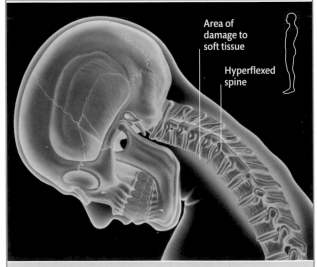

**WHIPLASH** – HYPERFLEXION

Area of damage to soft tissue

Hyperflexed spine

As the muscles are not poised to absorb the shock, the joints are forced to the extreme of their range: the ligaments absorb the impact of this. An X-ray will not reveal the strain on the ligaments, and internal bleeding may be very slow.

# SPINAL STENOSIS AND DEGENERATION

**The process of ageing** commonly affects the vertebrae, discs, and facet joints in the lower lumbar and cervical spine. Pain caused by general facet joint degeneration is sometimes referred to as osteoarthritis. When the discs thin and bony spurs called osteophytes develop around the vertebrae, this is known as spondylosis. When osteophytes protrude into the spinal canal, this results in a condition called stenosis.

## CAUSES

Some people who suffer from spinal stenosis are born with a particularly narrow spinal canal. For most people, however, problems with narrowing of the spine start sometime after the age of 50, around which time spinal degeneration advances to a moderate level. If bony spurs form on your vertebrae and protrude into the spinal canal, they may pinch the nerve roots, reducing blood flow and causing pain. Osteoarthritis and spondylosis are mostly silent ageing processes, which may be initiated or accelerated by injury. Overdoing heavy physical work may cause pain due to the extra strain.

## SYMPTOMS AND DIAGNOSIS

If you have spinal stenosis you may feel pain in your back, buttocks, and in one or both legs after standing or walking. Some people also have "pins and needles" and numbness or weakness in their legs, particularly when walking and running. Stenosis-related pain tends to be in the lower part of the back and legs, as the spinal canal in the neck area is naturally wider, and less susceptible to stenosis. Your doctor will make a diagnosis by performing a physical examination, and may order a scan. If you have osteoarthritis or spondylosis, you may feel pain in your back and stiffness on waking. You doctor will make a diagnosis with an X-ray (»pp.82–83): this diagnosis may not be useful for identifying causes of pain, as most people over the age of 60 will have these changes without experiencing pain.

## RISKS AND RECOVERY

If you are born with a narrow spinal canal, you are at risk of your spinal nerves becoming compressed, leading to long-term back problems and sciatica. The main risk of osteoarthritis and spondylosis is increasing immobility; your doctor or physical therapist will try to prevent or minimize this.

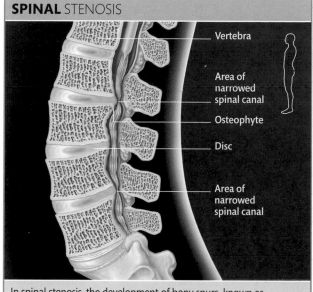

**SPINAL** STENOSIS

Vertebra

Area of narrowed spinal canal

Osteophyte

Disc

Area of narrowed spinal canal

In spinal stenosis, the development of bony spurs, known as osteophytes, lead to narrowing of the spinal canal. This can result in severe pain.

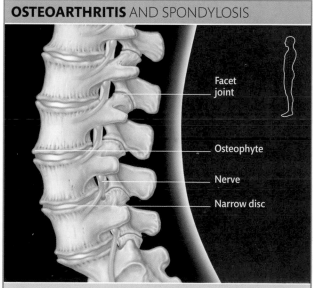

**OSTEOARTHRITIS** AND SPONDYLOSIS

Facet joint

Osteophyte

Nerve

Narrow disc

As the spine ages, the discs gradually dry out and become thinner. Bony spurs (osteophytes) may also develop around the intervertebral and facet joints, causing stiffness. Rarely, a spur will sit in an awkward place, causing pain by pressing on a nerve.

# SCOLIOSIS

**Scoliosis, or curvature** of the spine, is a deformity of growth that causes the spine to twist to one side. It can be so mild that it is barely noticeable and creates few or no symptoms. However, scoliosis may result in a severely deformed posture, although it rarely causes much pain. In severe cases, there may be difficulty with breathing and walking.

## CAUSES

If you have a slight difference in leg length – around 10 per cent of the population have a difference in leg length of 1cm (⅜in) or more – your spine may start to curve sideways to compensate. However, the curvature in such cases is usually quite mild and rarely causes problems. True structural scoliosis starts either in infancy, when it can become very severe, or in early adolescence, when it becomes more obvious during the growth spurt.

## SYMPTOMS AND DIAGNOSIS

If your child's back appears crooked when standing or bending to one side and slightly forwards, or if one shoulder blade appears to be more prominent than the other, you should consult your doctor so he can perform a physical examination. A spinal brace or other support may be prescribed for your child to wear while still growing, in order to help prevent any excessive deformity. If this does not have the desired effect, surgery may be required to straighten the back (**»pp.88–89**). Twisting of the spine also means that the muscles that surround it will have to work harder to maintain posture, and this can cause mild postural pain.

## RISKS AND RECOVERY

Failure to recognize the increasing deformity during a child's growth period means that the progression may not be prevented nor the timing of corrective surgery optimized. Over a long period of time, the unequal distribution of stresses and strains on the back that result from having even mild scoliosis may lead to a persistent general ache in the back, shoulders, or neck in later years. It is also likely that people with lumbar scoliosis will suffer from painful degeneration of the joints between the vertebrae later in life.

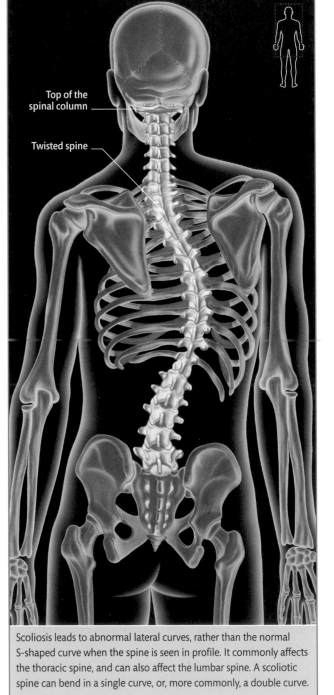

**SCOLIOSIS**

Top of the spinal column

Twisted spine

Scoliosis leads to abnormal lateral curves, rather than the normal S-shaped curve when the spine is seen in profile. It commonly affects the thoracic spine, and can also affect the lumbar spine. A scoliotic spine can bend in a single curve, or, more commonly, a double curve.

# COCCYDYNIA

## COCCYDYNIA

The coccyx is the bone at the base of the spine. It is located just above the cleft in the buttocks, and curves forward so that it points towards the front of the body.

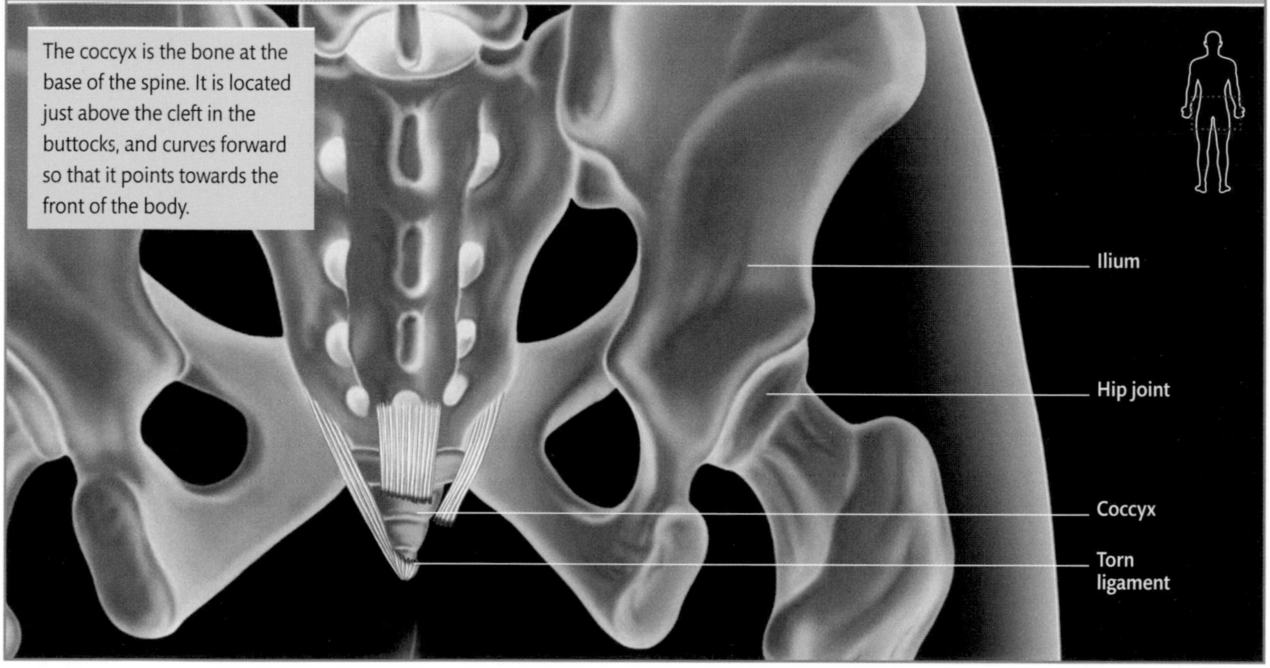

Ilium

Hip joint

Coccyx

Torn ligament

**Pain or soreness** occurring in and around the coccyx – the three to five fused vertebrae at the base of the spine that are often referred to as the tail bone – can vary from general discomfort to bouts of sudden sharp or nagging pain. Also known as coccygeal pain, this condition tends to be brought on or made worse by sitting down.

## CAUSES

A number of very different sets of circumstances appear to be responsible for triggering episodes of tenderness and pain in and around the coccyx region. Muscle spasms that have been brought on by prolonged tension and stress might be a trigger, for example, as might a damaged ligament that has been caused by a heavy blow or fall. In a large number of cases, coccydynia is the result of sitting in more or less one position for a very long period of time. Many women also suffer bouts of pain around the coccyx after giving birth. It is always important to have these symptoms checked by your doctor.

## SYMPTOMS AND DIAGNOSIS

You will find it uncomfortable and often very painful to sit down, with the pain getting worse the longer you stay in one position. There may also be some inflammation and bruising in the coccyx area. Occasionally, bowel movements can be painful, and sex, especially for women, may be difficult or uncomfortable. Your doctor will make a diagnosis by performing a physical examination, and may order X-rays if he suspects you have broken bones.

## RISKS AND RECOVERY

Coccyx pain can be difficult to treat, so it needs an expert eye and awareness of the full range of related conditions that can occur; as such, the main risks stem from inadequate treatment. If your pain persists for several months and is consistently severe enough to make daily life difficult, a local injection of cortisone may reduce any inflammation and alleviate your symptoms. In extreme cases, where a fall or blow has damaged the coccyx, you may need surgery to remove any loose bone fragments and possibly the last few segments of the coccyx, but this is usually a last resort.

# PIRIFORMIS SYNDROME

**The piriformis muscles** are one of several sets of muscles that rotate your hips outwards, helping to keep you stable and upright when moving around. There are two of these muscles, one running across from either side of the sacrum to the top of each thigh bone. Piriformis syndrome occurs when one of these muscles tightens and irritates the sciatic nerve.

## CAUSES

The piriformis muscles run over the sciatic nerve, and can easily put pressure on it if they become too tight or go into spasm from strain or overuse. This irritates the nerve, causing pain. In around 15 per cent of people, the sciatic nerve actually runs directly through the piriformis muscle: these people are particularly predisposed to piriformis syndrome.

## SYMPTOMS AND DIAGNOSIS

You will feel a dull, annoying pain in your buttock that usually radiates down your leg, often accompanied by tingling or numbness. This tends to get worse when you sit down, particularly for any length of time, or climb stairs or a steep slope. You may also have difficulty walking. Some sufferers find sex painful, and some experience pain in the rectum when defecating. Your specialist is likely to be able to diagnose the condition from a description of your symptoms and a physical examination, but he may also arrange an MRI scan to rule out other possible causes of your pain.

## RISKS AND RECOVERY

With suitable physical therapy and exercises, most people make a full recovery within 4–8 weeks. Any activities involving strenuous, repeated forward movements of the legs, such as running, cycling, and rowing, can put particular strain on the piriformis muscles, so you should exercise caution when performing them. If your symptoms are very severe and persist after a range of methods have failed to bring you relief, you may be offered a piriformis block or a botulinum injection into the muscle (**»pp.86–87**).

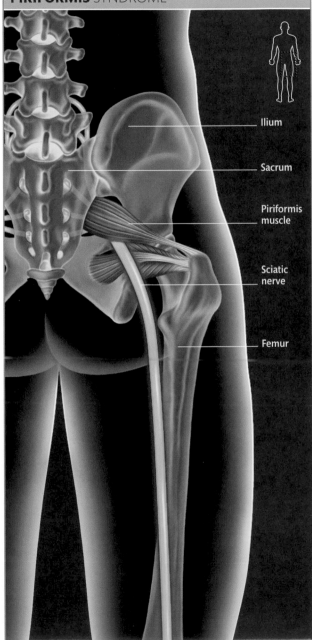

**PIRIFORMIS** SYNDROME

Ilium

Sacrum

Piriformis muscle

Sciatic nerve

Femur

The piriformis muscle is one of the small muscles deep in the buttocks. It runs from the base of the spine (sacrum) and attaches to the thigh bone (femur). The sciatic nerve runs very close to this muscle.

# GLUTEUS MEDIUS DYSFUNCTION

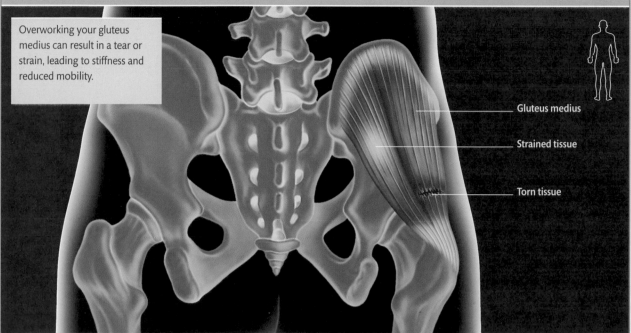

**GLUTEUS MEDIUS** DYSFUNCTION

Overworking your gluteus medius can result in a tear or strain, leading to stiffness and reduced mobility.

Gluteus medius

Strained tissue

Torn tissue

**The gluteus medius** is one of the main buttock muscles that are responsible for holding the pelvis stable and supporting your body on your legs when standing, walking, or running. It also helps control the sideways movement of your legs. If the gluteus medius is strained in some way, it can become tender and tight and less able to function normally.

## CAUSES

Stress or tension alone, if it continues with some intensity over a long period of time, can make your gluteus medius tighten up. Apart from the pain this causes, the muscles may become shortened and less flexible. In addition, referred pain from the spine or hip can cause dysfunction in the muscle. However, the most common cause of injury to the gluteus medius is overworking or stretching them beyond their normal range. Athletes, particularly runners, hurdlers, and long jumpers, frequently overuse their gluteus medius and

sometimes cause them to tear from failing to adequately stretch or warm up before any activity, particularly in cold weather. A less common cause of gluteus medius trauma is a direct impact, such as a heavy fall onto the buttocks, which usually leads to bruising and irritation of the underlying bursa (a protective fluid-filled sac).

## SYMPTOMS AND DIAGNOSIS

Apart from buttock and hip pain on one or both sides of your body, and possibly leg pain, you may feel stiff, be slightly unstable when standing, and find moving your hip awkward. Your doctor will carry out a physical examination to establish the cause of your problems.

## RISKS AND RECOVERY

Minor strains and bruises will usually heal on their own within a few weeks, but if action is not taken fairly promptly to rehabilitate overtight or stretched muscles, recovery may be slower. Muscles held in a state of tension for too long will fail to regain their former range of movement and response.

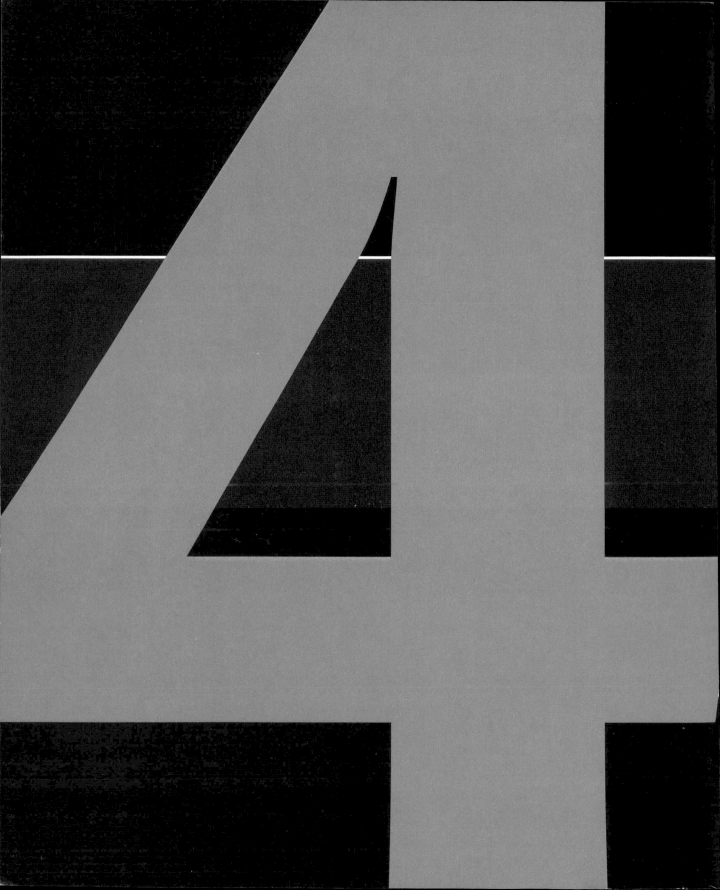

# WHERE TO FIND HELP

**Obtaining a specific diagnosis** can sometimes be a lengthy process requiring the expertise of a number of different specialists. This chapter gives you an insight into the various types of consultation you may be given, while providing useful information on the wide range of medical and complementary treatments now available.

# CONSULTING YOUR DOCTOR

**If this is your first attack** of back pain, you should consult your doctor. Back pain is rarely an emergency, but getting a diagnosis and guidance will help you better manage any future episodes.

Your doctor will probably begin by asking you some, or all, of the following questions:

■ Did the pain come on suddenly or build up gradually?
■ Where do you feel it, and where does it radiate to?
■ Is the pain sharp, dull, heavy, or burning?
■ Which positions or movements seem to ease it, and which tend to make it worse?
■ Is the pain constant?
■ Do you feel any numbness or pins and needles?
■ Have you had similar attacks before?
■ What kind of job do you do?

## DESCRIBING YOUR PAIN

Many adjectives can be used to express the quality and severity of your pain. Some, such as "sharp", "shooting", or "pulsating", may describe the physical sensation; others, such as "gnawing", "burning", or "stinging", may describe your perception of the pain; and others, such as "mild", "moderate", or "severe", may describe its intensity. As different types of pain have different causes, depending on the tissues involved, how you describe your pain will give your doctor a clue to its cause.

A general, dull ache is often the result of tense muscles or irritation deep inside the spinal joints. A sharp, shooting pain is probably due to a pinched nerve and, as with sciatica (**»p.46**), you may feel it somewhere other than the injury site.

If you are experiencing a diffuse burning sensation, it is likely to be caused by a problem with your sympathetic nervous system (**»pp.14–15**), which controls involuntary activities such as digestion and circulation of the blood.

## DIAGNOSIS AND TREATMENT

After examining you (**»below**), your doctor should be able to make a preliminary diagnosis. Since 94 per cent of back pain is purely mechanical, five per cent is nerve-root pain, and only one per cent has a possibly serious cause that requires further specialist investigation, it is likely that your doctor will be able to offer you reassurance of recovery.

## PHYSICAL EXAMINATION

After you have answered all your doctor's questions he will give you a physical examination. He will probably ask you to undress to your underwear in order to observe your back as you move and bend. He will also feel your spine for problem areas.

Your doctor will feel your spine for signs of misaligned vertebrae

Your doctor will apply gentle pressure to check for sore or painful areas

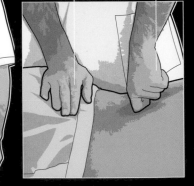

Sit with your legs relaxed and hanging freely

**Testing your reflexes**
Your doctor may test the reflexes of your knees, ankles, and feet. To test your knees he will use a small hammer to strike the patellar tendon; this should make your

**Feeling for tenderness**
Your doctor will feel for tender areas by pressing down on your spine and the surrounding muscles while you lie

You may be advised to rest or take it easy for a short period of time while taking simple painkillers or anti-inflammatory drugs (**»pp.84–85**), followed by gradually increasing activity. Your doctor is likely to tell you to be careful not to overdo things, but to stay active and not worry about, or fear, the pain. As you begin to get moving again, you should always bear in mind that "hurt does not usually mean harm". If you have any concerns about how far to push yourself, you can always return to your doctor, or other health professional who might be treating you, for further advice.

If your pain is severe, you will probably need a strong analgesic (**»pp.84–85**). Never be afraid to ask for stronger painkillers if you feel that you need them (talk to your doctor if you have any concerns regarding addiction). If you experience recurrent back pain and your job entails lifting or carrying heavy objects, ask your doctor to liaise with your employer about a gradual return to work, with modified or lighter duties.

## FURTHER INVESTIGATIONS

If your pain is especially severe or prolonged, or if it recurs frequently, your doctor may suggest further investigations. Initially, you may be referred to a local clinic or hospital for a blood test or X-rays, or your doctor's surgery may have on-site facilities to provide these services. Any further treatment will depend on the results of these tests.

### Blood tests

The various tests that are carried out on your blood sample may reveal an infection, inflammation, or even a tumour. They may also show that you are anaemic, indicating the possibility of an underlying disease.

### X-rays

Soft tissues, such as muscles, ligaments, discs, and cartilage, do not show up on X-rays. Since problems with these tissues are the cause of most back pain, X-rays are often helpful only for ruling out specific causes for your back pain, such as bone damage and disease, tumours, and advanced ankylosing spondylitis (**»p.63**).

X-rays can also reveal any degenerative changes that may be present, usually in people over 30, including osteophyte formation (**»p.73**) and narrowing of the discs or the foramina (the gaps between the vertebrae). However, findings of this type may not always be directly linked to the pain that you are experiencing.

## SLUMP TEST

Your doctor will use this test to rule out any serious diseases of the spine before checking for more common conditions. It will also tell him about the mechanics of your spine, pelvis, and lower limbs.

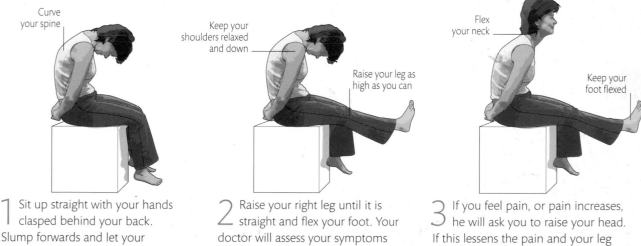

1 Sit up straight with your hands clasped behind your back. Slump forwards and let your head drop towards your chest.

2 Raise your right leg until it is straight and flex your foot. Your doctor will assess your symptoms based on your response.

3 If you feel pain, or pain increases, he will ask you to raise your head. If this lessens the pain and your leg straightens further, this suggests there is a neural element to your condition.

# CONSULTING A SPECIALIST

**If your condition** is not improving after 6–8 weeks of treatment from your doctor, you may be referred to an orthopaedic specialist. You may be referred earlier if your condition worsens or you develop other symptoms.

The first thing a specialist is likely to do, especially if he feels that surgery may be necessary, is arrange for further tests to assess your condition. If you have been in severe pain for many weeks and show clear signs of nerve damage to one or more of the sciatic nerves, he may also arrange for you to be given a spinal injection (**»pp.86–87**) for pain relief.

## BLOOD TESTS

Checking the levels of vitamin D and certain minerals – such as calcium and phosphate – in your blood can reveal whether you have a bone disease. If ankylosing spondylitis (AS) is suspected (**»p.63**), your specialist may also look for the presence of the HLA-B27 protein, which affects the immune system and is often common in the blood of AS sufferers.

## X-RAYS

If you have a spinal deformity, as would be the case if you were suffering from scoliosis (**»p.74**), an X-ray may help to assess the exact extent of any excessive or abnormal curvature, and would therefore help your therapist to plan a course of

### SPECIALIZED X-RAYS

**CT scans**

CT (computerized tomography) scanners send out several X-ray beams at once, each from different angles. This produces a more detailed image than standard X-rays and, until the advent of MRI, CT scans were widely used. In fact, CT scans show calcification in soft tissues and bone damage more clearly than MRI. However, CT scanning can take up to 40 minutes, during which you have to lie in a narrow tunnel (similar to MRI); it also involves exposure to radiation.

**Bone scans**

This involves injecting radioactive material into a vein, which is absorbed by your bones, making areas of high tissue renewal – a sign of possible infection, a tumour, or a healing fracture – visible when X-rayed or scanned. The procedure is safe and painless. Problem areas can be detected up to three months earlier than they can via routine X-rays.

treatment. Standing X-rays may also be used to check if your legs are slightly different lengths, or if your pelvis is misaligned in some way: both conditions are common causes of postural problems that can lead to muscle strain and back pain.

## MAGNETIC RESONANCE IMAGING (MRI)

MRI scanning (**»opposite**) has revolutionized the investigation of problems affecting the spine and musculoskeletal system. It allows the specialist to get a close look at the soft tissues in and around your spine – such as discs, nerves, and the spinal cord – that do not show up on X-rays.

During the scan, you lie on a narrow bed inside a tunnel, surrounded by a series of large magnets, and an image is produced that is effectively a photograph of a cross-section of your body. By combining a series of these cross-sections, a computer can create a detailed picture of your anatomy, clearly revealing muscles, ligaments, organs, and blood vessels. MRI scanning also has the benefit of being totally non-invasive and does not involve any potentially harmful radiation.

MRI scanning of a section of your spine will usually take about 30 minutes to complete, so it is important to tell your doctor if you are at all worried that you might feel claustrophobic during the procedure. You may be offered a sedative or, if possible, an open scan.

## MOIRÉ FRINGE ANALYSIS

This technique can show up specific problems with your posture and differences in leg length, helping your specialist to determine exactly how much correction is needed.

During the process, a polarized light is used to project a contour pattern on to your back. If the pattern is not symmetrical, orthotic lifts (**»p.113**) of varying thicknesses are placed under one foot (or buttock, if you are sitting) until symmetry is achieved.

## DISCOGRAPHY

The aim of this test is to identify the exact source of your discogenic pain (**»p.67**). You will be given a local anaesthetic to allow the specialist to insert a long needle into the suspect disc or discs, whereupon a small amount of dye will be injected into the centre of the disc. This disc will then be X-rayed, and you will be asked to describe any symptoms that the procedure itself provokes. If the X-rays show that the injected dye has spread throughout the disc and your pain is reproduced simultaneously, it is a positive result if adjacent tested discs are not painful. Your specialist may recommend surgical fusion (**»pp.88–89**) or replace this disc, which will relieve your pain.

## ELECTROMYOGRAPHY

By monitoring the electrical activity coming from a particular muscle or set of muscles, both when you are still and when you are moving, electromyography can identify any damage to the nerves controlling those muscles. This procedure involves inserting very fine needles, which are wired up to a monitor, into the muscles that are being investigated in the leg, foot, or calf. As the nerves controlling these muscles all emerge from the spinal cord, any that are not functioning properly may indicate pressure on the nerve roots. Electromyography has no side-effects and, apart from a slight pricking sensation as the needles are placed in position, the entire procedure is painless.

## MRI SCANNING

The highly detailed images of your internal organs and structure produced by MRI scanning have revolutionized the investigation of the spine and musculoskeletal system. You lie on a motorized bed that then moves into the scanner tunnel, which is surrounded by a series of powerful magnets that create the individual scans.

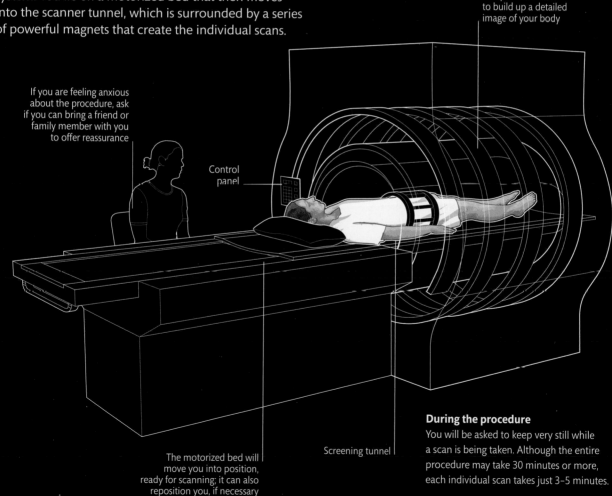

Signals relayed to the computer are used to build up a detailed image of your body

If you are feeling anxious about the procedure, ask if you can bring a friend or family member with you to offer reassurance

Control panel

The motorized bed will move you into position, ready for scanning; it can also reposition you, if necessary

Screening tunnel

**During the procedure**
You will be asked to keep very still while a scan is being taken. Although the entire procedure may take 30 minutes or more, each individual scan takes just 3–5 minutes.

# TREATMENT WITH DRUGS

**Doctors use a wide range of drugs** to relieve back pain and to treat its causes. These drugs range from simple over-the-counter painkillers to more complex medications that have been formulated to tackle specific conditions.

## SIMPLE PAINKILLERS

Painkillers such as aspirin, ibuprofen, codeine, and paracetamol are useful for coping with mild to moderate pain. They are widely available and do not require a prescription.

## COMBINATION DRUGS

Aspirin, codeine, ibuprofen, or paracetamol, mixed in varying combinations with another pain-killing medication such as co-codamol or co-dydramol, can be very effective in relieving pain. Drugs of this type are available on prescription.

## STRONGER PAINKILLERS

You need powerful pain-relief if you are in severe pain, are unable to find comfort in any position and cannot sleep, and, particularly, if your pain continues for more than 24 hours. Also, if you suffer from severe sciatica or brachialgia caused by nerve-root compression, there is evidence that good pain relief in the early stages helps to speed up recovery.

Examples of powerful painkillers include narcotics, such as morphine and buprenorphine, and non-narcotic opioids, such as tramadol. Non-narcotics have fewer side-effects,

but are often less effective than narcotics (which can cause constipation and drowsiness). Some doctors are also reluctant to prescribe strong narcotics because there is a risk of a patient becoming addicted to them. If you have any concerns about this, always discuss them with your doctor.

## MUSCLE RELAXANTS

When you suffer from acute neck pain or lower-back pain, your muscles tend to tighten up to protect the painful area from further injury, so you may be prescribed muscle relaxants. If you are stressed or apprehensive, your muscles may remain tight for longer than necessary after the injury has occurred and can remain fixed like this, even after healing has begun. Massage or relaxation therapy (**»pp.98–99**) can help, or you may be given diazepam or a similar muscle relaxant for two or three days. The drawback of these drugs is that they make you drowsy and slow you down mentally; furthermore, drugs such as diazepam are usually recommended only for short-term use due to the risk of dependency.

## ANTI-INFLAMMATORY DRUGS

A large number of doctors now routinely prescribe these drugs to treat painful joints. Their main effect is to soothe areas of inflammation, which plays an important role in alleviating pain. However, anti-inflammatory drugs can have side-effects, including drowsiness, skin rashes, nausea, gastric irritation, diarrhoea, and occasionally internal bleeding. Uncommon side-effects include increased risk of heart attack and stroke. Other side-effects may be due to allergy.

## STEROIDS

These synthetic cortisone-type agents are very similar to the steroid hormones that your body produces naturally. They are particularly good at reducing inflammation and can help to soothe some of the conditions that may affect any of the joints in your body, including those between the vertebrae in your spine. Unfortunately, the long-term use of oral steroids can have a number of distressing, and sometimes serious, side-effects, such as weight gain, acne, growth of body hair, diabetes, high blood pressure, reduced resistance to infection, and osteoporosis (**»p.65**). However, a small quantity of a cortisone-type steroid, administered via a local injection to reduce swelling and irritation around a nerve root, or to treat inflammation in a joint, usually has no side-effects.

---

### BONE REPAIR

The bones throughout your body are constantly breaking down and being rebuilt. If this balance is upset, as with osteoporosis (**»p.65**), your bones will become thin, brittle, and easily fractured or broken.

**Taking supplements**
One easy and effective way to build up and strengthen your bones is by ensuring you get enough calcium and vitamin D in your diet. Taking a good-quality vitamin and mineral supplement on a regular basis can help, but is not a replacement for a balanced diet.

**Bisphosphonate drugs**
For more serious problems, your doctor may recommend bisphosphonate drugs to slow the breakdown process and help prevent problems such as vertebral compression fractures (**»p.65**).

# DRUGS FOR BACK AND NECK PAIN

| TREATMENT | WHAT DO THEY DO? | WHAT MIGHT I BE GIVEN? |
| --- | --- | --- |
| **Simple painkillers** | ■ Relieve mild to moderate pain, acting both locally (at the site of the injury or problem) and centrally (via the brain) | ■ Aspirin<br>■ Codeine<br>■ Ibuprofen<br>■ Paracetamol |
| **Combination painkillers** | ■ Relieve mild to moderate pain, acting centrally (via the brain) | ■ Mostly combinations of paracetamol and codeine in varying dosages |
| **Stronger painkillers** | ■ Relieve moderate to severe pain | ■ Dihydrocodeine tartrate |
| **Strong non-narcotic opioids** | ■ Relieve severe pain | ■ Meptazinol<br>■ Tramadol |
| **Narcotic painkillers** | ■ Relieve severe pain (acting via the brain) | ■ Morphine<br>■ Buprenorphine |
| **Muscle relaxants** | ■ Provide relief by sedation (acting via the brain) and causing the muscles to relax | ■ Baclofen<br>■ Dantrolene<br>■ Diazepam<br>■ Methocarbamol |
| **Non-steroidal anti-inflammatory drugs (NSAIDS)** | ■ Reduce pain by inhibiting enzymes at the site of injury or inflammation | ■ Celecoxib<br>■ Diclofenac<br>■ Etoricoxib<br>■ Fenbufen<br>■ Ibuprofen<br>■ Meloxicam<br>■ Naproxen |
| **Steroids (cortisone-type agents)** | ■ Counteract inflammation | ■ Betamethasone<br>■ Dexamethasone<br>■ Hydrocortisone<br>■ Methylprednisolone<br>■ Prednisolone<br>■ Triamcinolone acetonide<br>■ Triamcinolone hexacetonide |
| **Low-dose tricyclic antidepressants** | ■ Suppress nerve pain, relieve muscular tension, and help to allieviate insomnia | ■ Amitryptyline<br>■ Dosulepin |
| **Anti-convulsants** | ■ Soothe chronic nerve pain | ■ Carbamazepine<br>■ Gabapentin<br>■ Pregabalin |

# TREATMENT WITH INJECTIONS

**Injections can bring rapid relief** from pain by delivering an appropriate drug directly to the source of the trouble. This also means that the drug acts largely on the exact area where it is needed, lowering the risk of any side-effects.

Targeting your symptoms by injection can make the drugs used much more effective. If you were to swallow the drugs in the form of pills or liquid medicine, they would have to pass through your entire digestive system and into your bloodstream before they would begin to have any impact. When drugs are injected, you may notice their effect very

quickly indeed – sometimes relief is almost instantaneous. However, you should not always expect an injection to bring you immediate benefit. It can take 7–10 days or longer for a particular drug to have a marked therapeutic effect on the specific damage or injury that is causing your back or neck pain.

## HAVING TREATMENT

It may take your doctor just a few minutes to give you some of the injections discussed in the table below, such as trigger point or ligament injections to help relieve tense muscles and sprained ligaments. However, some procedures, such

## INJECTIONS FOR BACK AND NECK PAIN

| TREATMENT | WHAT DO THEY DO? |
| --- | --- |
| **Trigger-point injections into muscle** | ■ Extreme muscular tension that is causing pain can be successfully eradicated with local injections of anaesthetic. |
| **Ligament injections** | ■ A sprained ligament may heal quicker with a local injection of steroid combined with an anaesthetic. |
| **Prolotherapy** | ■ Weakened ligaments, particularly in the lower back, can be restored to normal strength by injecting a fibroproliferative agent such as a vein sclerosant into them. This stimulates the production of fibrous tissue and new collagen, leading to tighter ligaments. |
| **Epidural injections** | ■ Backache and sciatica caused by disc protrusions may benefit from injections of anaesthetic and some steroid into the epidural space – between the outer lining of the dural sheath and the bony walls of the spinal canal. The anaesthetic blocks the pain, while the steroid reduces inflammation of the dural sheath. |
| **Nerve blocks** | ■ An epidural may fail to relieve pain if a nerve is trapped in the exit foramen. An injection of anaesthetic and steroid directly to the nerve root will block the nerve, shutting out the pain it is transmitting, and reduce inflammation. |
| **Facet joint injections and radiofrequency denervation** | ■ Severe backache related to facet joints can be treated with an injection of steroid and anaesthetic. A temporary response can be followed up by heating the nerve that leads to the joint with an electrically charged needle – a technique known as radiofrequency facet denervation. This can provide a lasting cure. |

as epidural injections and nerve blocks, can take 30 minutes or longer to carry out, and may require you to attend a specialist clinic.

## SUCCESSFUL RECOVERY

The success of many forms of treatment involving injected drugs – especially in the long term – also depends to some extent on you following your doctor's advice on how to look after your back, both between injections and after you have completed your course of treatment. This may involve limiting your activities – avoiding lifting and carrying heavy objects, for example, or taking part in certain sports – and making sure that you do not overexert yourself in general. Your doctor or specialist may also give you some remedial exercises to do.

## DIAGNOSIS BY INJECTION

As well as being used to alleviate symptoms and speed up recovery, your doctor may use injections as a diagnostic tool. Observing the effect of a local anaesthetic injection may help to determine exactly which area of the spine, or its associated muscles or other structures, is generating the pain you are feeling.

Diagnosis by injection involves injecting the region under investigation, such as a facet or sacroiliac joint, with lidocaine or a similar anesthetic drug. If this gives you almost immediate temporary relief from your pain, your doctor can infer that the injected area of your back must be involved in causing your symptoms.

Your doctor can use an X-ray-guided diagnostic injection, along with your medical history, a physical examination, and perhaps imaging such as X-rays or MRI scans, to plan further treatment.

| WHAT DOES IT INVOLVE? | WHAT RESULTS SHOULD I EXPECT? |
|---|---|
| ■ Your doctor will inject a small dose of anaesthetic directly into the muscle at the site of the pain. Trigger-point injections are often used alongside stretching exercises and a cooling spray to alleviate pain. | ■ The muscles should start to relax, causing any tension-related pain to fade away. |
| ■ Having identified your sprained ligament with his fingers, your doctor will inject a drop of the steroid and anaesthetic mixture at closely spaced points along the length of the ligament. | ■ You may be sore or ache for several days and must avoid heavy lifting and carrying, bending, and sitting in one position for long periods, because the steroid initially weakens the ligament. After 10–14 days, the ligament should return to normal. |
| ■ This usually involves a course of three weekly injections, which can be painful, and you may be given sedation or analgesic gas such as Entonox. Before performing the injection, your doctor will ask you to lie on your front over a pillow or cushion so that your lower back is slightly rounded. | ■ The site of the injection will feel sore and bruised for 2–3 days. Do not expect much improvement until 8 weeks after the first injection, as it takes time for new ligament tissue to grow. Keep bending and lifting to a minimum during this time. After 4–5 weeks, your doctor may advise you to walk about 5km (3 miles) a day to aid your recovery. You should feel the full benefits after around 3 months. |
| ■ Your doctor will ask you to lie on your front over a pillow while he gives you the injection, which is delivered slowly over a ten-minute period. You may feel slight pressure in the base of your spine, but very few people experience pain. After the injection, you must rest for 10 minutes on your front, followed by 10 minutes on your back, before you are ready to go home. | ■ Immediately after the injection your pain should ease. It may never return; it may go away for a few hours, return for a few days but fade away by the end of the week; or it may gradually fade over 7–14 days. If the injection brings only partial relief after two weeks, your doctor may offer you alternative treatment, such as a nerve block (**»below**). |
| ■ Your doctor will ask you to lie on your front while he injects the nerve root with a small amount of local anaesthetic mixed with corticosteroid. Nerve blocks are usually given using an X-ray image to guide the needle. | ■ Results are variable, with 50 per cent of people responding very well. If the relevant nerve root has been accurately located, the anaesthetic and steroid will provide good pain relief. In some cases, prolonged or even permanent relief is obtained. |
| ■ Your doctor will inject directly into the facet joints, using X-rays to guide the needle. You may find it a little painful. In radiofrequency facet denervation, the current applied via the needle heats the nerve to the facet joint, just enough to destroy the fibres that are transmitting the pain. | ■ You will probably be sore for a few days after the injection. Pain relief should be permanent, but if you have osteoarthritis these injections may bring you only a few pain-free months. If it recurs, radiofrequency facet denervation may bring more permanent relief. |

# TREATMENT WITH SURGERY

**Spinal surgery** has a high success rate, regardless of the patient's condition and age. This is due to increasingly accurate diagnostic tools, as well as advances in surgical techniques.

You will usually be offered surgery only if other treatments have failed. Most people benefit from undergoing surgery, and although they may not be completely cured of backache, they remain largely free of symptoms for at least ten years after their operation.

Some conditions, however, are surgical emergencies on which it is best to operate without trying other treatment first. A good example is when disc herniation (**»p.70**) puts so much pressure on your cauda equina (spinal nerve roots) that

you experience pain, coupled with loss of sensation, weak muscles and sciatica in one or both legs, and bladder and bowel weakness or incontinence. If these symptoms occur, you are likely to be given an MRI scan, followed by surgery.

## COMMON OPERABLE CONDITIONS

Disc herniation – especially if it causes sciatica – is one of the most common conditions to be treated surgically. But unless it is severe, your doctor is more likely to monitor your condition for several weeks, while treating you with less invasive methods such as medication and therapeutic injections, before suggesting surgery. Other back conditions that may demand surgery include spinal stenosis (**»p.73**) and severe spondylolisthesis (**»p.64**).

## SURGERY FOR BACK AND NECK PAIN

| TREATMENT | WHAT DOES IT DO? |
|---|---|
| **Discectomy** | ■ Relieves pressure on nerve roots that have been trapped by disc herniation and brings quick relief from nerve pain in the leg or arm. It is performed when other forms of treatment have failed to bring any significant level of pain relief. About 15 per cent of disc herniations will require surgery. |
| **Decompression** | ■ Brings relief from nerve pain by removing or reducing any pressure on your spinal cord, or the nerve roots leading from it, that is caused by spinal stenosis. |
| **Spinal fusion or disc replacement** | ■ If discectomy or decompression fails to relieve severe ongoing back or neck pain, or if you suffer from disabling discogenic or facet pain that is unresponsive to all other treatment, fusion may be suggested to stabilize the spine. As the operation stops all movement in the affected area, leaving it rigid, it is performed only when all other types of treatment have been unsuccessful. <br> ■ The modern alternative is disc replacement, which restores disc height while allowing some normal mobility. This puts less strain on adjacent motion segments and slows their degeneration. |
| **Surgery for scoliosis** | ■ In severe cases of scoliosis, you may need surgery to straighten your spine. The operation is usually done in early adolescence, when most severe spinal curvature develops. |
| **Surgery for coccydynia** | ■ Relieves long-term pain in and around the coccyx area. It is only carried out when other, less invasive, forms of treatment have failed to bring any long-term pain relief. |

Sometimes tumours or infections in and around the spinal column can produce similar symptoms to a disc herniation. These would need urgent surgery or antibiotics.

## SURGERY ON THE NECK

The problems that occur in the neck are much the same as those in the lower spine, but doctors are usually reluctant to recommend surgery. This is because the spinal canal is narrower in the neck, increasing the risk of damage to the spinal cord, which could lead to paralysis or nerve damage, or could even be fatal.

However, with conditions where pressure on the nerves could cause permanent damage to the spinal cord (cervical myelopathy), an urgent operation may be needed. These conditions include a disc protruding into the spinal canal, a dislocated vertebra, bony spurs, or a large tumour.

## PREPARING FOR SURGERY

The prospect of spinal surgery can be frightening. However, most operations are successful, and there is a lot you can do towards achieving a positive outcome and rapid recovery.

Make sure that you are as healthy as possible before your operation. Your doctor will assess your suitability for surgery, but you may also be asked to improve your diet, lose some weight, exercise, or stop smoking. A healthy diet strengthens your immune system, which helps wounds - including surgical incisions - to heal faster, and may prevent infection. Being overweight puts extra pressure on your spine, which can make the operation harder to perform and make recovery slower and more painful. Overall, the fitter you are, the quicker you are likely to be enjoying a more active, pain-free life.

Remember to ask your doctor or specialist as much as you can about your operation. If you know what to expect, you are likely to be less anxious, and this will help you to recover faster too.

| WHAT DOES IT INVOLVE? | WHAT RESULTS SHOULD I EXPECT? |
|---|---|
| ■ Your surgeon will remove the protruding part of the disc and any loose fragments of cartilage, and will check that no nerve roots remain trapped. | ■ Pain relief is usually dramatic. You should avoid heavy lifting or carrying for the first few weeks after the operation, and avoid heavy manual work for at least 3 months. |
| ■ Your surgeon will chip tiny amounts of bone from the lamina of the vertebra to widen your spinal canal. He will also check whether blood circulation to your dural sheath is impaired due to pressure within the spinal canal. If it is, the operation will also fully restore this circulation. | ■ You should be able to walk around within a day of the operation, but will need to stay in hospital for about 2–3 days to recover from the operation. You should avoid any strenuous exercise and lifting for about 3 months. |
| ■ Your surgeon will take bone from another part of your body, usually the pelvis, and graft it either over a facet joint or into the space between two vertebrae (having first removed any damaged disc). Alternatives include metal cages inserted in between the vertebrae. Several sections of the spine may be fused at the same time and screws inserted to hold the area rigid while the fusion solidifies. <br> ■ Disc replacement with a prosthesis involves placing a disc prosthesis between the vertebral bodies: usually two metal end plates and a pliable inner core are inserted through the abdomen after the contents of the disc space have been removed. | ■ This operation takes from 6 months to a year to achieve its full effect, allowing you to perform normal daily activities without fear of pain. You should be able to return to a sedentary job within 2 weeks, but should not take up work that involves any heavy lifting or carrying for at least 2 years. |
| ■ Your surgeon will wedge a telescopic metal rod alongside the vertebrae of the abnormal curvature. He will then elongate this rod to open up the curve, before fusing this section of your spine (»above). Alternatively, your surgeon may remove the discs between the vertebrae in the abnormal curvature. He will then drill bolts through the vertebrae and attach them to a steel cable running along the curve, and pull your spine straight by tightening this device. | ■ For either operation, you will be in hospital for around 2 weeks, and off work for a month. You will have to avoid sport for 6–12 months. Both operations will leave you with a very stiff back, but free of the pain that was caused by the strain your abnormal curvature was previously putting on your back muscles. |
| ■ Your surgeon will remove the last two or three segments of your coccyx. If there has been a fracture that has not reunited fully, your surgeon may remove any loose bone fragments. | ■ You should be up and about within a few days of the operation, but you will not be able to sit up until the wound from surgery has healed. Usually, you may return to work, provided it does not involve heavy manual labour, within 2–3 weeks. |

# CONSULTING A PHYSIOTHERAPIST

**At your first meeting**, your physiotherapist will carry out a detailed physical examination, look at your medical history, and ask you about your general health and any medication you are currently being prescribed by your doctor.

Your physiotherapist will ask you to perform various basic movements, such as walking, standing, and sitting. She may ask you to stand on one leg to assess your balance, and to perform more specific movements to help her identify any abnormalities. She may then test your muscle flexibility and strength, and perform neurological and neuromuscular tests, before checking your joints and muscles for pliability and for any problems such as spasms, swelling, or changes in tissue temperature. On the basis of these tests, she will then choose one or more of the following methods to treat your condition.

## SPINAL MOBILIZATION AND MANIPULATION

These techniques are used to reduce pain and increase joint mobility, and are often used in conjunction with exercises and guidance on correcting body movements. If using spinal mobilization, your physiotherapist will perform a series of movements, with you either in a passive position or actively involved. Spinal manipulation can involve a combination of thrusting movements that are applied to a joint to push it beyond its physiological – but within its anatomical – limit of motion.

## THE MCKENZIE METHOD

Your physiotherapist will use this comprehensive approach to the spine to identify your underlying disorder. She will guide you through the process, which involves using repeated movements and positions to assess the way your body processes and responds to pain, and help you to actively

## ASSESSMENT BY A PHYSIOTHERAPIST

Your physiotherapist will assess how you use your body and evaluate how your pain is affected by underlying genetic and age-related factors, alongside the effect of everyday movements, and what you can do to avoid aggravating the pain. This involves your physiotherapist assessing your muscle length and balance, and how your muscles work together.

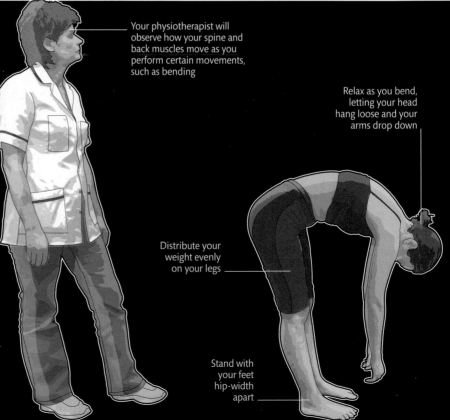

Your physiotherapist will observe how your spine and back muscles move as you perform certain movements, such as bending

Relax as you bend, letting your head hang loose and your arms drop down

Distribute your weight evenly on your legs

Stand with your feet hip-width apart

**Checking your flexibility**
By closely observing your posture – both standing and sitting – and how easily you perform a range of basic movements, your physiotherapist will be able to evaluate your condition and flexibility. She may ask you to perform bending movements forwards, backwards, and to either side.

manage your pain. She will also use the McKenzie method to help you "centralize" the pain in your lower back or neck, even if it initially extends to another part of your body. The aim is to reduce the range of your pain until it disappears altogether, while the new skills and behaviour patterns you learn will minimize the risk of recurrence.

## SOFT-TISSUE MOBILIZATION

Most physiotherapists also employ a wide range of soft tissue mobilization techniques. Soft-tissue refers to all tissue other than bone: tendons, ligaments, fascia, skin, fibrous tissues, synovial membranes, muscle, nerves, and blood vessels.

## MYOFASCIAL TRIGGER-POINT THERAPY

This involves your physiotherapist locating and deactivating painful trigger points (muscle "knots") using manipulation techniques from firm pressure to myofascial release (deep tissue work), often combined with Muscle-Energy Technique and Proprioceptive Neuromuscular Facilitation (**»p.92**).

## THE SCHROTH METHOD

A system of therapeutic exercises designed to correct abnormal curvature of the spine, the Schroth Method was devised by the physiotherapist Katharina Schroth (1894–1985) and developed further by her daughter Christa Lehnert-Schroth. It has been used in Germany since 1921, and by the 1960s was the standard non-surgical treatment for scoliosis (**»p.74**) in the country. German orthopaedic specialists routinely refer scoliosis patients for Schroth treatment. Access to a physiotherapist who is trained to offer this type of therapy is often limited in other countries, although its availability is beginning to match the growing demand.

### Muscle control

Schroth treatment is based on the idea that the muscles associated with the spine need to be retrained so that they are strong enough to pull it back into its normal vertical position. The exercises are tailored to the individual and are performed in front of a mirror so that the patient learns to control their corrected posture. Special breathing exercises enable their ribs to act as levers, assisting their strengthened muscles and helping to increase lung capacity.

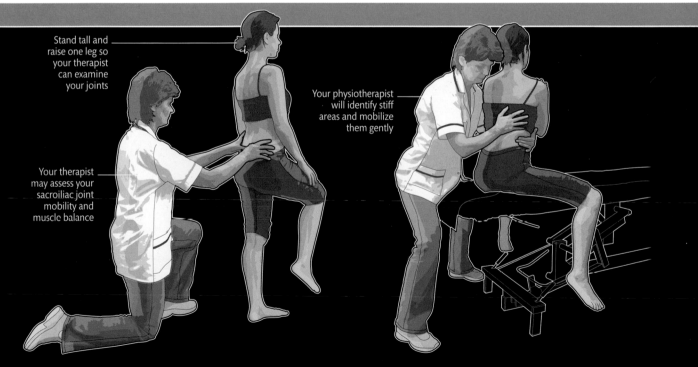

Stand tall and raise one leg so your therapist can examine your joints

Your therapist may assess your sacroiliac joint mobility and muscle balance

Your physiotherapist will identify stiff areas and mobilize them gently

**Palpation**
Your physiotherapist will ask you to stand, sit, or lie down, while she palpates (feels) your muscles and joints to assess your movement, muscle action, and pliability. She will also check for signs of poor balance, control of posture, and joint dysfunction.

**Assessing segmented mobility**
You may be asked to move your body in different directions. Your therapist will feel for any restrictions and check the range of your movements. This can also be used as a mobilizing technique to help you restore the rotational mobility of your spine.

## MUSCLE-ENERGY TECHNIQUE

Your therapist may use this to treat somatic dysfunctions (the impaired or altered function of body tissues), such as impaired movement or muscles in spasm. She will ask you to perform specific movements against her resistance, away from the restrictive barrier (the limit of the range of movement). As your range of function improves, she will repeat the process at each new restrictive barrier, with the aim of restoring full mobility.

## PROPRIOCEPTIVE NEUROMUSCULAR FACILITATION

This method involves a range of passive and active techniques that your physiotherapist may use to improve the flexibility, coordination, stability, and mobility of your joints, muscles, and other connective tissues.

## NEURODYNAMICS OR NEUROMOBILIZATION

Your physiotherapist may use this technique to treat disorders that involve your nerves, such as sciatica (**》pp.46–49**), with the aim of decompressing and mobilizing the affected nerves. It involves a combination of targeted stretching, mobilization, and the correction of your movements.

## ACUPUNCTURE

This is one of the many techniques used within physiotherapy as part of an integrated approach to pain management (**》pp.100–01**). Acupuncture can assist with the release of natural chemicals such as endorphins to ease pain, melatonin to promote sleep, and serotonin to enhance wellbeing. As your pain decreases and general wellbeing improves, your physiotherapist may introduce other manual therapies and rehabilitation exercises.

## THERAPEUTIC ULTRASOUND

Your physiotherapist may use ultrasound for a range of reasons, such as to increase blood flow, reduce muscle spasm, increase extensibility of collagen fibres, and speed up the healing of affected cells.

# TREATMENT

Your physiotherapist may employ a wide range of different devices and techniques, in conjunction with hands-on manipulation, to treat the problems you are experiencing with your back and neck.

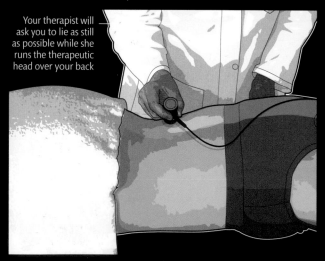

Your therapist will ask you to lie as still as possible while she runs the therapeutic head over your back

**Therapeutic ultrasound**
Your therapist will apply a water-based gel to the affected area and will move the therapeutic ultrasound head in a circular motion for about 5 minutes. The ultrasound will encourage the increased generation of new tissues to stimulate repair.

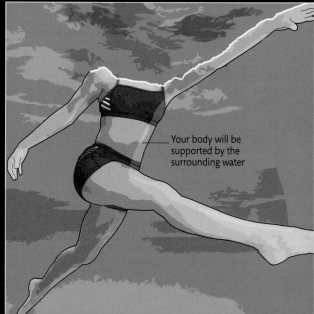

Your body will be supported by the surrounding water

**Hydrotherapy**
If you have musculoskeletal problems, exercise can improve your condition, but care needs to be taken to avoid damaging yourself further. Performing exercises in water is ideal as your weight is supported, so any stress and strain resulting from your activity will be minimized.

## FUNCTIONAL TRAINING

Predominantly using weight-bearing activities, functional training targets the core muscles of your lower back and abdomen. Your physiotherapist will guide you through a set of movements that mimic those performed in everyday activities, and tailor a set of exercises to build up your strength and mobility, and decrease your chances of injury. Functional training can also be used to improve performance and prevent injuries in sports and active leisure activities.

## SENSORIMOTOR TRAINING

This type of training is primarily concerned with your balance and postural control, and is used in the treatment of chronic musculoskeletal pain. Your physiotherapist will guide you through a range of static, dynamic, and functional stages using simple rehabilitation tools, such as wobble boards, resistance bands, and foam pads. The overall aim of the training is to restore, or improve, nerve-signal communication between your brain and your muscles.

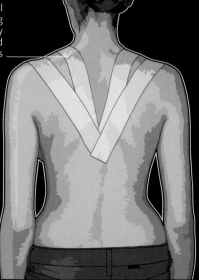

Your therapist will apply the strapping and the tape may need to be changed every 2–3 days

**Postural strapping technique**
Strapping will encourage correct posture of the upper back and neck. It may be used in the early stages of rehabilitation to take the strain off your neck and back.

## PHYSIOTHERAPY Q&A

**Q** | **How does physiotherapy work?**

**A** | Physiotherapists use a variety of manipulation and massage techniques to alleviate muscular tension, loosen stiff joints and ligaments to improve mobility, and increase blood flow to the damaged area to help speed up recovery.

In addition, your physiotherapist may devise and recommend exercise programmes to aid and maintain your recovery, as well as improve your posture and general fitness. They may also advise on correct movements for everyday activities, suggest coping strategies for those in severe pain, and recommend equipment that you can use at home to improve your condition.

**Q** | **Do I need a medical referral?**

**A** | No, but it is preferable for your doctor to make the referral as they have access to your medical history, are familiar with your personal background, and can provide your physiotherapist with useful information about your condition and general health. Furthermore, you might not be able to claim the treatment on your health insurance unless you have been referred by your doctor or specialist.

**Q** | **How long will a consultation last?**

**A** | Your first visit is likely to last between 30–45 minutes. Follow-up sessions will usually take around 20–30 minutes.

**Q** | **What should I expect during the consultation?**

**A** | Your physiotherapist will start by asking you a lot of questions about your symptoms and general state of health. This will include asking for details of any medication you may be taking, whether it is for your back condition or not.

Your physiotherapist will then conduct a thorough physical examination, which will involve checking the flexibility of your spine, testing your reflexes, and feeling your back for signs of muscular tension and tenderness. She may then offer you a brief massage or some manipulation. Follow-up appointments will involve her carrying out a programme of manipulation and exercise that she has devised from her diagnosis.

**Q** | **How many treatments will I need?**

**A** | Some people will only require one or two visits to be substantially clear of pain. Others will need far more. You should notice some benefit after the first few sessions; if not, physiotherapy may not be the right treatment for you.

**Q** | **Does it hurt?**

**A** | Possibly a little, but probably no more than the condition for which you are seeking treatment. You should feel better when you leave than you did at the start of the consultation. The next day, you may feel sore, but this should disappear in a day or two.

**Q** | **What should I wear?**

**A** | Wear comfortable clothes that are easy to remove. Your physiotherapist will ask you to undress to your underwear in order to assess your condition and make a diagnosis.

# CONSULTING AN OSTEOPATH

**Osteopaths adopt a holistic approach** to treatment, focusing not only on relieving your back and neck pain, but also on improving your overall health and general level of fitness.

Your osteopath may use a range of different manipulation techniques, some of which may be used together. All of them will be aimed at correcting the problems with your muscles and joints that he considers to be related to the pain you are feeling. Your osteopath may also give you advice on your diet and a programme of exercises aimed at improving your posture.

Osteopathy for treating spinal disorders focuses largely on improving or correcting any abnormal joint movement that a particular injury, or other problem, has caused.

Manipulation is aimed at loosening and freeing, rather than realigning, a faulty joint, and it includes rhythmic mobilizing of the joints to restore the optimal range of movement. Your osteopath may also massage an affected area to help relax the muscles there, relieving some of the pain and discomfort before beginning manipulation.

## MAKING A DIAGNOSIS

After taking a full medical history, discussing your symptoms, and perhaps performing an assessment of your posture, your osteopath will carry out a thorough physical examination. You will be asked to bend forwards, backwards, and to either side, describing any pain or discomfort that these movements provoke. Your osteopath will also ask you to lie down on your back: he will then lift up each of your

## TREATMENT BY AN OSTEOPATH

Your osteopath will usually begin by massaging your back for several minutes to relax the muscles and make you feel more comfortable. This will also stretch your

spine slightly, helping to reduce pressure on the discs. He will then start to manipulate the joints in and around the area that is causing you pain.

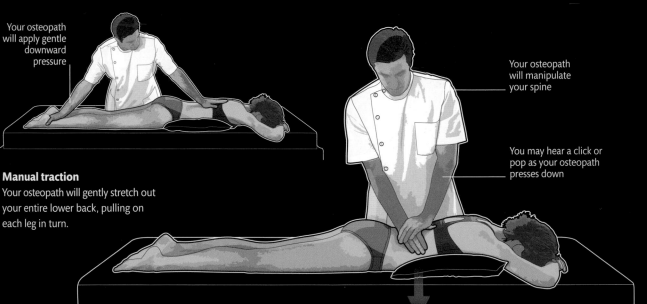

Your osteopath will apply gentle downward pressure

**Manual traction**
Your osteopath will gently stretch out your entire lower back, pulling on each leg in turn.

Your osteopath will manipulate your spine

You may hear a click or pop as your osteopath presses down

**Testing spinal mobility**
As you lie face down on the couch, relieving pressure on your spine, your osteopath will press down on each of your spinal joints in turn, attempting to move them as far as he can within their normal range

legs in turn to see how far he can raise them without causing you pain. He will also perform a physical examination both while you are lying on your front and while on your side.

## PLANNING TREATMENT

By observing the type of movements that cause you pain, your osteopath will be able to work out which part of your spine is malfunctioning. He should then be able to devise a programme of treatment to restore normal pain-free movement. If, for example, he decides that your pain is due to disc bulge, he may conclude that the disc will return to its normal position as soon as pressure from the upper part of your spine is no longer bearing down on it. Gentle manipulation while you are lying down, combined with manual traction, might then be sufficient to cure this problem. This is likely to involve several sessions of treatment, supported by therapeutic exercises performed at home.

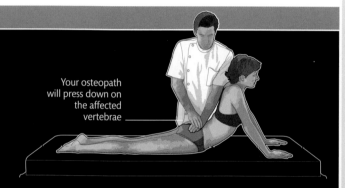

Your osteopath will press down on the affected vertebrae

**Lumbar extension**
As you lie on your front, your osteopath will ask you to arch your back by pressing yourself up with your hands, while keeping your hips on the couch. This will help him localize the downward pressure on the affected vertebrae.

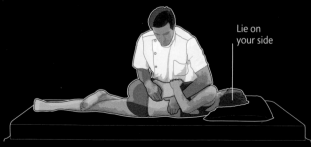

Lie on your side

**Rotary manipulation**
Your osteopath will ask you to lie on your side. He will then manipulate any stiff joints in your spine by using a gently rotating movement to help loosen them and increase their mobility.

## OSTEOPATHY Q&A

**Q** | **How does osteopathy work?**

**A** | Treatment is based on the idea that problems in any part of your body are all related to structural and mechanical problems of your musculoskeletal system. Your osteopath will feel your back muscles and spinal segments to check their tone and their response to movement. This will help him to make a diagnosis and plan a course of manipulation.

**Q** | **Do I need a medical referral?**

**A** | No, but if you have already consulted your doctor about your back problem, it would be courteous and probably helpful to tell him that you are planning to see an osteopath. Most doctors will be happy to give you a letter of referral, detailing information about your condition and any previous treatment. Furthermore, you might not be able to make a claim on your health insurance unless you have been referred by your doctor or specialist.

**Q** | **How long will a consultation last?**

**A** | Your first appointment will usually be about 45 minutes. Subsequent visits should last between 20 and 30 minutes.

**Q** | **What should I expect during the consultation?**

**A** | On your first visit, your osteopath will ask about your condition and medical history. He will also ask if you are currently taking any pain-relief medication or other drugs. If you were referred by your doctor, your osteopath should have details of your condition and any previous treatment. He will then examine you thoroughly, and possibly treat you briefly with some gentle manipulation or massage. Subsequent visits will be devoted to manipulation to alleviate your pain.

**Q** | **How many treatments will I need?**

**A** | Most people notice a difference after two to three sessions with an osteopath, but no two people are the same, and a range of factors will affect how quickly you progress. Once you are free of pain and feeling generally better, it may be useful to visit your osteopath every two or three months for maintenance treatment, particularly if you suffer from arthritic joints.

**Q** | **Does it hurt?**

**A** | This depends on your problem. In a few cases, osteopathy may cause some discomfort. It is, however, a very gentle form of manipulation, and osteopaths are trained never to use force when working on a joint. If one form of manipulation is not proving effective, your osteopath will usually try another.

**Q** | **What should I wear?**

**A** | Wear something comfortable and quick and easy to remove. Your osteopath will need to see as much of your body as possible to assess your condition, so you will usually be asked to undress down to your underwear. If you have neck or shoulder pain, it may only be necessary to remove your top.

# CONSULTING A CHIROPRACTOR

**A chiropractor can manipulate** your spine to help relieve the back pain caused by different types of spinal disorders.

Chiropractic treatment is based on the theory that mechanical problems with your musculoskeletal system, especially the spine, can affect the way your nerves function, which can lead to a variety of health problems. Chiropractors use similar methods and techniques to osteopaths and regard back problems as symptoms of problems with the way your entire musculoskeletal system is working. However, they differ from osteopaths in that they focus their treatment on correcting misalignments of the vertebrae that make up your spinal column. For example, a whiplash injury may cause stiff facet joints in your neck and back. This could put pressure on the nerves branching out from your spinal cord close to these damaged joints, causing pain, poor reflexes, and even a lack of feeling in your arms. A chiropractor would treat this by manipulating the problem areas of your spine in order to restore their normal mobility. This improves the alignment of your vertebrae and relieves the pressure on your nerves so that they function fully again. The treatment is not painful, but there may be some mild discomfort.

## MAKING A DIAGNOSIS

Individual chiropractors vary in their approach, but a well-qualified practitioner will always start by taking a full medical history from you, including details of any previous treatment

## TREATMENT BY A CHIROPRACTOR

Your chiropractor will ask you to lie on a specialized couch divided into four sections that can be raised or lowered independently of each other. This enables her to use sharp, thrusting movements to manipulate your spine without causing further damage. She can also lower the appropriate section of the couch as she thrusts down on your back, helping to minimize the force she has to use to achieve a significant movement of your vertebrae.

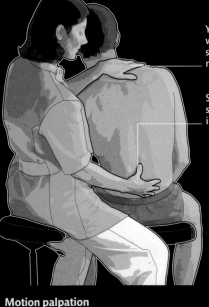

Your chiropractor will hold your shoulders and neck still

She will feel your spine for signs of injury or damage

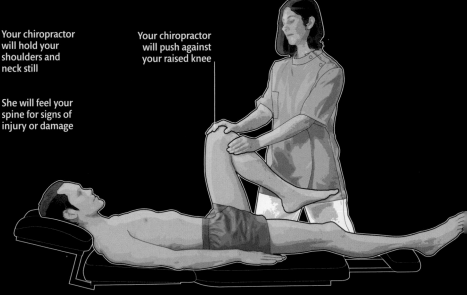

Your chiropractor will push against your raised knee

### Motion palpation

Your chiropractor will ask you to sit with your legs hanging freely while she moves her hand up and down your spine, using her thumb to check for misaligned vertebrae and to feel for any spinal joints that appear to be stiff or "locked"

### Assessing flexibility

You will lie on your back with your head slightly raised. Your chiropractor will then ask you to bend one leg and lift it off the couch. She will press gently against your raised knee, pulling the muscles in your lower back and around your hip joint to see how flexible they are. She will then repeat this with your other leg.

you may have had, followed by checks on your blood pressure, muscle reflexes, and the flexibility of your spine. Your chiropractor may ask you to bend forwards and backwards and to twist your body and head from left to right; you should mention any pain you feel when doing so. Your chiropractor may also take X-rays of your back to help detect any misaligned vertebrae or other structural problems.

## FURTHER TREATMENT

Your chiropractor may give you remedial exercises to do at home and advise you on posture and back care. You are likely to feel some relief after your first visit, but this may not last. You may need at least 2–3 sessions before you start to feel the long-term benefits: if you still do not experience any relief, then this treatment is probably not appropriate for your back pain.

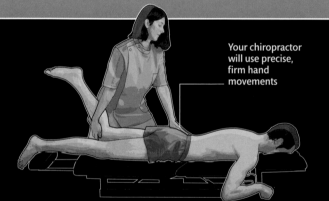

Your chiropractor will use precise, firm hand movements

**Relieving tension**
By lifting and bending each leg in turn, your chiropractor will stretch your thigh and hip muscles, reducing tension in the base of your spine.

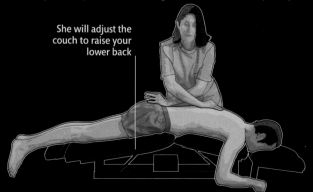

She will adjust the couch to raise your lower back

**Stretching the tissues**
As you lie with your back curved over the raised segment of the couch, your chiropractor will gently stretch the soft tissues in your lower back.

## CHIROPRACTIC Q&A

**Q** | **How does it work?**
**A** | The nerves that branch out from your spinal cord reach into every part of your body, carrying messages from the brain that control and coordinate all your movements and bodily functions. If your spinal vertebrae move out of alignment for some reason, the nerve roots next to them can become pinched or trapped, so that they and the parts of your body they control cease to function fully. This can lead to considerable pain and, theoretically, other health problems. Your chiropractor will manipulate any "misaligned" vertebrae, restoring them to their correct position and relieving any pressure they may have been putting on your nerve roots.

**Q** | **Do I need a medical referral?**
**A** | No, but it may be a good idea to keep your doctor informed about your treatment, especially if you have previously consulted him about your problem. Your doctor is also likely to offer you a letter of referral, containing information on your condition and any previous treatment that your chiropractor will find helpful. Be aware that you might not be able to claim the treatment on your health insurance unless you have been referred by your doctor.

**Q** | **How long will a consultation last?**
**A** | Your first visit will usually last for half an hour. Subsequent treatment sessions are generally about 15–20 minutes each.

**Q** | **What should I expect during the consultation?**
**A** | At your first consultation your chiropractor will discuss your symptoms and general health; she will also ask if you are currently taking any medicines, whether they are prescribed for your back pain or not. She will then examine you to check the movement of your back, neck, and limbs, as well as the alignment of your spine. She may also take some spinal X-rays to assist with diagnosis and planning treatment. If you are in great pain, your chiropractor may also give you some immediate treatment to help ease it. Over the next few sessions, she will carry out a programme of spinal manipulation designed to treat your condition and improve your overall spinal health.

**Q** | **How many treatments will I need?**
**A** | A range of factors can affect how quickly you progress, but you should notice some improvement after 2 or 3 visits. Further treatment may eliminate all pain.

**Q** | **Does it hurt?**
**A** | No, although areas of your spine that have been "realigned" may feel a little sore for a day or two after treatment. However, this will quickly pass and you should start to feel much better.

**Q** | **What should I wear?**
**A** | Wear something that makes you feel comfortable and relaxed. You will be asked to undress down to your underwear, so choose something that is quick and easy to remove.

# USING MASSAGE

**Massage is an excellent way** of relaxing tense, aching muscles. You may choose to visit a professional therapist, but even a friend or partner can give you a soothing massage. All they need are sensitive hands and a calm, reassuring manner.

Most people enjoy a massage, and, given the option, many would choose massage over a course of tranquillizers to help them to relax and feel better. Massage therapy is a very effective treatment for the type of back and neck pain that is triggered by muscular tension (**»p.62**).

## EFFECTS OF MASSAGE

Massages relax the muscles and stimulate circulation of the blood. When a muscle is tight, whether through injury or stress, it contracts, limiting the flow of blood through it. This causes the fibres that make up the muscle to become dry and sore. When a muscle that is contracted and tense is massaged, the blood flow is increased, and this in turn helps to lubricate and soothe the muscle fibres. Tight

muscles gradually affect the skeletal system by putting excessive tension on the adjacent bones and joints. Massage helps to lengthen the muscles and eliminate any abnormal tension – after a massage a person often looks taller and straighter.

## APPLYING PRESSURE

A massage does not have to be vigorous or painful in any way, but if it is to be effective in banishing muscular tension and relieving stress, it is unlikely to be completely pain-free. Particularly tense areas in the back, neck, and shoulders may be "trigger points" – areas that are often painful when any pressure is placed upon them. You may initially experience discomfort when these tender spots are massaged, even gently. But as your massage session progresses, you should feel the tension and discomfort melt away, leaving you relaxed and refreshed.

Your massage should help you to identify your main areas of muscle tension and this knowledge, as well as the massage itself, can help you to relax. If a muscle goes into spasm in response to any pressure applied during your massage, then you should tell your therapist, friend,

## TREATMENT WITH MASSAGE

Massage not only helps you to relax, it also stimulates the pituitary gland at the base of your brain to secrete natural, pain-relieving chemicals known as endorphins into your bloodstream.

Your therapist will rub oil over her hands to minimize friction

Your therapist will place a pillow or rolled-up towel under your feet to prevent cramp

To start, your therapist will place her hands flat on your back

**Aromatherapy**
Aromatherapists massage using essential oils, extracted from aromatic plants. Each oil has a distinct effect: some can be relaxing, others invigorating.

**Preparing to massage**
After your therapist has rubbed massage oil into her warmed hands, she will place them flat on your back and hold them there for 15–30 seconds.

or partner that the massage is too vigorous. Ask them to use less pressure, or, if you are finding the pressure unbearable, ask them to stop.

## PREPARATION

Choose a well-heated room and a comfortable, firm surface to lie on. Most beds are too soft for a massage, and it is usually better to lie on a blanket or towel on the floor.

The person giving you a massage should ensure that their hands are warm. It will enhance the experience if they rub a little massage oil into their palms.

## HAVING A MASSAGE

Your therapist, friend, or partner should use firm, rhythmic strokes to massage your back or neck, making and breaking contact smoothly and gently while concentrating on the areas of muscle that seem most tense. If you suffer from pain in one particular area, ask the person massaging you to focus on that area. They should work from the top of the spine downwards, starting with long strokes from the shoulders down to the mid-back, or starting from the mid-back and working down to the buttocks. Unless the person is a professional, he or she should work on the areas either side of your spine, never on the spine itself.

### Starting to massage
Your therapist may begin with slow, long, rhythmic stokes, using the palm of her hand to spread the oil over your back, and stretch and relax your muscles.

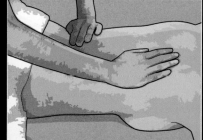

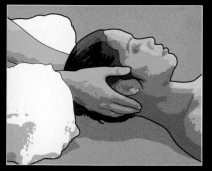

### Neck relaxer
Your therapist will ask you to lie on your back. Then, holding your head and the back of your neck with both hands, she will pull very gently towards her to stretch and relieve tension in your neck muscles.

## MASSAGE TECHNIQUES

Various strokes are involved in giving a massage. These are used either at different stages of a massage or on different areas of the body. Some of the best methods for massaging the back are outlined below. Start gently and gradually increase the pressure. When receiving a massage, tell the person massaging you which technique is most relaxing.

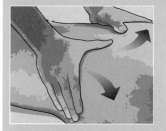

**Long strokes**
Start with gentle, sweeping strokes and large circular movements over a wide area to spread the oil. Use the whole hand, flat on the skin.

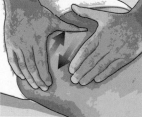

**Kneading**
Squeeze the flesh gently between the fingers and thumbs in rippling movements, or between the heel of the hand and the fingers.

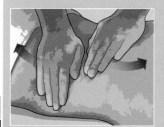

**Circling**
Press firmly, making circular movements. Try to build up a rhythm without losing contact.

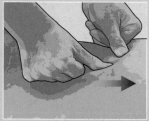

**Thumb pressure**
Use for bands of tense muscle, pressing firmly with your thumbs in a long, smooth stroke.

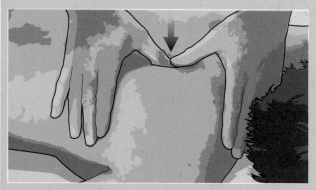

**Hand or finger pressure**
Place one thumb on the "knotted" muscle and the other on top. Press firmly and hold for 30 seconds. Repeat at other particularly tender sites. You can use fingers instead of thumbs.

# CONSULTING AN ACUPUNCTURIST

**Acupuncture is based** on the idea that energy, or "chi", flows through your body in channels called meridians. When these meridians become "blocked", so that chi cannot flow freely, you may become ill. Acupuncture practitioners believe that treatment can help to restore the flow of chi, thereby curing your illness.

The treatment involves inserting needles into specific points of your body. If your back pain is being caused by trigger points (**»p.62**), your acupuncturist may perform trigger-point needling, also known as intramuscular stimulation, in which the needles are inserted into trigger points. This may bring relief from long-standing pain and help improve your mobility.

Acupuncture works best when combined with physical therapy (**»pp.90–93**), as it reduces pain, enabling other methods to balance the body and restore function. There is no guarantee of relief – individual responses to acupuncture vary – but patients with a positive attitude towards the treatment are thought to get the best results.

## REASONS FOR CHOOSING ACUPUNCTURE

You may consult an acupuncturist at any time, although it is always wise to seek a medical diagnosis first. Most people will have tried or been offered more orthodox therapies for their condition before they decide to consult an acupuncturist. You may want to consider acupuncture for the following reasons:
- if rest, physiotherapy, manipulation, or analgesics are not helping to resolve an acute episode of pain.

## TREATMENT WITH ACUPUNCTURE

On your first visit, an acupuncturist will take a detailed case history of your symptoms and ask you about such things as your reaction to changes in the weather and your food and drink preferences. The acupuncturist will take your pulse and look at your tongue and complexion before deciding on a treatment. She may occasionally use a traditional Chinese remedy called moxa to clear blocked channels and re-establish the flow of energy.

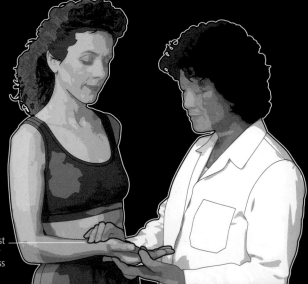

Your therapist will feel your wrist to assess your health

**Assessing your health**
In acupuncture, the qualities of the pulses at your wrist are thought to reveal a lot about the health of your main "meridians". Apart from the health and speed of each pulse, your acupuncturist will feel for pulse qualities such as hard or soft, rough or smooth, hollow or solid.

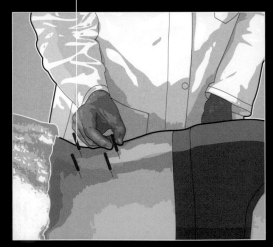

Your therapist will insert needles into strategic areas of your back

**Receiving treatment**
As you lie on a couch, your acupuncturist will insert sterilized needles into particular points on your body. This may be painless or create a fine, stinging sensation that lasts for a second or two. After the needles are inserted, the acupuncturist will leave you to relax for 10–15 minutes.

■ if you want to reduce pain and inflammation arising from osteoarthritis in your facet joints that does not respond to improved posture, exercises, or traction; or as an alternative to local injections to the joints (**》pp.86–87**).

■ if you have chronic back pain (**》pp.40–45**) or sciatica (**》pp.46–49**), which is not suitable for surgery, has failed to be relieved by surgery, or for which you have declined surgery.

■ if chronic "pain patterns" have set in. Acupuncture may help to break the cycle, perhaps by helping to close the "pain gate" (**》p.145**).

The use of acupuncture is not always based on scientific evidence, but can be an effective treatment for certain conditions such as lower-back pain (**》pp.36–45**). Try to find a licensed acupuncturist with a good background of training and experience in the field, who is also medically qualified and registered with a recognised administrative body (**》pp.216–17**).

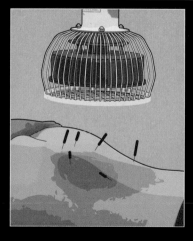

**Infrared treatment**
Some therapists hold an infrared biolamp above the needles to help ease back pain. The biolamp sends electromagnetic energy to the site of pain.

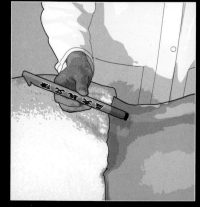

**Moxibustion**
Your acupuncturist may hold a lighted moxa roll over the acupuncture point to heat it. This assists the flow of chi by increasing blood flow to the area. She may also insert needles into the relevant points and burn small cones of moxa over them.

## ACUPUNCTURE Q&A

**Q| How does it work?**

**A|** The aim of acupuncture is twofold: firstly to identify the imbalance of energy that is causing a disease; and secondly to alter the energy flow until a harmonious balance is restored. In general, acupuncture may help back problems by reducing muscle tension, thereby relieving pain and improving mobility.

**Q| Do I need a medical referral?**

**A|** No, you do not need a medical referral to receive acupuncture treatment, although it is always advisable to seek a medical diagnosis of your back or neck problem before starting any course of treatment for it, including acupuncture.

**Q| How do I choose an acupuncturist?**

**A|** There are several organizations that work to defined codes of practice, which acupuncturists can register with if they hold certain qualifications (**》pp.216–17**). You can contact one of these organizations to find a qualified acupuncturist locally.

**Q| What should I expect during the consultation?**

**A|** Most of the treatment you receive will consist of your acupuncturist inserting sterilized needles into particular points on your body. Your acupuncturist will then leave you to relax for 10–15 minutes with the needles in place. Occasionally, your acupuncturist may burn a healing herb called moxa close to the acupuncture points to help re-establish the flow of chi: this process is known as moxibustion.

**Q| How long will a consultation last?**

**A|** Most acupuncture consultations will last for 30–60 minutes. Your first consultation will usually take around an hour, as your acupuncturist will need to ask you questions about your condition and general health, and will check your pulse for signs of blockage to the flow of chi along your meridians. Subsequent sessions will usually be shorter.

**Q| How many treatments will I need?**

**A|** Due to the lack of clinical evidence for the efficacy of acupuncture, it is difficult to be specific about how long a course of treatment will take. The length of the treatment will depend upon your condition, and how well you respond. Some people may feel an improvement after just a few sessions, while others may need a slightly longer course of treatment; some patients may never feel any benefit.

**Q| What should I wear?**

**A|** Wear loose, comfortable clothing. If your acupuncturist needs to work directly on your back, she will ask you to remove your top.

**Q| Does it hurt?**

**A|** No, although you may feel a slight stinging sensation when your acupuncturist inserts a needle. However, this feeling should only last for a few seconds.

# RELAXATION TECHNIQUES

**Learning to relax completely**, regardless of the stresses and strains of your everyday life, could be your key to banishing back pain forever. There are a number of techniques that will teach you to recognize and reduce muscular tension, and most can be learned fairly quickly and easily.

## MEDITATION

The aim of meditation is to bring your mind under control and focus it in such a way that you are freed from stressful fears and emotions. It can also slow your heartbeat and lower your respiration rate. Scientific studies have shown that by synchronizing the electrical patterns from your brain, meditation can induce alpha brainwaves, which are associated with feeling calm.

Initially, it is easier to learn meditation from a teacher. Look for a local centre or organization that will teach you the basic techniques. Some family doctors also run meditation groups in their practices and health centres.

The type of meditation most suitable for you depends partly on personal choice, and partly on your condition. Passive forms of meditation include transcendental, Buddhist, and yoga techniques. In the first, you raise your consciousness by silently and rhythmically repeating a word or sound. Yoga and Buddhist meditation involve deep breathing while concentrating on a single object or thought.

There are also active forms of meditation that involve spontaneous movement, adopting various postures, deep breathing, and facial contortions. If you have recurrent, mild to moderate back pain that is caused partly by muscular tension, this may help you to loosen up, both emotionally and physically. If you have severe back pain, however, it may not be the best choice.

## HYPNOTHERAPY

Hypnosis can help to influence the way that you perceive your pain. Under hypnosis your control over your conscious mind is suspended so that you are more open to new ideas and ways of processing feelings and sensations as suggested to you by your hypnotist. By talking about something that you associate with comfort and pleasure, your hypnotist can help you enter a state of deep relaxation, in which your pain subsides or vanishes completely. Even when you come out of your hypnotic trance and are again fully conscious, your pain is still likely to be considerably reduced. However, not

## SIMPLE MEDITATION

Choose a quiet room without any distracting background noises. Sit or lie down in a position that you find comfortable. Put a folded towel under your knees and a pillow under your head. Close your eyes and relax the muscles in your head and neck, then gradually move down your body to your toes, relaxing one area at a time. Do not worry about how well or deeply you relax; this will come with practice.

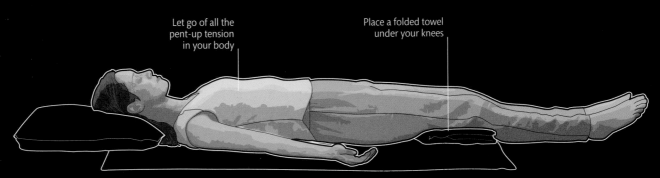

Let go of all the pent-up tension in your body

Place a folded towel under your knees

**Single focus meditation**
Breathe deeply and slowly through your nose. Become aware of your breathing and, as you breathe out, say the word "one" silently and slowly to yourself. Breathe easily and naturally like this for 10–20 minutes. Do

not dwell on distracting thoughts, allow them to drift from your mind, and return to repeating "one". When you finish, sit or lie quietly for several minutes, first with your eyes closed and then with them open

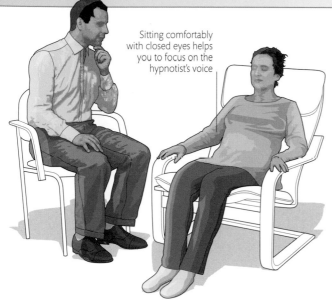

Sitting comfortably with closed eyes helps you to focus on the hypnotist's voice

## Hypnotherapy
A skilled hypnotist can help you to access the subconscious workings of your mind. This may change the way that you perceive your pain, giving you some control over how intensely you feel it.

everyone responds well to hypnosis. It usually works best on people who find it fairly easy to relax, let go of their concerns and worries, and put their trust in others.

## AUTOGENIC TRAINING
One of the most popular relaxation techniques, autogenic training involves sitting in a relaxed position while you silently repeat designated phrases, using them to stimulate visualizations. This prompts your body and mind to switch off from day-to-day concerns and to focus on calming thoughts, promoting deep relaxation and the release of pent-up tension.

## PROGRESSIVE MUSCLE RELAXATION
Also known as the Jacobson technique, this practice involves lying in a comfortable position, closing your eyes, and contracting and relaxing various muscles in your body. Your aim is to focus completely on the soothing sensation this should evoke and to shut out life's daily stresses (»p.149).

## DIAPHRAGMATIC BREATHING
It is common for people to tense their chest and back, making their breathing fairly shallow, limiting oxygen intake and affecting health. By learning to use your diaphragm – the large muscle below your lungs – to control your breathing, you will breathe more deeply, helping you to relax.

## RELAXATION TECHNIQUES Q&A

**Q** | **How do relaxation techniques work?**

**A** | Most relaxation techniques teach you how to shut out the pressures of daily life that are causing you stress, and to focus on releasing the pent-up tension in your body that this stress creates. Some, such as hypnotherapy, can help you to alter the way that you actually perceive your pain.

**Q** | **Do I need to consult a specialist practitioner, or can I learn to practise these techniques myself at home?**

**A** | It depends on the method you choose to help you relax. Many can be used, and in some cases successfully learned, without needing a specialist therapist or teacher to assist you. For example, you may find it easy to master some basic meditation techniques by simply reading about them and trying them out at home. However, you are more likely to get useful results from meditation if you learn a specific method from someone who has been teaching and practising meditation for years.

With hypnotherapy, it is best to start by having several sessions with an experienced medical hypnotist. He is likely to teach you some simple self-hypnosis techniques that you can practise at any time to help you relax, or whenever you have a particularly painful episode of back or neck pain.

**Q** | **How long do these methods take to have an effect?**

**A** | No two people are the same, and a range of factors will affect how much or how quickly you respond to any benefits a particular technique may bring. These will include how quickly you manage to master the relaxation technique you choose to practise, the severity of your back problems, and your temperament. Patience is generally an important factor in achieving a positive outcome. If you are used to being in an almost constant state of tension, it is likely to take you some time to learn how to cast this off and be able to relax completely.

**Q** | **Is any pain relief likely to be lasting?**

**A** | In many cases, yes it is. Once you have mastered your chosen relaxation technique, you should practise it regularly, as well as when you are feeling particularly tense and stressed. This will give you a more relaxed and calm approach to life generally, so that your muscles are less tense and any pain this tension has been generating will reduce or disappear.

**Q** | **Does it help to have a certain type of personality?**

**A** | Yes. Someone who is fairly easy-going and open to new ways of thinking and acting, will be more likely to benefit, or will benefit more quickly, from using relaxation techniques. This is especially true of hypnotherapy, which may have little or no effect when used on someone who is extremely tense or resistant to change and new ideas.

# OTHER THERAPIES

**Many clinics and hospitals** use electric currents to alleviate pain in a treatment known as neuro-stimulation. This can block pain and has been shown to trigger production of the body's own pain-inhibiting hormones. Other less orthodox therapies, such as aromatherapy and traction, may also help to relieve pain.

### NEURO-STIMULATION

This treatment uses electricity to stimulate the large nerve fibres that block the passage of pain messages to the brain, as well as reducing the action of the small fibres that relay pain messages to the brain from an injury or problem site. It also increases the level of endorphins and encephalins, pain-relieving hormones that circulate around the cerebrospinal fluid in the spinal canal (**»pp.14–15**).

### Transcutaneous stimulation (TENS)

TENS involves passing a pulsating current through electrodes that are placed on your skin. The rate of the pulse and the voltage can be varied according to the nature of your pain. This is the most common method of stimulating nerves electrically. TENS is a safe procedure, although there are certain restrictions on its use, such as if you have a cardiac pacemaker implanted or if you are in the first three months of pregnancy.

About 50 per cent of patients find that TENS reduces their pain. Some have short-lived relief, but experience continuing benefit in the long-term from using a TENS machine. An advantage of TENS is that it reduces the need for analgesics and narcotics. Drugs may be effective in dealing with acute pain, but over a long period of time they are likely to suppress the body's natural ability to produce the pain-relieving endorphin and encephalin hormones.

## NEURO-STIMULATORS

Various devices are used in neuro-stimulation treatment to manage back pain. They are all designed to generate a low-voltage electrical current that helps to block the transmission of pain messages to the brain.

Small, lightweight units, such as TENS machines, are suitable for self-administration at home, but a doctor should always be consulted on the long-term use of neuro-stimulation for chronic back pain.

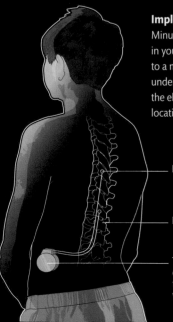

**Implanted stimulators**
Minute electrodes are implanted in your spinal canal and connected to a miniature generator by wires under your skin. The position of the electrodes depends on the location of your pain.

Electrode

Lumbar vertebra

The generator is controlled by a remote transmitter placed on your skin

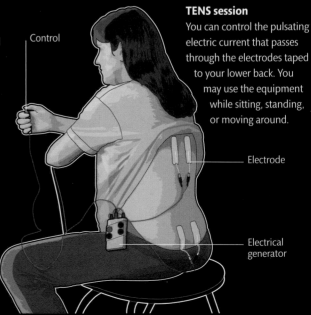

Control

**TENS session**
You can control the pulsating electric current that passes through the electrodes taped to your lower back. You may use the equipment while sitting, standing, or moving around.

Electrode

Electrical generator

## Implanted stimulators

If your pain is severe enough, your therapist may suggest that you have a procedure that involves having a battery-powered neuro-stimulator implanted in your spinal cord. Less common than TENS, this treatment is generally restricted to cases where back surgery has failed to bring relief. It is usually very effective and is particularly good if you have irreparable nerve damage. However, it should be used intermittently, as constant use can prevent the body from producing pain-relieving hormones.

Implants do not completely relieve pain – you will still feel sharply localized pain. People who remain on narcotic medicines after an implant may not obtain relief from pain, and prescribed courses of medication may affect the results of the implants. Their pain can be reduced by nutritional supplements and antidepressant drugs, which increase production of endorphins and encephalins.

## Other spinal implants and deep brain stimulators

Alternative types of spinal implant include epidural catheters, which provide a continuous infusion of local anaesthetic for up to a week to allow for active rehabilitation. Opiates can also be given via a slow-release system implanted under your skin at much lower doses than you would have to use by mouth, and therefore present fewer risks. These can be used in the long term to control severe pain.

A few people with very severe and widespread pain are treated with an electrode implanted in the brain that stimulates the production of endorphins and encephalins. This operation is performed only in extreme cases, as there is a slight risk of brain damage.

## COMPLEMENTARY THERAPIES

The therapeutic options for back pain are hugely varied, and include practices designed to tackle not just physical problems, but also psychological ones.

## Traction

Used to pull the spinal joints apart very gently, traction enables the muscles in the back to relax fully and reduces pressure on the discs. Inversion tables – with which you literally turn yourself upside down – are a popular form of traction as they can be used at home without the assistance of a therapist. They are safe, but you should consult your doctor or therapist before using one. Do not use one if you have suffered from strokes, raised blood pressure, or glaucoma.

## Aromatherapy and reflexology

Both aromatherapy and reflexology are used to treat back pain, although there is little evidence for their efficacy. Aromatherapy uses essential oils, which are either inhaled or massaged into the skin: the effect of the oils is varied, from relaxing and calming to energizing and uplifting.

Reflexologists apply pressure and massage-like techniques to specific points on your hands and feet, known as "reflex points", which they believe correspond to different parts of the body. Easing these is thought to have a beneficial effect on the area in which you are experiencing pain.

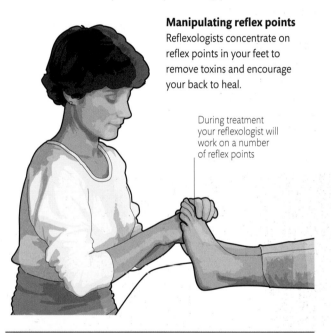

**Manipulating reflex points**
Reflexologists concentrate on reflex points in your feet to remove toxins and encourage your back to heal.

During treatment your reflexologist will work on a number of reflex points

## TALKING THERAPIES

Whatever the actual cause of your back or neck pain, you will almost certainly experience a psychological effect of some kind, especially if your pain is chronic. While there are a number of coping strategies that you can implement yourself (»pp.142-49), many people find that talking with a therapist can help.

The term "talking therapies" encompasses psychoanalysis, counselling, and Cognitive Behavioural Therapy (CBT). An increasingly popular practice, CBT is a practical, humanistic therapy, in which you and your therapist will uncover, examine, and talk through any negative thought patterns and irrational fears you may have and help you to break free from them. The emphasis is on learning to cope, and on developing strategies to help you do this – by accepting your present limitations and working within them – therefore enabling you to regain control of your body and manage your pain effectively.

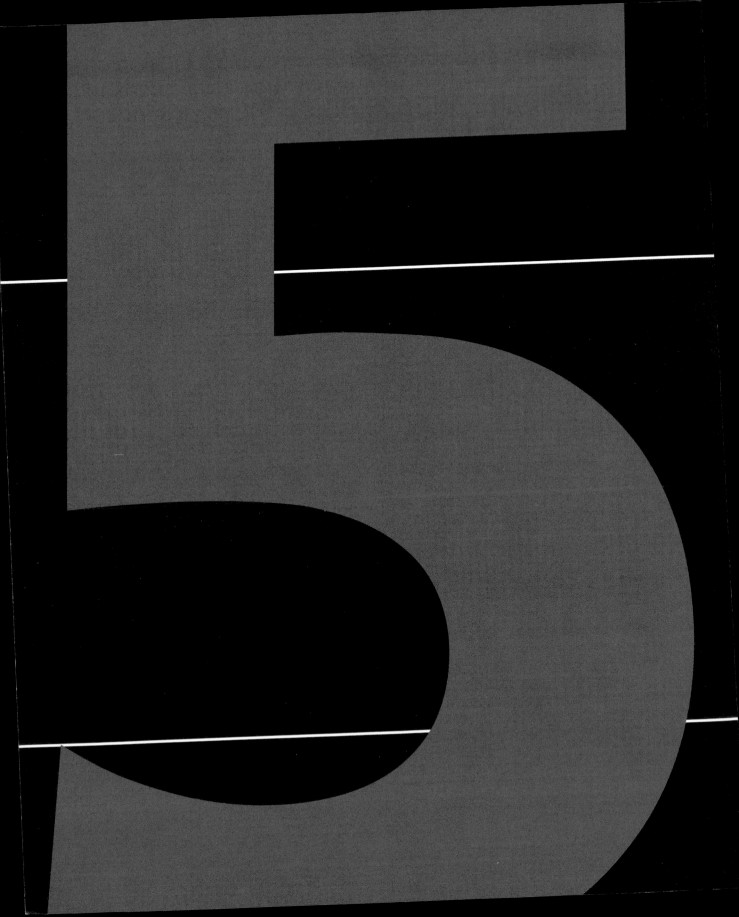

# BACK AND NECK MAINTENANCE

**Back and neck problems** can occur for a number of reasons – from those you cannot control, such as genetics and ageing, to those you can do something about, such as lack of fitness or poor posture. This chapter explains the role of your back and neck in movement, identifies key risk factors, and provides you with useful advice on basic lifestyle strategies you can adopt to improve your chances of avoiding or reducing pain.

# HOW THE BACK WORKS

**The spine supports** your entire body – it is responsible for almost every movement you make: you walk not only with your legs, but with your whole back, and you reach for, grasp, lift, and carry objects not just with your arms, but also with your back.

The structure and function of the spine are virtually identical in all mammals. One significant difference between humans and other animals, however, is that during evolution our centre of gravity shifted so that, when we are upright, gravity is exerted vertically throughout the length of our body. As a consequence, the human spine, together with its muscles and ligaments, has become a vertical shock absorber, with curvatures to provide the necessary resilience.

The spine must be firm enough to support your body when standing erect, yet strong and flexible enough to provide a source of movement for your upper and lower limbs. It is structured to allow for a whole host of complex movements, such as bending, reaching, lifting, and twisting. These movements are possible thanks to an elaborate and highly sophisticated relationship between discs, vertebrae, ligaments, and muscles (**»pp.10–17**).

Between each vertebra is a disc which provides cushioning and absorbs the shock that is created when you walk, run, and move (**»p.13**). Ligaments – slightly elastic bands of fibre – help to hold the vertebrae together, and in doing so allow a range of limited movements in any one direction, according to their length (**»pp.16–17**).

A group of muscles surrounds each joint of the vertebrae, and the ends of these muscles are firmly attached to a different vertebra, either directly or by a tendon. Close to the joints of the vertebrae, smaller muscles provide subtle alterations of movement when they contract, and it is these that control spinal posture. When you contract your muscles to move your spine, the ligaments and discs, which are specialized ligaments, allow the spinal column to bend.

## HOW THE DISC ALLOWS MOVEMENT

If you think of the vertebrae in a spinal joint as two pieces of wood and the nucleus pulposus as a soft rubber ball bearing, as shown, it is easy to see why the disc forms such a mobile joint.

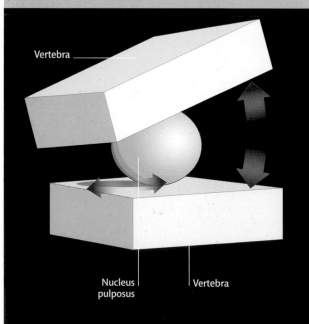

Vertebra

Nucleus pulposus

Vertebra

## THE ROLE OF LIGAMENTS

Ligaments extend right down the spinal column to support the vertebrae, hold the spinal joints together, and allow lateral movement.

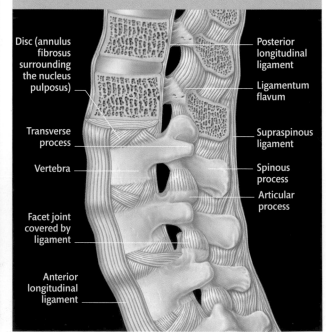

Disc (annulus fibrosus surrounding the nucleus pulposus)

Transverse process

Vertebra

Facet joint covered by ligament

Anterior longitudinal ligament

Posterior longitudinal ligament

Ligamentum flavum

Supraspinous ligament

Spinous process

Articular process

## MOVEMENT IN THE BACK

The human spine is the central support system for the entire body and plays a role in almost all our movements. To understand how all the separate parts of the back interrelate to allow movement, it is helpful to divide the spine into three main sections – the neck (cervical), mid-back (thoracic), and lower back (lumbar) – and look at how each segment functions in relation to the others (**»pp.10–11**).

■ **The cervical spine** (or neck) is made up of the first seven vertebrae in the spine. It is the most flexible part of the spine, as it controls movement in the neck. It must be strong enough to support the head, which is a considerable weight – an adult's head can weigh as much as 6–9kg (14–20lb). It must also be sufficiently flexible to allow you to turn your head so you can look and listen.

At the same time, you must be able to maintain a level gaze so as not to upset your organs of balance: these delicate sensors are located deep in each inner ear and are finely tuned to the forces of gravitation and rotation. This steady gaze is achieved through complex feedback mechanisms in the neck muscles, and these organs of balance allow the brain to account for movement while interpreting visual information at the same time.

■ **The thoracic spine** (or mid-back), is the longest portion of the spinal column and is made up of the middle 12 vertebrae. The primary function of the thoracic spine is to protect the organs of the chest by providing attachment of the ribcage. However, this bulky add-on greatly restricts the amount of movement in this portion of the spine. The movements that occur in the mid-back are limited mostly to rotation and a small amount of flexion and extension.

■ **The lumbar spine** (or lower back) is a more mobile part of the spine. It consists of five vertebrae and lies below the thoracic spine. This section of the spine is a lot more flexible than its neighbour and is the part that you use for many basic activities, such as bending backwards and forwards, walking, and running. Since it is connected to your pelvis, which is relatively immobile, this is where most of the stresses and strains occur.

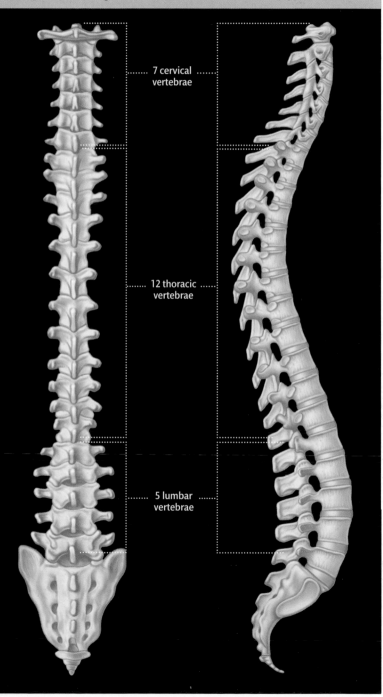

7 cervical
vertebrae

12 thoracic
vertebrae

5 lumbar
vertebrae

# WHO IS MOST AT RISK?

**It is difficult to isolate** any particular feature that predisposes people to back trouble, but factors such as age, gender, posture, fitness, occupation, and even genetics all play a part.

Numerous surveys and statistical reports from around the world reveal common findings about who is most at risk of back pain.

### YOUR AGE

You are more likely to have back trouble between the ages of 30 and 50. Fewer people under 18 and over 60 are affected. This is likely to be down to a combination of factors: the social and occupational demands of the middle years are often the most intense – from labour-intensive work and raising small children, to reduced sports activities, and a propensity to gain weight. The discs in your spine are most vulnerable between the ages of 30 and 50. Young people have strong, resilient discs, but they dry out with age (**»below**).

### YOUR GENDER

Women seem to be slightly more prone to back trouble than men. The cause for this is not known, but pregnancy, childbirth, and childrearing may take their toll on the spine (**»pp.136–39**). Men take more time off work because of back trouble and are twice as likely to undergo back surgery, but this may reflect the type of work they do.

### YOUR POSTURE

Poor posture accounts for a high proportion of back and neck pain. Commonplace activities that are likely to cause problems include leaning over a desk with your head craned forward and your back rounded, working with your arms raised – even if only slightly – for long periods of time, lifting heavy weights while bending from your waist instead of at your knees, and sitting in a chair set to the wrong height or without adequate back support. Slouching awkwardly in a chair or walking with your hands in your pockets may also place a strain on your back and/or neck.

## PHASES OF DISC DEGENERATION

Discs are composed largely of fibre, proteins, and water, but they dry out with age. The gradual process of desiccation is hardly noticeable until around the age of 30, when the outer layers of the discs (the annulus fibrosus) begin to degenerate. Inside the annulus fibrosus is a gelatinous substance known as the nucleus pulposus.

This gel acts as a cushion between each vertebra, and as the body ages, the gel dries out, leading to stiffer discs in old age. Although disc protrusions are less common in the elderly, thinner discs can cause problems, particularly for facet joints, and can lead to a reduction in the width of the spinal canal.

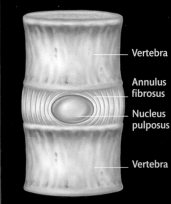

Vertebra
Annulus fibrosus
Nucleus pulposus
Vertebra

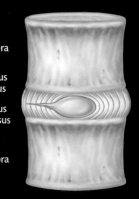

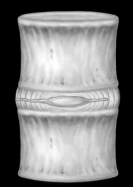

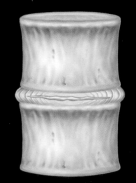

**Stage 1 (age 20–30)**
The nucleus pulposus of the disc is still healthy. During this period, hardly any fluid is lost from the pulpy gel.

**Stage 2 (age 30–40)**
The outer fibres are stiffer, with cracks developing in the annulus. The fluid content of the nucleus constantly decreases.

**Stage 3 (age 40–50)**
There is a progressive loss of fluid from the pulpy gel of the nucleus. The inner layers of the annulus have collapsed.

**Stage 4 (age 50 onwards)**
The disc becomes both thinner and drier, with a very much smaller nucleus. The annulus is stiff and inelastic.

## YOUR FITNESS AND STRENGTH

Research suggests that insufficient exercise increases the risk of back problems. If you are fit, your muscles will be strong and flexible, and you will recover more quickly from any injury or illness than an unfit person. Your bones will be stronger, too, and if you remain fit as you grow older, your bones will retain their strength for longer.

Abdominal muscles are often under-used in daily activities. If they are strong, they help to support the spine by increasing pressure in the abdomen, which reduces stress on the lower spine. If your abdominal muscles are weak, your back will take more weight, making you prone to lower-back pain. Tight hamstrings may also predispose you to back pain: because these muscles lengthen when you bend forwards, so that your hips do most of the bending, when they are tight, your back has to bend further, increasing the risk of back injuries.

A stiff back may not cause trouble. However, therapies that aim to alleviate back pain through making the back more supple are often successful (»p.142).

## YOUR OCCUPATION

Many industrial surveys investigate back trouble among the whole workforce, including workers with specific and very different tasks. In the building industry, for example, the crane driver, crane-watcher, and unskilled labourer all belong to the same trade but experience widely differing loads on their spines. The evidence shows that workers who are required to lift heavy weights manually are most at risk from back trouble, with unskilled and older labourers being particularly vulnerable.

However, people such as office workers, who are engaged in sedentary jobs, are just as much at risk as manual workers. Poor sitting posture is the main culprit: hunching over a computer keyboard for hours on end, sitting in a chair that is not properly adjusted to the individual, and cradling the phone between the ear and shoulder all increase the likelihood of developing back or neck pain (»pp.124–27).

Other workers who are also at risk of suffering from back strain include hospital workers, in particular nurses and porters, who are often on their feet, lifting and carrying heavy weights.

Driving long distances sitting in a poor position and with limited movements puts pressure on the spine. Truck drivers, bus drivers, tractor drivers, and aeroplane pilots tend to develop lower-back pain at an earlier age and show increased X-ray evidence of degenerative disease of the spine.

## HAZARDOUS ACTIVITIES

Often, the risks involved in any hazardous activity can be minimized by learning to lift and carry correctly, and by using appropriate equipment. The following factors increase the chances of incurring back problems:

- **Lifting weights** manually and lifting unacceptably heavy weights (a maximum of half your body weight for occasional handling, and of 40 per cent of your body weight for continuous lifting, was recommended as early as 1927). Equally, lifting an unexpectedly light weight can cause you to lose your balance.
- **Twisting, reaching, stooping**, prolonged bending, and any other similar movements.
- **Static work postures** – for example, driving (»pp.134–35), assembling electronic parts, sewing, and typing.
- **Inadequate seating** without a backrest, arm supports, or swivel action, as well as inappropriate working heights (»pp.124–27).
- **Poor viewing distance** for desk workers, as well as tools or controls that are not within easy reach.
- **Rapid, repetitive handling** tasks coupled with lack of attention.
- **Vibration** from operating machinery and driving heavy vehicles or trains.

## BACK PAIN AND SPORT

Regular physical activity is an important part of a healthy lifestyle. People who lead an active life are less likely to suffer from back pain. Joints, bones, and muscles require motion to stay in good condition, and so moderate activity or low-impact exercises can help prevent and reduce instances of back pain if practised regularly.

- **Yoga** improves spinal flexibility and strengthens the muscles in your body. Practise yoga gently, slowly, and safely within your level of capability. If you have a spinal condition, avoid strenuous backbends, inverted poses, and spinal twists. If a pose causes discomfort, perform a modified version, move on to the next one, or stop and rest.
- **Pilates** focuses on the development of abdominal strength and pelvic stability, and strengthens core muscles. Having core strength means that the muscles of your trunk are strong and flexible, and properly support your spine.
- **Moderate walking** is a great source of back pain relief as it gently exercises all the muscles around your lower back. It also increases your heart rate and blood flow. Make sure you walk briskly rather than stroll.
- **Swimming** is gentle on the joints. It helps prevent and heal muscular strains and can help with lower-back pain.

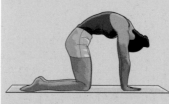

**Yoga stretch**
Regularly performing simple exercises like this one (»p.187) helps to ease aches and pains in your lower back and lubricates your spine.

# IMPROVING YOUR POSTURE

**There is no single ideal posture**, since humans come in all shapes and sizes. The ideal posture for you is one in which your back is put under the least strain, and in which your spine is naturally and gracefully curved.

Whether you are standing or sitting, the muscles in your back should be relaxed without being slack, and your spine should be gently S-shaped.

## GOOD STANDING POSTURE

How you stand and hold yourself makes a big difference not only to the way you look but also to the way you feel. When standing, your body should look symmetrical: it should be aligned equally both side-to-side and back-to-front (**»right**). Correct posture imposes less stress on the spine, so wear and tear is minimized.

The essence of good posture is awareness of fitness. Exercising and stretching your muscles, maintaining good core stability, and how you use your body when still or moving will also help. Fitness helps you stay mentally and emotionally balanced, which will help you avoid tensing your muscles and can help to improve your posture.

## BAD STANDING POSTURE

In the context of back pain, posture is poor when it puts your spine under unnecessary strain. Although "poor posture" is generally used to mean slack posture, an excessively rigid posture can be equally bad for your back (**»right**). This results in tense muscles and may even restrict your breathing. Poor posture causes tension in various parts of your body, and your back is more vulnerable to injuries and back pain because your back muscles, ligaments, discs, and spinal joints are all put under extra stress.

## CORRECTING BAD POSTURE

If you suffer from aching shoulders and neck, relax these muscles and avoid hunching or tensing. If you are overweight, it increases the stress on your spine because it causes your pelvis to tilt forwards unnaturally and moves your centre of gravity further forwards. As a result, your back muscles have to work harder, increasing the compression in your lower back. It is therefore important to lose weight and strengthen the muscles of your core.

If you are struggling to stick to a diet, try to do more exercise, perhaps by walking or cycling to work rather than driving. As you start to lose weight, your posture will improve. Do not be tempted to use a corset – it is no substitute for exercise.

If you are pregnant, your growing baby's extra weight will put an additional load on your spine, so good posture is imperative. Keep your abdomen pulled in to reduce the curvature in your lower back and pull in your buttocks so that your centre of gravity is over your hips. Avoid locking your knees when standing as this can increase the amount of curvature in your lower back, leading to lower-back pain.

Poor posture can also be caused by foot and ankle irregularities, but these can be corrected with orthotics (**»opposite**). You should also avoid wearing high heels, as this can increase the curve of your spine and cause back pain.

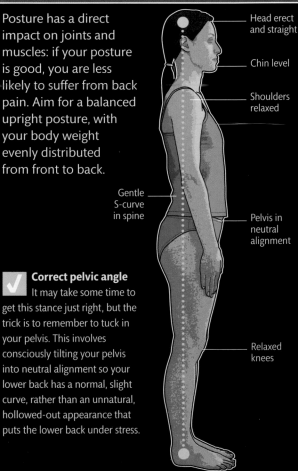

## STANDING POSTURE

Posture has a direct impact on joints and muscles: if your posture is good, you are less likely to suffer from back pain. Aim for a balanced upright posture, with your body weight evenly distributed from front to back.

Head erect and straight

Chin level

Shoulders relaxed

Gentle S-curve in spine

Pelvis in neutral alignment

Relaxed knees

✓ **Correct pelvic angle**
It may take some time to get this stance just right, but the trick is to remember to tuck in your pelvis. This involves consciously tilting your pelvis into neutral alignment so your lower back has a normal, slight curve, rather than an unnatural, hollowed-out appearance that puts the lower back under stress.

## ORTHOTICS

Orthotics is a branch of medicine that deals with the design, manufacture, and fitting of devices to help support and rectify congenital or acquired problems in your limbs and torso. These orthopedic devices come in various forms, such as back and knee braces, and shoe insoles.

One common problem that can be helped by orthotics is pronation (where your feet roll inwards, causing the misalignment of your knee joints and hips). Pronation leads to aches and pains in your lower back where your muscles over-compensate for this weakness. A customized corrective shoe insert can help to realign the joints, easing tension and discomfort in your lower back.

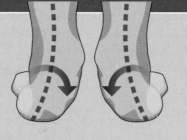

**Excessive pronation**
Here, the arches of the feet have collapsed, causing the feet to roll inwards. This condition results in the misalignment of the ligaments, muscles, and tendons in your feet, legs, and back. Left untreated, it can lead to progressive foot and back problems.

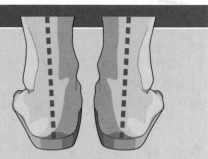

**Corrected pronation**
Orthotic insoles help to correct the misalignment and support your feet properly. They can be bought over the counter or custom-made for you.

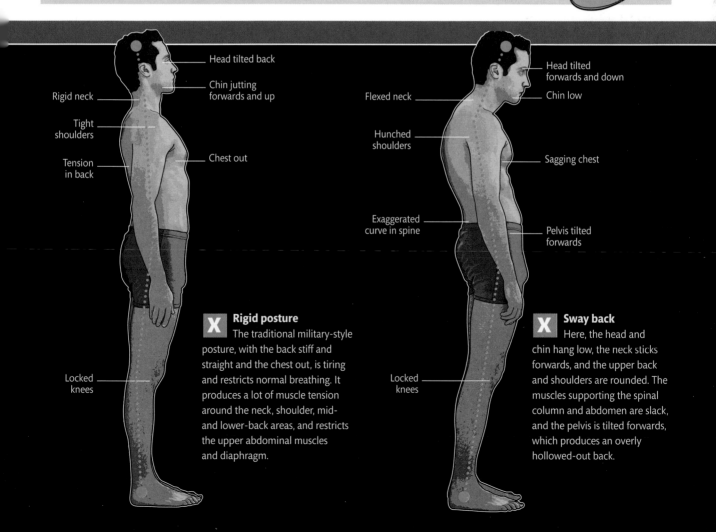

**X Rigid posture**
The traditional military-style posture, with the back stiff and straight and the chest out, is tiring and restricts normal breathing. It produces a lot of muscle tension around the neck, shoulder, mid- and lower-back areas, and restricts the upper abdominal muscles and diaphragm.

Head tilted back
Chin jutting forwards and up
Rigid neck
Tight shoulders
Tension in back
Chest out
Locked knees

**X Sway back**
Here, the head and chin hang low, the neck sticks forwards, and the upper back and shoulders are rounded. The muscles supporting the spinal column and abdomen are slack, and the pelvis is tilted forwards, which produces an overly hollowed-out back.

Head tilted forwards and down
Chin low
Flexed neck
Hunched shoulders
Sagging chest
Exaggerated curve in spine
Pelvis tilted forwards
Locked knees

## GOOD SITTING POSTURE

Sitting for prolonged periods of time can trigger pain in your lower back: this is because sitting imposes more strain on your spine than standing or walking. Adopting a correct sitting posture is not difficult and will reduce the stress placed on your back.

## RELAXING IN A CHAIR

Good sitting posture does not mean sitting up straight for long periods. You must relax in order to avoid straining your muscles. Anyone attempting to sit bolt upright will gradually slip into a relaxed, slouched position.

When you relax at home, choose a comfortable chair with enough space to let you change your posture: to avoid strained, tense muscles, you must be able to move around while watching television or reading. Cushions placed behind your lower back will help to support your spine.

## SITTING AT A DESK

Most office workers tend to be desk-bound, which involves sitting at a workstation for most of the day. If you must sit down for long periods of time, use a well-designed chair to reduce the risk of developing either back or neck pain and headaches (**»pp.124–27**), and stretch regularly (**»pp.118–19**).

### HEAD AND NECK ALIGNMENT

If, when sitting, you find that your shoulders are rounded or you tend to lean over a desk with your head bent forwards, the muscles in your upper back, shoulders, and neck can easily become fatigued. The result can be a painful neck or headaches. Whenever your neck feels tense or you find you are holding your head forwards with your chin out, try to reduce the curve in your neck by pulling your chin back and making the crown of your head the highest point. Neck retraction exercises (**»p.172**) reduce tension by bringing the weight of your head over your spine, so that your neck muscles have less work to do.

## SITTING POSTURE

Sitting actually puts more strain on your back than standing, and many of us spend most of our day sitting. That is why it is important to get into good habits early on to help avoid neck and back pain. It is easy to slouch when sitting, so try to catch yourself whenever you do this and make a conscious effort to sit up.

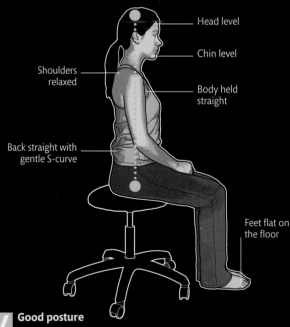

Head level

Chin level

Shoulders relaxed

Body held straight

Back straight with gentle S-curve

Feet flat on the floor

**✓ Good posture**
Sitting correctly helps to keep your bones and joints in correct alignment, and decreases the stress on your spine. Train yourself to be aware of your posture, especially if you have to sit for prolonged periods of time.

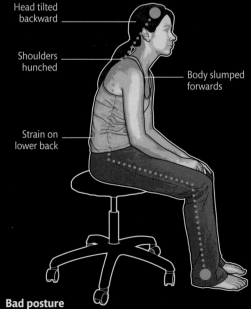

Head tilted backward

Shoulders hunched

Body slumped forwards

Strain on lower back

**✗ Bad posture**
Slouching is one of the most common forms of bad posture. It leads to musculoskeletal pains, backache, joint pains, and tension headaches. It also restricts breathing as your diaphragm is compressed.

## PRESSURE ON THE SPINE

These postures show how the pressure within the lumbar discs varies in different positions. Pressures are shown as a percentage relative to standing, which is 100 per cent.

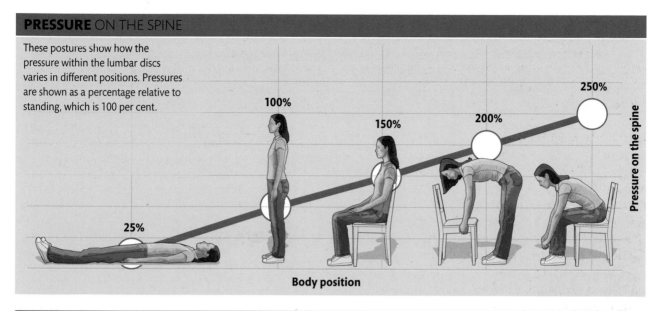

100%
150%
200%
250%
25%

Pressure on the spine

Body position

## THE ALEXANDER TECHNIQUE

The Alexander Technique aims to treat and prevent a range of disorders by improving posture. It is based on the principle of relaxing muscles – the neck and shoulder muscles in particular – and of adopting the posture that puts the least amount of stress on your spine.

Actor F. Matthias Alexander developed this technique after progressively and inexplicably losing his voice during performances. He found that, just before delivering a speech on stage, he tended to pull his head backwards and down in a manner that cut off his voice. He realized that posture exerts a constant influence on both physiology and psychology.

A qualified Alexander teacher will help you undo any postural habits that have become second nature. She will teach you techniques developed specifically for your own posture, which you should practise every day. The course may last just a few weeks or up to a year.

A course will not cure acute problems such as a disc prolapse (»p.70) or acute facet dysfunction (»p.68), but can help with "trapped nerves" by making more space. However, once an acute attack is over, the technique helps to prevent a recurrence. It is especially useful for avoiding postural pain, and if you are elderly, it may prevent acute episodes of back pain by teaching you to use your back properly.

### The technique in practice

Your Alexander teacher will help you eliminate postural defects by studying the way you sit, stand, and move. Your teacher will then tailor the lesson accordingly and may work with you sitting, standing, or lying down, depending on what she feels is required. She will encourage you to imagine that you are being pulled upward from the crown of your head.

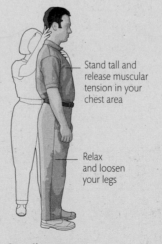

Stand tall and release muscular tension in your chest area

Relax and loosen your legs

Let your head, neck, and torso all work together

### Standing posture

Keep your spine straight when standing, rather than leaning forwards and pulling your head back.

### Sitting posture

Achieve good sitting posture by encouraging the right amount of curve in your neck, mid-back, and lower back.

# EXERCISE AND SPORT

**Exercise is crucial** for the health of your back. Working out regularly helps to keep your joints supple and strengthens your muscles, allowing your spine to move with ease and comfort.

Research shows that people who are physically fit are healthier and more resistant to back pain and injury. Performing a regular programme of stretching and strengthening exercises (**»pp.160–213**) can help to improve not only your general fitness levels, but also the strength and mobility of your muscles. Developing good stability and functional movement in the muscles of your abdomen and trunk (your "core") can be particularly useful when it comes to improving your posture. Playing sport regularly offers a range of benefits, helping you to improve your fitness, stamina, and endurance levels, lowering your heart rate and blood pressure, burning fat, and reducing stress, all of which can help reduce your chances of back and neck pain.

## MOST COMMON CAUSES OF INJURY

The key to avoiding injury is to listen to what your body is telling you and not push yourself too hard. The following factors are the most common causes of sporting injuries:

■ **Failure to warm up**, resulting in your muscles being less responsive and prone to strain.
■ **Overtraining**, which increases the risk of chronic injury by putting continuous pressure on your body.
■ **Excessive loading** on the body, which applies forces to your body tissues for which they are unprepared.
■ **Poor exercise technique**, leading to overloading on body tissues – especially if carried out repeatedly.
■ **Not taking safety precautions**, or ignoring the rules of the sport, so increasing the risk of an accident.
■ **An accident**, often the result of an impact or collision, and usually occuring suddenly.
■ **Inappropriate equipment**, so your body may not be adequately supported or protected from shock.
■ **Recurring injury**, which can weaken your body and make it more susceptible to other injuries.
■ **Genetic factors**, which are intrinsic (belonging to you) and influence the shape and structure of your joints.
■ **Muscle weakness and imbalance**, including poor core stability, which can lead to strains.
■ **Lack of flexibility**, which will decrease your range of motion and limit some of your body's capabilities.
■ **Joint laxity** (a condition which, if you have it, you should already be aware of), which can make it difficult for you to control and stabilize your joints.

## WHAT SORT OF EXERCISE SHOULD YOU DO?

The type of exercise you choose depends on your personal needs and preferences. All exercise is good, but to get the most out of your routine, it is advisable to practise a variety of both cardio and low-impact sports. High-impact cardio work, such as skipping and running, can be tough on the joints, especially the knees, so choose low-impact cardio exercises instead. These include walking at a good pace, step aerobics, and using equipment such as kettlebells or dumbbells in your daily exercise workout. Swimming, yoga, and Pilates are low-impact sports, and are ideal for improving the health and suppleness of your back.

## CHOOSING THE RIGHT GEAR

Ill-fitting or unsuitable equipment increases the chances of injury. Consider the following tips before buying:
■ Footwear should be suited to your chosen sport and must provide sufficient support and cushioning for your feet and ankles. Seek specialist advice, and always try before you buy.
■ Clothing should be constructed from a material suited to the purpose, such as breathable fabric for warm-weather sports or insulated fabric for cold- and wet-weather sports.
■ Sport-specific equipment, such as rackets, skis, and bicycles, should be custom-fitted to your body's dimensions and weight, and suited to your level of ability.

## HOW TO AVOID INJURY

Before doing any exercise, make sure you have the necessary footwear, clothing, and equipment (**»above**). Once you are fully prepared, begin your routine with a 10-minute warm-up (**»opposite**). Warming up helps your body prepare itself for exercise, both mentally and physically, and is the key to unlocking tight muscles. Some people miss out this important part of their routine altogether, but doing so is likely to increase your chances of incurring an injury.

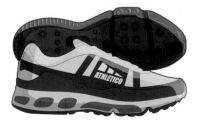

**Sports footwear**
It is important to buy the correct footwear for your chosen sport as there are marked differences in the way various trainers support your feet.

## WARM-UP EXERCISES

A good warm-up prepares your body for exercise and reduces the risk of injury. Every warm-up should include the following routines:

■ **Low-impact cardio work** includes exercises that involve your whole body (rather than a specific part of your body); big movements, like going from standing to crouching down and back up again; and ballistic movements, like swinging a kettlebell or a dumbbell. These low-impact, high-intensity exercises will increase your heart rate and blood flow, and warm up your muscles without being tough on your joints. You should begin your warm-up with up to 10 minutes of low-impact cardio work.

■ **Gentle loosening exercises** help to loosen up your body if you have been in a sedentary state, and may include rotations of the ankles, hips, wrists, and shoulders, and gentle jogging on the spot. The duration and intensity of the exercises depend on your level of fitness, but should last between 5 and 10 minutes, and produce a light sweat.

■ **Dynamic stretching** contributes to muscular conditioning as well as flexibility. It is best suited to high-level athletes and should only be performed once your body has reached a high degree of flexibility.

■ **Sport-specific exercises** consist of activities and exercises related to your chosen sport, and should be performed at a more vigorous level of exertion than the first stages of your warm-up routine.

### Whole body move

Low-impact, high-density moves such as this multi-jointed squat involve your whole body and work large groups of muscles without pounding the joints.

## COOL-DOWN EXERCISES

Cooling down after exercise is equally important as warming up. It restores your body to its pre-existing state in a controlled manner, helps your body repair itself, and can lessen muscle soreness. Never skip your cool-down, which should consist of the following components:

■ **Gentle walking** allows your heart rate to slow down and recover its resting rate, decreases your body temperature, and aids in the removal of waste products (such as lactic acid) from your muscles. You should spend between 5 and 10 minutes walking after exercise.

■ **Static stretching** involves gradually easing yourself into a stretch position and holding this position. It helps to relax your muscles and tendons and allows them to re-establish their normal range of movement. Perform only one or two stretches per muscle group, and hold each position for 20–30 seconds. Take care not to overstretch as this may injure your muscles.

### Static stretch

Static stretches should be performed after you have exercised to help your muscles relax. Try to do a selection of both seated and standing stretches to mobilize a whole range of muscles.

---

If you have not exercised for a while, make sure you consult your doctor before you start a new regimen. Set yourself clear, realistic goals, and aim to increase the duration and intensity of your exercise routine gradually. You should aim for slow but safe progress.

## EXERCISING AFTER INJURY

If you suffer an injury, your body will let you know. Sharp pain is likely to accompany an acute injury, while a dull, nagging pain is usually a sign of the onset of a chronic injury. If you experience pain at any time, modify your activity to reduce strain, and have a period of rest. If the pain recurs, seek professional advice.

However, it is important for you to return to an active lifestyle as soon as the worst of the pain is over. Exercising your back is important for recovering from acute backache, and may help those with chronic back pain. After an acute attack, begin exercising as soon as you can move without undue pain. You may ache and feel slightly stiff, but do not let this put you off. Some of the exercises in this book are designed to help with specific back problems, while others are for more general back care (»pp.160–213). Try to exercise once or twice a day, but if this is not possible, practise a few exercises at least once a day. If you are unsure whether you are doing an exercise correctly, seek advice from your physiotherapist or a qualified and registered trainer.

# THE BENEFITS OF STRETCHING

**A gentle stretching routine**, when practised regularly, can help prevent episodes of back pain. Make it part of your daily routine, whether you do any other form of exercise or not.

Stretching increases your range of motion and lengthens and loosens your muscles, making them more flexible and thus helping prevent injury. Simple stretching exercises should be carried out once or twice a day (**»opposite**). These exercises are designed to prevent back pain by increasing movement in your spine and reducing stiffness and pressure on your discs, ligaments, and facet joints. Relax your body and breathe deeply and rhythmically, inhaling before each stretch and exhaling during the movement. Perform the same number of stretches on both sides of your body, and if you feel any pain, stop and come back to it another day.

## WHEN TO STRETCH

Ideally, you should aim to stretch daily. If you plan to stretch every day, choose a convenient time and either incorporate the stretches into your regular exercise routine or just carry them out on their own. Find a time that works best for you – perhaps first thing in the morning or when you get home in the evening. Try to integrate stretching into your day whenever possible: during long periods working at the computer, get into the habit of taking regular stretching breaks; or take 5 minutes to perform a short routine after a flight or a long drive. Even short bursts of stretching can be really invigorating.

## PHYSICAL BENEFITS

Incorporating regular stretching into your routine brings many physical benefits, such as:
- Reducing the risk of injury by improving flexibility and balance.
- Helping to balance muscle lengths, which aligns the body, improving and correcting posture.
- Improving flexibility and mobility so that sitting, walking, and standing become easier.
- Promoting relaxation and reducing stress.
- Energizing body and mind.

## STRETCHING DURING PREGNANCY

Gentle stretching is generally safe and beneficial during pregnancy (**»pp.136–37**) and after birth. Relaxin, a hormone produced during pregnancy, relaxes the ligaments in preparation for childbirth, but it may also put you at risk of stretching beyond your normal range. Check with your doctor or midwife before you begin stretching.

## STRETCHING Q&A

**Q | Why should I follow a stretching programme?**

**A |** We all know that regular exercise is beneficial to our wellbeing, but if you do not have time for a full workout, then follow the simple stretching programme opposite. These exercises are usually performed as a warm-up or cool-down at the start or end of a session, but can also be performed on their own if time is tight. Controlled stretching improves and maintains flexibility and mobility, corrects bad posture, reduces the risk of injury, relieves pain, and even helps counteract the effects of ageing.

**Q | Is stretching like yoga or Pilates?**

**A |** Many people think of yoga or Pilates when they think of stretching. Yoga increases flexibility for the positions of meditation, whereas Pilates concentrates on improving torso strength and control. Stretching is different, in that it aims to align the body, improve posture, and encourage better mechanical movement of the joints, thus reducing wear and tear.

**Q | What happens when I stretch?**

**A |** Strong muscles, tendons, bones, and ligaments are essential to maintain a healthy body. When you go into a stretch, you feel the pull of your muscles on your bones. Tendons connect muscles to bones, and the pull of stretching helps the tendons to remain flexible, preventing injuries. Ligaments connect bone to bone and hold the skeleton together. When stretching, the aim is to elongate the muscles and tendons while protecting the ligaments. Focused stretching aligns the spine and balances the muscle groups that would otherwise become shortened by gravity over time.

**Q | Does everyone benefit from stretching?**

**A |** Yes. Everyone, both young and old, male or female, and regardless of fitness level, can benefit from stretching. As well as working various muscle groups in the body, stretching energizes the mind, body, and spirit. Stretching consists of simple, straightforward exercises that can be performed almost anywhere.

## SIMPLE STRETCHING PROGRAMME

This sequence of stretching exercises will work both your upper-back and lower-back muscles (exercises 1–6 and 7–12 respectively). If you spend a lot of time sitting at a desk, the first 6 exercises will provide a welcome break to your day: do them 5 or 6 times a day. The remaining exercises are for the lower-back and should be carried out twice a day, morning and evening.

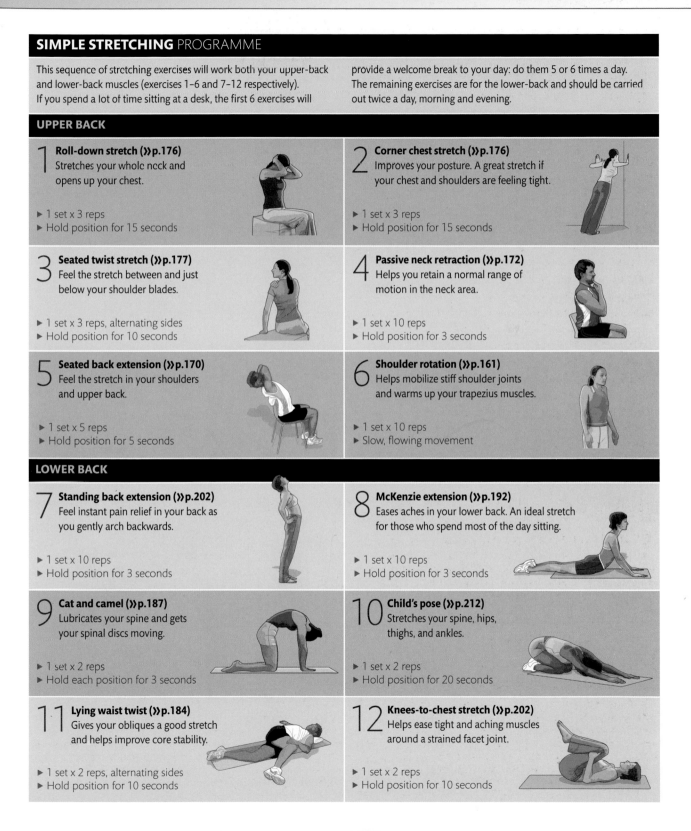

### UPPER BACK

**1 Roll-down stretch (》p.176)**
Stretches your whole neck and opens up your chest.

▸ 1 set x 3 reps
▸ Hold position for 15 seconds

**2 Corner chest stretch (》p.176)**
Improves your posture. A great stretch if your chest and shoulders are feeling tight.

▸ 1 set x 3 reps
▸ Hold position for 15 seconds

**3 Seated twist stretch (》p.177)**
Feel the stretch between and just below your shoulder blades.

▸ 1 set x 3 reps, alternating sides
▸ Hold position for 10 seconds

**4 Passive neck retraction (》p.172)**
Helps you retain a normal range of motion in the neck area.

▸ 1 set x 10 reps
▸ Hold position for 3 seconds

**5 Seated back extension (》p.170)**
Feel the stretch in your shoulders and upper back.

▸ 1 set x 5 reps
▸ Hold position for 5 seconds

**6 Shoulder rotation (》p.161)**
Helps mobilize stiff shoulder joints and warms up your trapezius muscles.

▸ 1 set x 10 reps
▸ Slow, flowing movement

### LOWER BACK

**7 Standing back extension (》p.202)**
Feel instant pain relief in your back as you gently arch backwards.

▸ 1 set x 10 reps
▸ Hold position for 3 seconds

**8 McKenzie extension (》p.192)**
Eases aches in your lower back. An ideal stretch for those who spend most of the day sitting.

▸ 1 set x 10 reps
▸ Hold position for 3 seconds

**9 Cat and camel (》p.187)**
Lubricates your spine and gets your spinal discs moving.

▸ 1 set x 2 reps
▸ Hold each position for 3 seconds

**10 Child's pose (》p.212)**
Stretches your spine, hips, thighs, and ankles.

▸ 1 set x 2 reps
▸ Hold position for 20 seconds

**11 Lying waist twist (》p.184)**
Gives your obliques a good stretch and helps improve core stability.

▸ 1 set x 2 reps, alternating sides
▸ Hold position for 10 seconds

**12 Knees-to-chest stretch (》p.202)**
Helps ease tight and aching muscles around a strained facet joint.

▸ 1 set x 2 reps
▸ Hold position for 10 seconds

# EATING FOR HEALTH

**Eating a healthy, balanced diet**, and staying hydrated, combined with doing the right exercises at the right intensity and volume, all contribute towards the health of your back.

If you are overweight, you run the risk of putting stress on your spine, so it is a good idea to think about your eating habits and cut down on unhealthy foods. This, coupled with a regular exercise regime, will lighten the load on your back.

### FOOD, CALORIES, AND BODY WEIGHT

The weight of your body is made up principally of your skeleton, organs, and the muscle, fat, and water that the body carries. Muscular development, body fat, bone density, and the amount of water in the body can all be changed by diet and exercise.

The basic facts about weight gain and loss are simple: you will gain weight if you consume more calories than you burn, and you will lose weight if you eat fewer calories than you need to fuel your basic body functions and lifestyle needs. It is a well-known fact that carrying excess body weight puts a greater strain on your joints, including the joints in your spine, placing them under unnatural pressure and ultimately resulting in back pain.

Some foods contain many calories for a given weight and are thus "energy-dense" – see Energy Density table (**»below**) – while others, such as dietary fibre or roughage, minerals, and vitamins, contain few or no calories, but are still necessary components of your diet.

### CALCULATING CALORIES PER FOOD PORTION

Most food products you buy in supermarkets feature a total calorie count per 100g (3½oz) of food. To calculate the calorie intake for the amount of food you actually eat, simply multiply the calorie count for 100g by the percentage of grams (or ounces) consumed. For instance, if you eat 150g (5oz) of food, multiply the calorie intake for 100g by 150 per cent.

| **ENERGY** DENSITY | |
| --- | --- |
| **Fat** | ▶ 9 calories per gram (255 calories per ounce) |
| **Carbohydrate** | ▶ 4 calories per gram (113 calories per ounce) |
| **Protein** | ▶ 4 calories per gram (113 calories per ounce) |
| **Water, vitamins, and minerals** | ▶ Zero calorific value |

## WHAT IS THE RIGHT LEVEL OF BODY FAT?

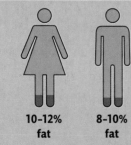

**10-12% fat**    **8-10% fat**

**Athletic**
Athletes in training, especially at the elite level, will have significantly less body fat: around 8-10 per cent for men and 10-12 per cent for women. High levels of fat in relative terms are a serious disadvantage to most athletes, especially in disciplines where "making weight" for a specific competitive class is a priority.

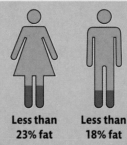

**Less than 23% fat**    **Less than 18% fat**

**Average**
It is generally accepted that men should have less than 18 per cent of their body weight as fat and women 23 per cent or less. A certain amount of body fat is essential for good health. There is plenty of evidence to indicate that carrying less than 5 per cent body fat compromises your immune system, making you prone to illness and infections.

**40% fat**    **35% fat**

**Hazardous**
Carrying more fat than the average person is not particularly hazardous to health until you accumulate 35 per cent (men) and 40 per cent (women) of total body weight as fat. Such levels constitute obesity and have a detrimental effect on health. Too low a level of body fat can also be hazardous, because fat is an important store of energy for aerobic activity.

## RECOMMENDED DAILY NUTRIENT INTAKE

There is no universally "correct" balance of daily nutrient intake; the proportions of the main nutrients you need depend on your individual characteristics and lifestyle. However, your food intake should consist, roughly, of:

■ 60 per cent carbohydrates. These are your main source of energy and are found in fruit and vegetables, bread, pasta, rice, and wholegrain foods.

■ 25 per cent fat. A good source of energy if consumed in moderation. Unsaturated fat can help lower cholesterol and is found in oily fish, nuts, seeds, and vegetable oils.

■ 15 per cent protein. Proteins are vital to the growth and repair of muscle and other body tissues. They are found in meat, poultry, fish, eggs, cheese, nuts, and seeds.

## YOUR BODY FAT LEVEL

Body Mass Index (BMI) is a measure of whether you are a healthy weight for your height. It is used to determine obesity in both male and female adults and can be calculated using the following equation:

If using metric measurements:

$$BMI = \frac{\text{weight in kilograms}}{\text{height in metres} \times \text{height in metres}}$$

or, if using imperial measurements:

$$BMI = \left( \frac{\text{weight in pounds}}{\text{height in inches} \times \text{height in inches}} \right) \times 703$$

The results should be read as follows:

**Underweight:** 18.5 or under
**Normal:** 18.6–24.9
**Overweight:** 25–29.9
**Obese:** 30–39.9
**Clinically obese:** 40 or higher

Although the results are very accurate, BMI does not distinguish between the weight of muscle and that of fat, so that if you are overly muscular (muscle weighs more than fat), the result will not be precise and you will be classified as overweight. So while it is a useful gauge for the general public, BMI needs to be interpreted with caution by anyone with significant muscle mass.

## YOUR ENERGY REQUIREMENTS

Your Basic Energy Requirement (BER) is the amount of energy you need to maintain your basic life processes, such as breathing and circulation, when at rest. In addition to your BER, you need energy to live your lifestyle and sustain your personal everyday work and activity patterns. The nature of your job is important: if you do a lot of manual, labour-intensive work, you will have a different energy requirement from someone who leads a more sedentary lifestyle and who works at a desk all day. You can calculate your approximate daily energy requirement by using the table below. The figure you end up with relates to the number of calories you should be consuming per day to retain your present body weight.

### CALCULATING YOUR ENERGY REQUIREMENTS

Locate your age range and enter your weight into the appropriate equation to find your BER. Then, multiply this figure by the factor associated with your type of lifestyle – sedentary, moderately active, or very active. The figure you arrive at is the level of calorie intake that will allow you to maintain your present body weight. If you take in more calories than your daily energy requirement (including the exercise you get), you will gain weight. If you take in fewer calories than your daily energy requirement (including exercise), you will lose weight.

| Male | | |
|---|---|---|
| ▶ 10–17 years | ▶ 17.5 x weight in kg<br>▶ (8 x weight in lb) | ▶ + 651 |
| ▶ 18–29 years | ▶ 15.3 x weight in kg<br>▶ (7 x weight in lb) | ▶ + 679 |
| ▶ 30–59 years | ▶ 11.6 x weight in kg<br>▶ (5.2 x weight in lb) | ▶ + 879 |
| ▶ 60+ years | ▶ 13.5 x weight in kg<br>▶ (6 x weight in lb) | ▶ + 487 |
| **Female** | | |
| ▶ 10–17 years | ▶ 12.2 x weight in kg<br>▶ (5.5 x weight in lb) | ▶ + 746 |
| ▶ 18–29 years | ▶ 14.7 x weight in kg<br>▶ (6.7 x weight in lb) | ▶ + 496 |
| ▶ 30–59 years | ▶ 8.7 x weight in kg<br>▶ (3.9 x weight in lb) | ▶ + 829 |
| ▶ 60+ years | ▶ 10.5 x weight in kg<br>▶ (4.7 x weight in lb) | ▶ + 596 |

**Sedentary** multiply by 1.5
**Moderately active** multiply by 1.6
**Very active** multiply by 1.7

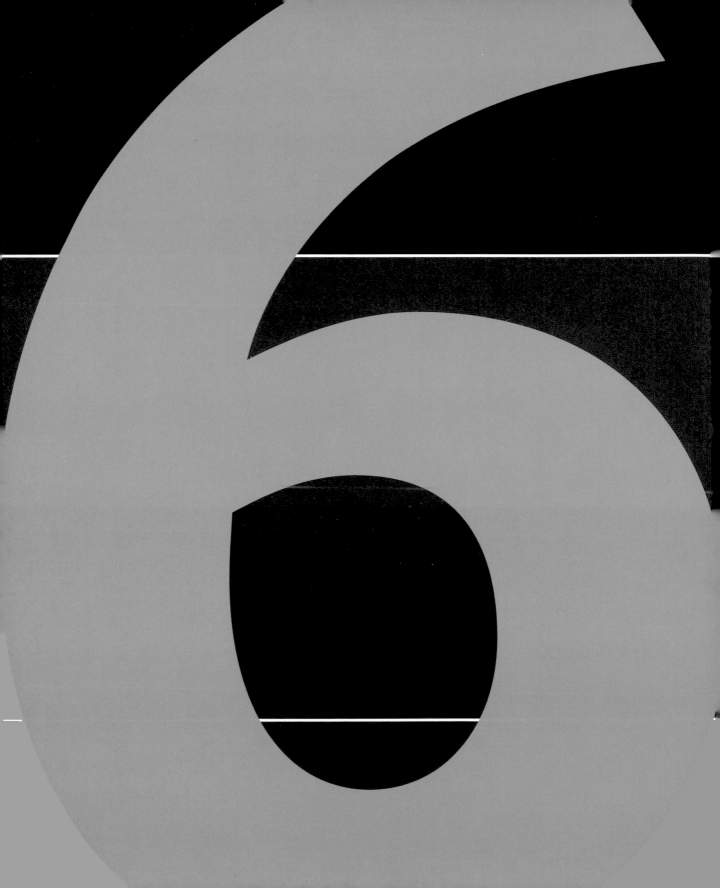

# STRATEGIES FOR PREVENTING PAIN

**Day in day out** you may perform any number of movements that involve your back and neck without a second thought. Over time, however, poor posture or incorrectly performed movements can cause or exacerbate back and neck conditions, whether in the form of a sudden twinge or long-term chronic joint damage. This chapter guides you through a range of common activities at work and home, showing you the correct position or movement for each.

# AT THE OFFICE

**If your work involves sitting** at a computer day after day, it is important to set up your work station correctly to give your back maximum support. Maintaining good posture is essential to protect your back, neck, and shoulders, and to avoid muscle tension and headaches.

Sitting imposes more strain on the spine than standing or walking, so a well-designed chair is very important if you spend long hours at a desk. If you are prone to lower-back pain, make sure that your chair is at the correct height for your leg length – your feet should be flat on the floor. Keep your seat horizontal, and sit close enough to the desk so that you can use your keyboard without having to stretch your arms out. To avoid tension in your shoulders and neck, the height of the desk should allow you to touch the keyboard with your fingers while keeping your arms bent just slightly below the horizontal. Rest your arms on the desk, keeping them parallel to the floor, but avoid leaning on them. You should change position regularly and take breaks away from your desk.

## HEAD AND NECK ALIGNMENT

If you spend time leaning over a desk with your back rounded and your head bent forwards, the muscles in your upper back, shoulders, and neck are likely to become fatigued.

## SITTING IN AN ERGONOMIC CHAIR

Adjust the height of your chair so that your feet are flat on the floor, and tilt the back slightly downwards to support you when you lean forwards to work. Ideally, the chair should also tilt backwards so that you can relax. The seat should be angled so that your hips are slightly higher than your knees.

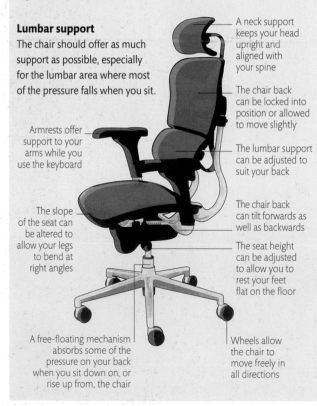

**Lumbar support**
The chair should offer as much support as possible, especially for the lumbar area where most of the pressure falls when you sit.

A neck support keeps your head upright and aligned with your spine

The chair back can be locked into position or allowed to move slightly

The lumbar support can be adjusted to suit your back

Armrests offer support to your arms while you use the keyboard

The slope of the seat can be altered to allow your legs to bend at right angles

The chair back can tilt forwards as well as backwards

The seat height can be adjusted to allow you to rest your feet flat on the floor

A free-floating mechanism absorbs some of the pressure on your back when you sit down on, or rise up from, the chair

Wheels allow the chair to move freely in all directions

## WORKING ON A DESKTOP COMPUTER

Even when you have set up your workspace so that the desk, chair, keyboard, and monitor are in the right place for you, you still need to be conscious of your posture. Good posture will ensure your back is supported and your spine aligned. It will help prevent backache as well as shoulder and neck pain that can lead to headaches.

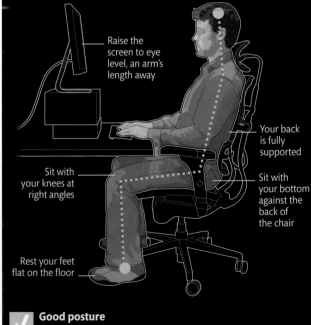

Raise the screen to eye level, an arm's length away

Your back is fully supported

Sit with your knees at right angles

Sit with your bottom against the back of the chair

Rest your feet flat on the floor

✓ **Good posture**
With your spine supported by an ergonomic chair, your back, shoulders, and neck are aligned. Your body appears alert and ready to work but at the same time it is relaxed with no areas of tension.

The result can be a painful neck or headaches. Chronic neck tension can also cause migraines. Whenever your neck feels tense or you are holding your head forwards with your chin out, reduce the curve in your neck by pulling your chin back and making the crown of your head the highest point. Neck retraction exercises (**»p.172**) reduce tension by bringing the weight of your head more directly over your spine, so that your neck muscles have less work to do.

## UNDER THE DESK

Keep your feet flat on the floor and your knees slightly below your hips. Ensure that there is adequate space from the back of your knees to the edge of the chair – roughly the width of three fingers – to allow your legs to move freely. Avoid crossing your legs as this results in a poor hip position.

## USING A COMPUTER

The following simple rules will help you avoid some of the common problems associated with working at a computer:
■ Place your monitor and keyboard directly in front of you.
■ Use a support to keep your hands and wrists aligned.
■ Set up your monitor so that the screen is an arm's length away from you and the toolbars at the top are at eye level.
■ Use a hard-copy holder to avoid constantly looking down.
■ Instead of leaning towards the screen in order to read the type, zoom in to enlarge the text – and have your eyes tested.
■ Keep the mouse near but with space to move it freely.
■ Touch the keys lightly and touch type if you can, to avoid having to look down at the keys.
■ Keep your elbows vertically under your shoulders and close to the sides of your body, or on an armrest.

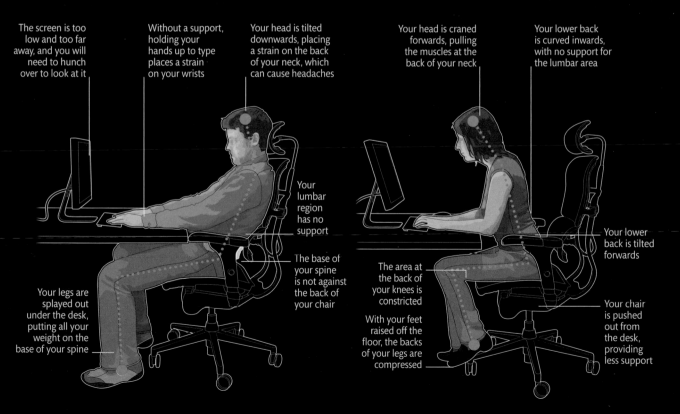

The screen is too low and too far away, and you will need to hunch over to look at it

Without a support, holding your hands up to type places a strain on your wrists

Your head is tilted downwards, placing a strain on the back of your neck, which can cause headaches

Your lumbar region has no support

The base of your spine is not against the back of your chair

Your legs are splayed out under the desk, putting all your weight on the base of your spine

Your head is craned forwards, pulling the muscles at the back of your neck

Your lower back is curved inwards, with no support for the lumbar area

Your lower back is tilted forwards

The area at the back of your knees is constricted

With your feet raised off the floor, the backs of your legs are compressed

Your chair is pushed out from the desk, providing less support

**X** **Poor posture – leaning back**
It is very easy to slump when you have been working at your desk for hours at a stretch. Here, the shoulders are rounded inwards and the head is leaning forwards, both of which can lead to upper-back pain.

**X** **Poor posture – leaning forwards**
Leaning into the monitor means that your neck and upper back have no support and your legs are constricted. The lumbar area is also unsupported and your knees are strained.

## USING A LAPTOP

Many people spend time using a laptop at home, but since laptops are designed to be portable and lightweight rather than adjustable, this can easily lead to back problems. It is common to use them while lying on the sofa or slumped with your back and neck in an awkward position. However, if you are spending hours working on a laptop, you need to take care to set up a healthy working environment, applying the same principles as you would to arranging your workstation in the office.

You will need a supportive office chair – ideally an ergonomic one that can be adjusted – and a desk or table that is the right height for you. Follow the advice given for sitting at an office desk (**>pp.124–25**) and avoid leaning forwards over the laptop. You should also take care not to slump at the shoulders or crane your neck, since both of these positions will lead to tension in your neck and shoulders, and pain in your upper back.

### Laptop set-up

If you position your laptop so that the screen is at the right height, then the keyboard will not be, and vice versa. The screen should be an arm's length away from you and at eye level, while your arms should be resting at right angles to your body when using the keyboard. If you need to work on your laptop for any length of time, a separate keyboard and mouse are easier to use and adjust to your needs, or you may wish to invest in a separate desktop computer. Laptop

## USING LAPTOPS AND OTHER PORTABLE DEVICES

Laptops, netbooks, and tablets are compact and easy to carry around but you cannot adjust them to make them comfortable to work on for long periods. You risk back problems if you use these devices without taking measures to ensure that you maintain good posture.

Ideally, you should set up at a desk, using a purpose-made stand – or a box, or books – to raise the device to the correct level, and a separate keyboard and mouse. Even when working away from your desk there are steps that you can take to protect yourself from injury.

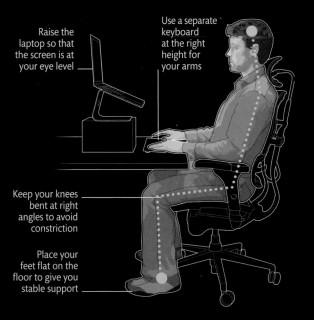

Raise the laptop so that the screen is at your eye level

Use a separate keyboard at the right height for your arms

Keep your knees bent at right angles to avoid constriction

Place your feet flat on the floor to give you stable support

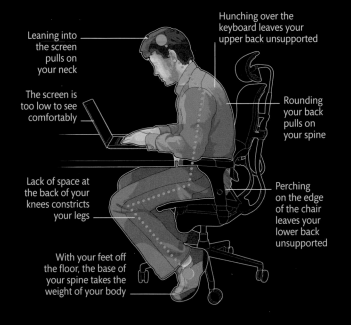

Leaning into the screen pulls on your neck

The screen is too low to see comfortably

Hunching over the keyboard leaves your upper back unsupported

Rounding your back pulls on your spine

Lack of space at the back of your knees constricts your legs

Perching on the edge of the chair leaves your lower back unsupported

With your feet off the floor, the base of your spine takes the weight of your body

 **Good posture**

Keep your head and neck aligned and your back straight. Face forwards and keep your arms bent at right angles at the elbow when using the keyboard. Make sure your spine is supported by keeping your back against the back of the chair.

**X Bad posture**

Without a laptop stand and separate mouse and keyboard it is difficult to sit upright while using a laptop. Your head cranes downwards and brings your neck and shoulders with it. Working on the keyboard can feel cramped, pulling on your shoulders and upper back.

stands are useful for raising your laptop to the correct height. Some of these are designed to be used when you are out and about, while others might form part of a more permanent set-up in your home – it is worth spending time finding out which stand works best for you.

## Using a laptop on the sofa

Of course, some of the time spent on your laptop will be for pleasure rather than work, but you still need to protect your back. Laptop cushions provide a comfortable and stable base for your machine and make it easier to use while sitting upright on a sofa. Keep your feet flat on the floor and your back against the back of the sofa. Use cushions to support your back, if needed.

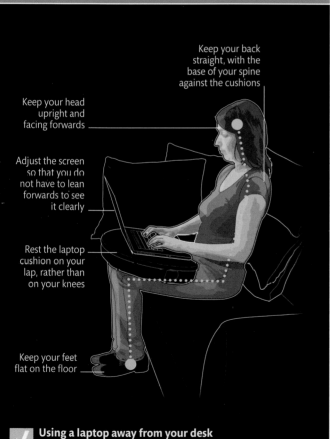

Keep your back straight, with the base of your spine against the cushions

Keep your head upright and facing forwards

Adjust the screen so that you do not have to lean forwards to see it clearly

Rest the laptop cushion on your lap, rather than on your knees

Keep your feet flat on the floor

### ✓ Using a laptop away from your desk
While it is best to work at a desk, if you have to sit on a sofa, use cushions to support your back and a laptop cushion to steady your machine. Sit upright with the laptop in front of you and your elbows under your shoulders. Avoid leaning forwards or to the side.

## USING A PHONE

If you make and receive phone calls while working at your computer, it is tempting to hold the handset between your shoulder and ear while you continue to work. However, gripping the phone with your shoulder can cause tension in your shoulder, neck, and upper back. Follow the suggestions below to avoid these problems:

■ Wear a headset rather than using a handset: this keeps your hands free so you can carry on working.
■ Sit facing your desk and keyboard while you talk – twisting round places unnecessary stress on your back.
■ Keep the keyboard within easy reach so that your arms and shoulders stay relaxed. Avoid over-reaching.

### ✓ Good practice
If you are going to continue working on your computer while you talk on the phone, be sure to use a headset. Sit upright and facing forwards, with your back against the chair to support your spine.

Use a headset even if you are making a short phone call

Relax your shoulders

Keep your arms relaxed, with your elbows under your shoulders

Position your keyboard within easy reach of both hands

### ✗ Bad practice
Gripping the phone between your shoulder and ear while you continue working is a very bad habit to get into. It can lead to neck, shoulder, and back pain, and can also cause headaches.

Tilting your head can cause neck strain

Gripping the phone can cause tension in your neck and shoulder

Hunching over puts a strain on your upper back

Stretching for the keyboard can create tension in your upper back

# LIFTING AND CARRYING

**When lifting a load**, it is common to round your back and take the weight on your spine. It is much safer to keep your back straight and let your more powerful abdominal and leg muscles do the work instead.

It puts strain on your spine if you round your back forwards or arch your back and stick your hips out when lifting. Both positions shift the weight down onto your lower back, which can lead to backache. Instead, you should straighten your back against the pull of the load, keep your hips in a flexed position, and use your leg muscles to take the strain.

If you are carrying something in front of you, take care not to increase the arch in your lower back or to lean backwards, and avoid pushing your hips forward. Your abdominal and back muscles should support your back,

while your leg muscles take the weight. If you are carrying something on your back, try to avoid leaning forwards to take the strain, as this places the weight on your curved spine rather than your muscles.

In general, keep your back straight and avoid lifting anything that is too heavy for you. As well as getting into the habit of using the muscles in your abdomen and legs, check your posture in the mirror to find out how your spine feels when it is straight and when your pelvis is in a neutral position.

## WARNING!

Don't try to lift something that is too heavy for you, as this could strain your back. If you are not sure of the weight, make an assessment by following steps 1 and 2 below, but just lifting the box a little way off the ground. If it is too heavy, get help to lift it.

## LIFTING A BOX

Before you lift a box, take a moment to assess how heavy it is. Squat down, keeping your back straight and using your leg muscles to lift the weight; come up smoothly. Keep the load close to your body when you lift and carry it.

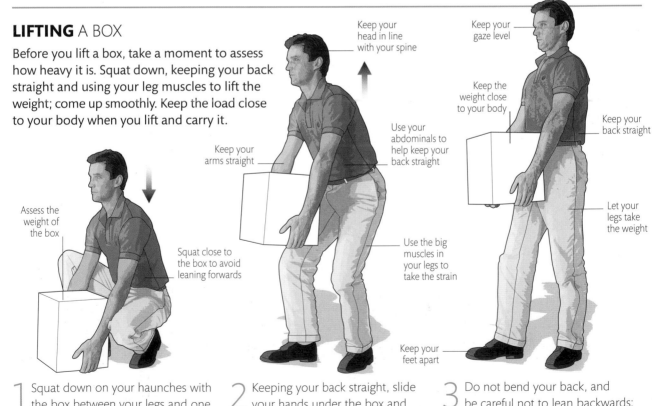

Assess the weight of the box

Squat close to the box to avoid leaning forwards

Keep your head in line with your spine

Keep your arms straight

Use your abdominals to help keep your back straight

Use the big muscles in your legs to take the strain

Keep your feet apart

Keep your gaze level

Keep the weight close to your body

Keep your back straight

Let your legs take the weight

1 Squat down on your haunches with the box between your legs and one foot on either side. Try to assess whether the box is too large, heavy, or awkwardly shaped before you attempt to lift it.

2 Keeping your back straight, slide your hands under the box and grasp it on either side. Stand up in one smooth motion, keeping the object close to you.

3 Do not bend your back, and be careful not to lean backwards; use your abdominal muscles to support your spine. Keep your weight equal on both legs.

## CARRYING BAGS

When you are packing shopping, distribute the items between several bags to balance the weight, then spread the load so that you are carrying an equal weight in each hand. When carrying a single heavier item, such as a laptop or file, a bag that you can wear across your body or a backpack is a good idea. Choose one with a wide strap and keep the weight close to your body. Remember to swap the bag from one shoulder to the other occasionally. Take care when putting them on and taking them off – use a table as a halfway point.

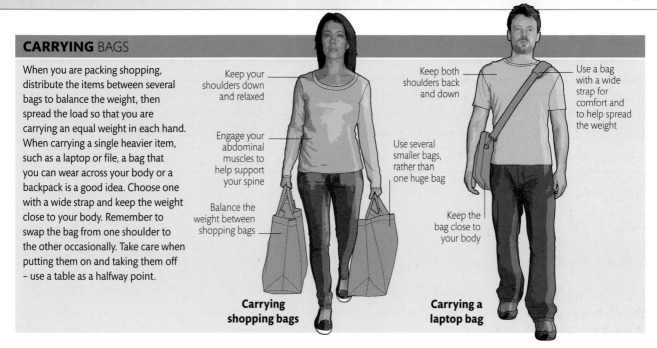

Keep your shoulders down and relaxed

Engage your abdominal muscles to help support your spine

Balance the weight between shopping bags

**Carrying shopping bags**

Keep both shoulders back and down

Use a bag with a wide strap for comfort and to help spread the weight

Use several smaller bags, rather than one huge bag

Keep the bag close to your body

**Carrying a laptop bag**

## LIFTING A LONG LOAD

When you need to lift a longer load, begin by making an assessment of the weight and, if you can't get someone else to carry the other end, assess whether it is safe for you to lift on your own. If it is, squat down with your legs astride one end of the load. You can either keep your legs in line or put one in front of the other. Try not to lean forwards, and keep your back straight throughout.

Keep your chin tucked in and your head in line with your spine

Keep your shoulders aligned

Assess the weight of the load and how best to lift it

Begin to lift the load

Keep your bottom low to maintain a stable base

Let your leg muscles do the lifting work

Ensure your weight is evenly balanced

1 Squat down with one end of the load between your feet. Slide both hands underneath the load and take a firm grip.

2 Raise the end nearest to you, tilting it away from your body until the load is balanced upright on the other end. Step forward if necessary.

3 Move your hand underneath the end of the load and bring it close to your body, resting the load against your shoulder.

4 Keeping the load vertical and, gripping it firmly, stand up slowly, keeping your back straight throughout.

# DOING HOUSEWORK

**Many household chores** involve bending and lifting. You can reduce the strain on your back by learning new techniques and using different ways to approach your tasks.

As a general rule of thumb, if some chores are causing you pain, vary your activity, rest frequently, and avoid too many repetitive movements.

In the kitchen, be aware of your posture when you are preparing food on the worktop. Ideally, the worktop should be slightly lower than your elbow. Stand close to it to avoid overreaching, and keep your back straight. It may feel more comfortable to have one foot in front of the other, or one foot resting on a small step or on the base of the cupboard. The sink should also be at elbow height, so you are not forced to stoop when washing up. If necessary, put the washing-up bowl on the worktop or on top of another bowl to get it to the right height.

To reach into high cupboards, you may find it useful to keep a low step in the kitchen. Take things down individually, and avoid overstretching so that you do not lose your balance. You may need to rearrange the contents of your cupboards to store the most-used items on the lowest shelves. Keep your back straight when you bend to the oven or dishwasher.

## WORKING AROUND THE HOME

Approaching everyday chores in a different way can help protect your back from strain. Prepare the area in advance so you have everything you need in position, and work slowly to avoid sudden twists or jolts to your back.

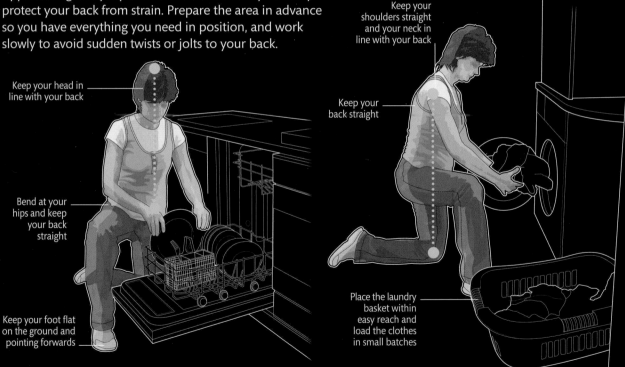

Keep your head in line with your back

Bend at your hips and keep your back straight

Keep your foot flat on the ground and pointing forwards

Keep your shoulders straight and your neck in line with your back

Keep your back straight

Place the laundry basket within easy reach and load the clothes in small batches

### ✓ Loading the dishwasher
Pile up your dirty dishes beside the dishwasher within easy reach. Kneel down on one knee, and keep your other leg perpendicular. Keeping your back straight, put the items in one by one, and avoid leaning too far forwards and overreaching. Use your leg muscles to take the strain. An alternative method is to squat down beside the machine with your legs apart and your knees in line with your ankles.

### ✓ Using a washing machine
If you have a front-loading washing machine, squat, sit, or put one knee on the floor while you fill or empty it. If you have a top-loading machine, avoid bending and twisting as much as possible by keeping your basket at the same height as the machine. Reach into the machine with one arm and raise the opposite leg for balance.

## CLEANING THE FLOOR

Stand facing the area you are cleaning, and try not to twist or reach too far forwards. Move the broom, mop, or vacuum cleaner and your body at the same time. If you are using an upright vacuum cleaner, keep it close to your body. Stand with one foot in front of the other with your knees bent, and, rather than bending, rock backwards and forwards. Avoid dragging the vacuum cleaner, and instead make short movements backwards and forwards. If you are using a cylinder vacuum cleaner, keep the hose fully extended. To clean under a table, bend at your hips and knees, keeping your back as straight as you can. When it comes to buying a new cleaner, choose a high-powered lightweight model with a long hose and a wide head.

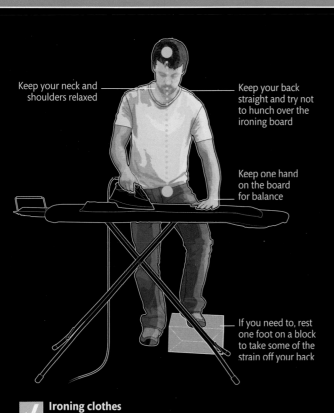

Keep your neck and shoulders relaxed

Keep your back straight and try not to hunch over the ironing board

Keep one hand on the board for balance

If you need to, rest one foot on a block to take some of the strain off your back

### ✓ Ironing clothes

Raise the ironing board up to around hip height to avoid stooping. You should be able to move your arms freely without having to lift your shoulders. Stand close to the board, and, with one foot facing forwards and the other in the direction the board is pointing, sway from one foot to the other as you iron. Alternatively, you can take the weight off your legs by perching on the side of an armchair or sofa while you iron.

## HOUSEWORK Q&A

**Q | What should I wear?**

**A |** Wear comfortable clothing so you can move around freely. Put on old clothes so you don't have to worry about them getting dirty or wet.

**Q | How should I reach for things in the fridge?**

**A |** When organizing your fridge, keep the items that you use regularly on the middle shelf to avoid having to do too much reaching and stretching. When you do have to bend, squat down or place one knee on the floor, and use the power in your legs to get up. When buying a new fridge, if space allows, choose one that sits above the freezer, rather than below it.

**Q | What is the best way to make a bed?**

**A |** Squat down or kneel by the bed when you tuck in the sheets. Buy fitted sheets and duvets to make it easier. Fit smooth-running casters if you need to move the bed.

**Q | How should I approach general cleaning tasks?**

**A |** Use long-handled implements to avoid overstretching. If necessary, kneel down to clean.

**Q | How can I make doing the laundry easier?**

**A |** Place the laundry basket on a stool nearby to avoid having to bend down to the floor. Small items can be placed in a mesh bag so that they are easier to get hold of. Wet laundry will be much heavier to deal with, so you may want to take it out of the washer one piece at a time. Keep the washing line at a sensible height so you don't have to strain to reach it.

**Q | If I suffer from ongoing back pain, how can I make household chores easier for myself?**

**A |** Consider making small adaptations to your home environment. For example, an ergonomically-designed kitchen may make cooking much easier.

**Q | How should I approach DIY?**

**A |** Don't twist your trunk when doing any lifting. Let other parts of your body, such as shoulders, pelvis, or thighs, take the weight. Don't overstretch. Avoid unnecessary effort – buy any tools that will make the task easier.

**Q | What if there are some chores I just cannot do?**

**A |** Ask friends and family for help, and consider paying a professional to do the more strenuous tasks for you.

# WORKING IN YOUR GARDEN

**Many garden tasks** involve crouching, bending, and lifting. You can minimize the strain on your back by working in an upright position, following the rules for lifting (**»pp.128–29**), and varying the tasks to reduce the strain on your back.

When lifting and carrying, use the strength in your legs rather than your back to move the weight. If you are performing any work that is high up, such as pruning trees or fixing fences, use a stepladder and long-handled tools so that you are not forced to overstretch. When mowing, face in the direction you are moving, engage your abdominal muscles, keep your back straight, and hold your head up. If you are weeding or planting, kneel down on a cushioned pad or sit on a low stool. If your back is very bad, you may want to convert your garden to raised beds, or grow plants in a greenhouse instead.

## WARNING!

Approach your activities in the garden as you would any form of exercise. Wear suitable clothing, perform simple stretching exercises to warm up beforehand, take regular breaks, and drink plenty of water. If necessary, ask someone to help.

## DIGGING THE GARDEN

This is a task that will put pressure on your back, whether you usually suffer from back pain or not. The key is to avoid lifting too much soil in one go. Work at a steady pace, and if you feel any twinges, rest before resuming. There are specially adapted spades available that have levers to make the task of digging and turning soil easier.

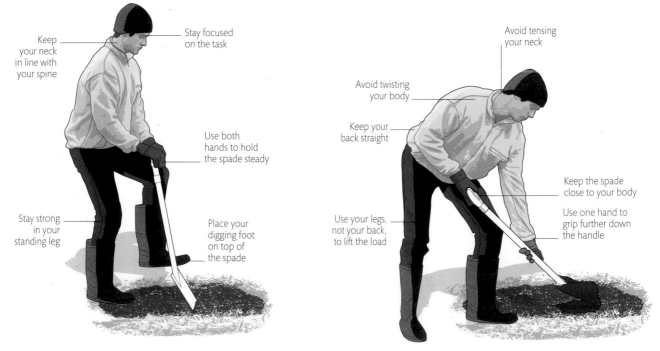

Keep your neck in line with your spine

Stay focused on the task

Use both hands to hold the spade steady

Stay strong in your standing leg

Place your digging foot on top of the spade

Avoid tensing your neck

Avoid twisting your body

Keep your back straight

Keep the spade close to your body

Use one hand to grip further down the handle

Use your legs, not your back, to lift the load

1 Keeping your back straight, push the spade into the ground using your body weight, rather than your muscle power. Bend at your knees and hips rather than your waist, and do not grip the spade too tightly. Before you start to lift the soil, cut around the sides of each spadeful.

2 Hold the handle at the end and use the spade as a lever to ease the soil out. Raise the soil using the handle of the spade near its base for leverage. Move your feet and turn towards where you want to place the load: do not stand in one position and twist your back.

## GARDENING TOOLS

Your tasks will be made easier if you work with the right equipment. Wear appropriate shoes to avoid slipping or falling, gardening gloves to protect your hands, and gardener's knee pads to protect your knees. Use long-handled tools to minimize bending. Look after your gardening tools so they work efficiently.

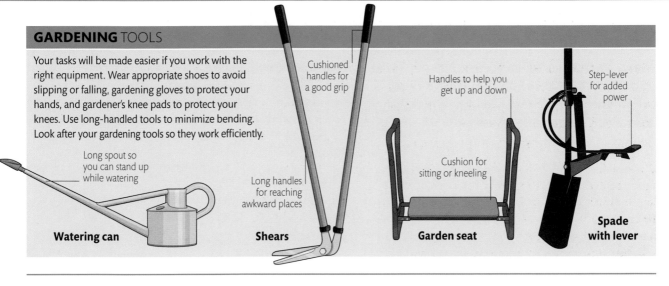

Cushioned handles for a good grip

Handles to help you get up and down

Step-lever for added power

Long spout so you can stand up while watering

Long handles for reaching awkward places

Cushion for sitting or kneeling

**Watering can**

**Shears**

**Garden seat**

**Spade with lever**

## SHOVELLING EARTH

Much of the advice for digging also applies to shovelling – the difference being that you crouch down low, and move the spade with a more shallow movement. In general, and where possible, you should wait for the right conditions: try to avoid digging or shovelling when the soil is wet and heavy or hard, dry, and compacted, as this will make your task more arduous, and could place more strain on your back.

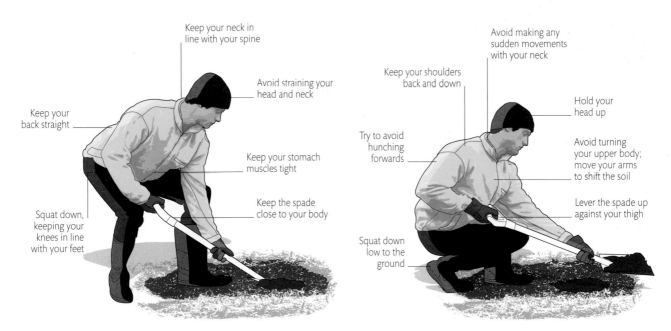

Keep your neck in line with your spine

Avoid straining your head and neck

Keep your back straight

Keep your stomach muscles tight

Squat down, keeping your knees in line with your feet

Keep the spade close to your body

Avoid making any sudden movements with your neck

Keep your shoulders back and down

Hold your head up

Try to avoid hunching forwards

Avoid turning your upper body; move your arms to shift the soil

Squat down low to the ground

Lever the spade up against your thigh

1 Squat down, bending at the knees and hips and keeping your back as straight as possible. Lean forward but maintain a low, stable centre of gravity. Slide the shovel along the ground, resting the back of your top hand against the inside of your knee or thigh to use as a lever.

2 Squat down to the ground and push the spade forwards in one smooth movement. When your spade is full, throw the soil to one side using a sideways movement, rather than lifting it. Do your best to move your arms but minimize the movement of your upper body.

# DRIVING YOUR CAR

**It can be agonizing** to drive your car if you suffer from a bad back or neck problems, unless your car is equipped with a good car seat and well-placed controls.

Even if you do not usually suffer from back or neck pain, driving is one of the activities that can encourage these problems, as you are not only subject to constant vibrations and sudden movements, but are often forced to sit in one position for a long time. Therefore you need to sit in a position that keeps your arms and legs relaxed and that provides proper support for your body, especially your back. Before driving off, always make sure that you are demonstrating good posture: adjust the height of your seat, the angle of the backrest, and the distance from the steering wheel. You should be able to look into your rear view and wing mirrors comfortably without straining your neck.

## IN THE DRIVER'S SEAT

Try to get into the habit of relaxing your neck and shoulder muscles while you are driving. It is helpful to become aware of times when you grip the wheel too tightly or hold it too high up with your arms outstretched. If your shoulders are hunching up towards your ears, develop a relaxed and steady breathing rhythm, and with each breath let go of the tightness in your muscles, slowly dropping your shoulders. Gently work your head and neck back into a more relaxed position against your headrest.

It is also advisable to take frequent breaks when making long journeys. Stop the car and walk around for a few minutes, perform some simple stretches, and roll your shoulders with small circular movements.

If you are buying a new car, look at the car seat design very closely; make sure that the seats are adjustable, and take a test drive to see whether you find them comfortable.

## GETTING OUT OF A CAR

Getting out of a car is usually harder than getting in, as your body may be stiff and immobile from the journey. To get into a car, simply reverse the process outlined below; the difference being that you turn away from the car and support yourself by holding onto the door, bend your knees, and lower your bottom onto the car seat. Once you are seated, shift your left leg and then your right leg carefully into the car.

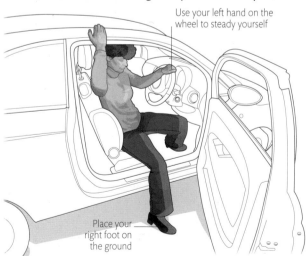

Use your left hand on the wheel to steady yourself

Place your right foot on the ground

1 Park away from the kerb and move the car seat back to give yourself plenty of room. Open the door, and, holding onto the wheel with one hand and the car roof with the other, use them as leverage, turning your body towards the door.

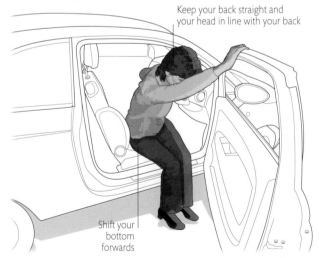

Keep your back straight and your head in line with your back

Shift your bottom forwards

2 Place your left foot on the ground next to your right foot. Once you are facing the door, shift your bottom forwards to the edge of the seat and place your right hand on the upper frame of the door. Keep your left hand on the steering wheel.

## CORRECT DRIVING POSITION

To avoid subjecting yourself to unnecessary strain when driving, work through this checklist next time you sit in your car:

■ **Make sure that** the cushioning of the car seat does not slope towards the middle, or too much weight will be borne by your pelvic bones instead of your thighs. The seat must be firm enough to resist the indirect forces you experience when using the pedals; however, if the seat is too hard, engine vibrations will be transmitted up your spine.

■ **Ensure that the backrest** gives good support to your lower back. Ideally, your car should have in-built lumbar support; if not, use a rolled-up towel instead, or cushions that can be attached by a strap. If you can, alter the angle of the backrest to an optimum of between five and ten degrees behind the vertical.

■ **Rest your head** on the headrest, relaxing your neck and shoulders while looking straight ahead. The headrest should be slightly padded, and adjustable both up and down, forwards and back. The top of the headrest should be at least level with your forehead in order to effectively reduce whiplash strain (»p.72).

■ **Make sure your feet** rest comfortably on the pedals. Check that the pedals are not too stiff (especially the clutch), too high off the floor, or set too far to one side.

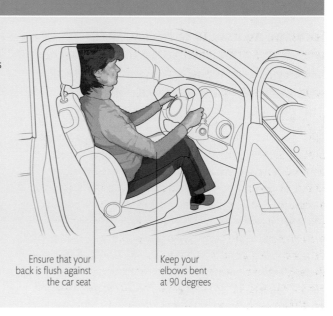

Ensure that your back is flush against the car seat

Keep your elbows bent at 90 degrees

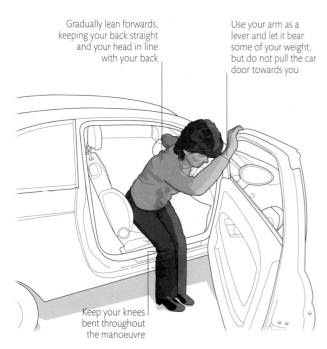

Gradually lean forwards, keeping your back straight and your head in line with your back

Use your arm as a lever and let it bear some of your weight, but do not pull the car door towards you

Keep your knees bent throughout the manoeuvre

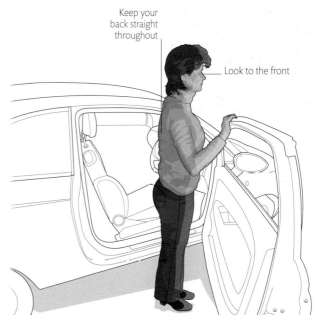

Keep your back straight throughout

Look to the front

3 Start to lean out of the car, using your outstretched arm to help control the movement. Keep your head lifted and your knees bent throughout; use your hips to move, rather than your lower back.

4 Bearing the weight in your legs rather than your back, gradually straighten from the knees until you are standing. While this procedure may take a little longer than usual, it is worth getting into the habit of exiting a car in this way.

# DURING PREGNANCY

**Most women will experience** back and pelvic pain during pregnancy, particularly in the third trimester, with the pain becoming more intense as the due date approaches. The pain is usually felt in the lower back, sacroiliac joint, buttocks, and legs.

Pregnancy may be the first time you experience back pain, although women who have been pregnant before are more likely to experience back pain during subsequent pregnancies. Keeping active while pregnant will help strengthen your back and pelvis, maintain your flexibility, and even assist your ability to cope with the stresses of labour: walking, swimming, yoga, and Pilates are all recommended exercises. Relaxation techniques, such as meditation, will help you cope with pain (**》pp.102–03**).

### THIRD TRIMESTER

In late pregnancy, the pelvic joints and ligaments relax, and the growing weight of your uterus will change your centre of balance. This means that you will have to stand with your shoulders further back than normal, and that you may be tempted to alter your posture to compensate for the extra weight. Your doctor or therapist may suggest that you wear a sacroiliac joint maternity belt to help take the pressure off your back.

If you are experiencing severe pain while pregnant, especially in your joints, you should consult your doctor or physiotherapist. You may have developed pelvic girdle pain, which is also known as symphysis pubis dysfunction. This can usually be treated with appropriate exercises, as recommended by your physiotherapist (**》pp.90–93**).

### POSTNATAL BACK CARE

Back pain is common in the few days following delivery, but it should ease soon afterwards. If your pain persists, you should seek medical advice, as it may indicate that you have an underlying problem that needs attention.

Once your baby has been born, you will have to learn new ways of lifting and adapting to the demands of caring for young children (**》pp.138–39**). You should not carry your baby in a sling, as this distributes the weight unevenly.

## STANDING POSTURE

The usual advice for good posture also applies when you are pregnant (**》pp.112–14**). It is a good idea to avoid wearing high heels during your pregnancy.

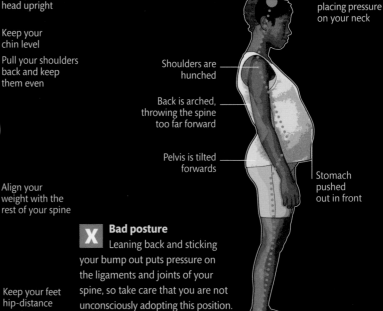

Keep your head upright

Keep your chin level

Pull your shoulders back and keep them even

Straighten your back and tuck your buttocks in

Align your weight with the rest of your spine

Keep your feet hip-distance apart

Head tilted, placing pressure on your neck

Shoulders are hunched

Back is arched, throwing the spine too far forward

Pelvis is tilted forwards

Stomach pushed out in front

 **Good posture**
Distribute your weight evenly on both your legs, and tuck your buttocks under to help keep your back straight. Make sure that you do not stand for too long unnecessarily.

**X Bad posture**
Leaning back and sticking your bump out puts pressure on the ligaments and joints of your spine, so take care that you are not unconsciously adopting this position.

# GETTING UP

When you are pregnant, your stomach muscles separate to allow your bump to grow, and your abdominal muscles cannot be used in the same way as before, so you need to learn a new technique for getting up. In the latter stages of your pregnancy you may find it difficult to establish a comfortable resting position, as your bump makes it painful to lie on your front or back. You should find relief by lying and sleeping on your side (»Step 1) with a pillow between your knees, and another pillow under your stomach.

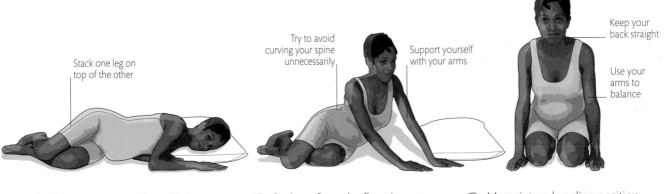

Stack one leg on top of the other

Try to avoid curving your spine unnecessarily

Support yourself with your arms

Keep your back straight

Use your arms to balance

1 Turn onto your side and bring your hands up beside your head, palms facing downwards.

2 Push up from the floor in one smooth movement, letting your arms bear your body weight.

3 Move into a kneeling position. To stand, push with your hands and bend your knee to bring one leg up, keeping your back straight.

## SITTING POSTURE

When sitting, your back should be flush against the chair back, and never arched. Make sure that the back of the chair is high enough, and use pillows to give your lower back plenty of support if necessary. Bear in mind that you may find driving a car uncomfortable when you are pregnant (»pp.134–35).

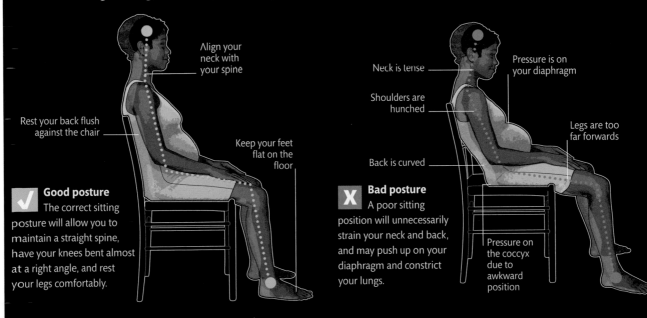

Align your neck with your spine

Rest your back flush against the chair

Keep your feet flat on the floor

Neck is tense

Shoulders are hunched

Back is curved

Pressure is on your diaphragm

Legs are too far forwards

Pressure on the coccyx due to awkward position

✓ **Good posture**
The correct sitting posture will allow you to maintain a straight spine, have your knees bent almost at a right angle, and rest your legs comfortably.

✗ **Bad posture**
A poor sitting position will unnecessarily strain your neck and back, and may push up on your diaphragm and constrict your lungs.

# CARING FOR YOUNG CHILDREN

**New mothers are particularly** vulnerable to developing back strain arising from weak and overstretched stomach muscles, poor posture, or faulty lifting. This is because it can take up to five months for the ligaments of your spine and pelvis to tighten up again after giving birth.

Looking after young children involves lifting, carrying, and stooping over beds. Pay special attention to the way you lift your child, and watch out for unpredictable behaviour, such as when they struggle against being picked up.

## CARRYING YOUR BABY

Lift and carry your baby carefully, always protecting your back. Squat rather than bend, and keep the child close to your body. Try to avoid carrying your child on one hip as this creates an imbalance in your posture. If you do have

to do this, make sure it is only for a few minutes. Whenever you can, carry your baby in a special baby carrier on your back to distribute the weight close to your centre of gravity. Slings worn at the front of your body tend to slacken and impose a strain on your back similar to that of pregnancy, except now your baby is heavier. As your baby grows, he or she will begin to wriggle and reach out to things, often unexpectedly, so be prepared for sudden movements.

At bath time, squat or kneel down on a rolled towel beside the bath. Stay close to the tub while you lower your baby into the water and when you take him out of the bath.

## PUTTING YOUR BABY TO BED

You should choose a cot with a side that can be lowered right down or a crib with low sides, since these save you having to bend over in an awkward way to pick up your baby. When you place your baby down, bend your knees and keep your back straight. Always lay your baby to sleep on his or her back.

## LIFTING YOUR BABY

You will want to be sure you are lifting your new baby securely, while also maintaining good posture to protect your back.

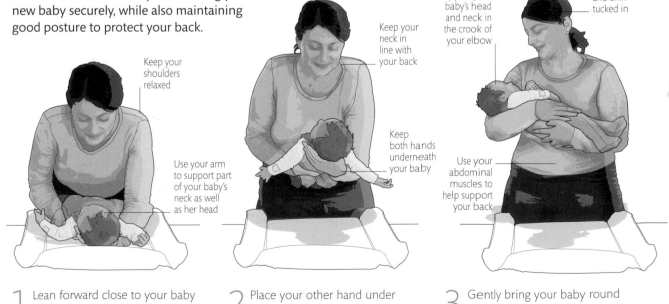

Keep your shoulders relaxed

Use your arm to support part of your baby's neck as well as her head

Keep your neck in line with your back

Keep both hands underneath your baby

Support your baby's head and neck in the crook of your elbow

Keep your head upright and chin tucked in

Use your abdominal muscles to help support your back

1 Lean forward close to your baby to pick her up, but keep your back straight. Slide your hand under your baby's head to support it.

2 Place your other hand under your baby's bottom so she is fully supported, and bring her close to your chest. Straighten up from your hips.

3 Gently bring your baby round to cradle her in your arms. Slide the hand behind her head around her body, and hold her close to your chest.

## CARING FOR YOUR BABY

Many tasks involved in caring for your baby can put a strain on your back, especially as he or she grows. To minimize bending and leaning over, set up a changing area at the right height for you and use a chair that will support your back while you breastfeed.

### Washing and changing

You can do these jobs on a work surface a little below elbow level, such as a chest of drawers, or you can kneel on the floor and change your baby on a low bed or sofa.

Try to avoid twisting as you lean over

### Breastfeeding

While you are nursing, sit in an upright chair rather than a soft couch, or use a chair that you can tilt backwards, such as a platform rocking chair. You might also use a footrest to elevate your feet and legs and push your back more firmly into the chair, and cushions to help create the support you need. Rather than bending over your baby, bring the baby to your breast. This will help avoid upper-back pain. Another option is to breastfeed in a side-lying position.

Cradle your baby close to your body

## LIFTING YOUR TODDLER

When you lift a young child, follow the rules of lifting: squat down and use your leg muscles to rise up again, keeping your back straight as you stand up. Keep the child close to your body rather than stretching out your arms, and avoid twisting.

Maintain a straight back as you reach out to your child

Keep your bottom low to help stabilize your body

Keep your arms close to your body

Avoid overarching the curve of your back

Come up smoothly in one motion

Keep your feet flat on the floor and hip-distance apart

Be prepared for sudden jerks and movements from your child

Engage your abdominal muscles

Keep your pelvic floor muscles tight

Bend your knees over your ankles

1 Squat down with both feet firmly on the floor. Keep your back straight, stomach muscles tight, and pull in your pelvic floor muscles. Bring your child close to you and lift him with both hands under his arms.

2 Bring him close to your body to avoid overreaching, and engage your abdominal muscles to help support your back. Be careful not to twist as you lift. As you stand up, let the strong muscles in your legs bear the load.

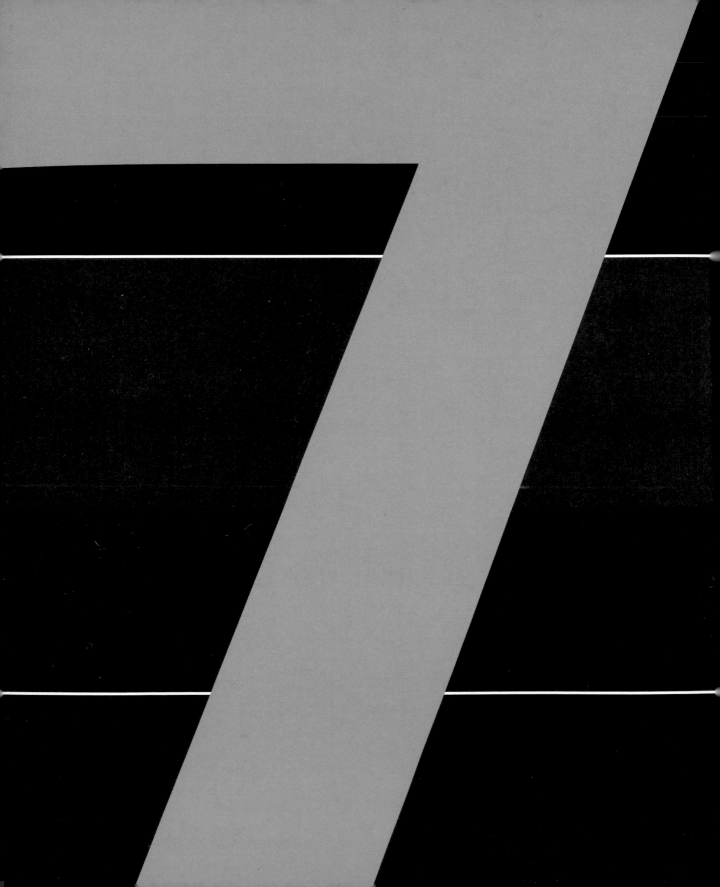

# STRATEGIES FOR COPING WITH PAIN

**Back and neck conditions all involve** a certain amount of pain, which can be both debilitating and depressing. This chapter aims to help you to manage your pain as effectively as possible, offering useful advice on a range of coping strategies, along with step-by-step guidance on basic movements to help you avoid aggravating your pain, particularly at an early stage of your recovery.

# COPING WITH PAIN

**Severe or long-term pain** causes changes of behaviour and mood which affect the intensity of your pain and your ability to tolerate it. There are several approaches to consider when treating chronic back pain: complementary therapies, psychological techniques, and conventional methods of pain-relief such as drugs or surgery. These methods are increasingly being combined.

## COMPLEMENTARY THERAPIES AND PSYCHOLOGICAL TECHNIQUES

| TREATMENT | WHAT DOES IT INVOLVE? | WHAT IS IT USED FOR? |
|---|---|---|
| Acupressure | A method of massage that, as with acupuncture, works on the principle of stimulating influential points and meridians. The difference is that these points are stimulated by pressure – often with the thumb or finger – rather than with acupuncture needles. | ■ Sciatica<br>■ Acute lower-back pain<br>■ Neck pain<br>■ Tension headaches |
| Acupuncture | This ancient Chinese medical practice uses needles inserted along energy lines of the body to stimulate energy flow until a harmonious balance is restored and pain is reduced. The Western approach involves deep needling at "trigger points" (focal areas of muscle spasm located by palpation), which is just as effective as the traditional Chinese approach (»pp.100–01). Acupuncture is often used when rest, manipulation, or analgesics are not helping to resolve an acute episode of pain. | ■ Acute lower-back pain and acute torticollis, whether caused by a disc protrusion or facet joint problem<br>■ Wear and tear (osteoarthritis) of the facet joints<br>■ Episodes of acute pain due to instability in the lower back<br>■ Mild sciatica without signs of damage to the nerve root, such as weakness or numbness<br>■ Sacroiliac strain |
| Massage | Involves the manipulation of the superficial and deeper layers of muscles and connective tissues. Releases muscular tension and promotes relaxation (»pp.98–99). | ■ Tense areas around the neck and shoulders<br>■ Bands of tense muscles in the back<br>■ Neck and upper- and lower-back pain |
| Hypnotherapy | Entails accessing the subconscious functions of the brain while under hypnosis, giving you the power to control and influence your subconscious thoughts and feelings, and your perception of pain. Hypnotherapy works best if you are receptive to the idea of the treatment (»pp.102–03). | ■ Chronic back and neck pain |
| Alexander Technique | A method of teaching improved posture based on the principle of relaxing the muscles and putting the least amount of pressure on the spine, to help you stand, sit, and move more efficiently (»p.115). | ■ Postural pain<br>■ Acute episodes of back pain in the elderly<br>■ Recurring back pain |
| Meditation and mindfulness | Aims to bring the mind under control and focus it in such a way that you are freed from stressful fears and emotions. It can help you to recognize and reduce stress in your body, and to overcome the anxieties and fears that cause it (»p.102). | ■ Chronic pain<br>■ Back pain where muscles are chronically tense<br>■ Recurrent back pain resulting from postural tension |
| Relaxation | A technique that heightens your awareness of tension in your body and teaches you how to release it. There are many relaxation techniques, including deep breathing exercises, which help to relax your muscles and lower your blood pressure, heart rate, and respiration (»pp.148–49). | ■ Muscle tension that develops into spasms<br>■ Acute and chronic back and neck pain<br>■ Postural pain<br>■ Tension headaches |

## MEDICAL SOLUTIONS

| TREATMENT | WHAT DOES IT INVOLVE? | WHAT IS IT USED FOR? |
|---|---|---|
| Combination analgesics | These generally work on the brain. They can be used to reduce general aches and pains temporarily but do not reduce inflammation or treat it directly. They are safe to use if the dose limit is not exceeded and if they do not contain large doses of codeine, which is likely to impair consciousness. Examples include combinations of codeine and paracetamol (»pp.84–85). | ■ General mild to moderate pain<br>■ Inflammatory conditions such as facet-joint irritation or swelling around the dural root sleeve |
| Anti-inflammatory drugs | Ease symptoms of pain and stiffness and decrease inflammation. Examples include ibuprofen and diclofenac (»pp.84–85). | ■ Musculoskeletal pain and joints that have become painfully inflamed<br>■ Inflammation caused by local internal bleeding in cases where the muscles, ligaments, or joints have been damaged; regular doses of ibuprofen will help<br>■ Protruding disc(s) |
| Strong analgesics (narcotics) | Used in moderate doses, prescribed narcotics relieve pain and also induce sleep. Examples include morphine and buprenorphine, and synthetic opioids such as tramadol (»pp.84–85). | ■ Severe back pain that lasts for more than 12–24 hours<br>■ Severe sciatica or brachialgia caused by nerve-root compression |
| Muscle relaxants | Work to relax tense muscles. An example is diazepam (»pp.84–85). | ■ Acute neck pain or lower-back pain, where the muscles tighten up to protect the painful area from further injury |
| Amitriptyline and anti-convulsants | Low doses of tricyclic antidepressants are effective for nerve pain, especially neuropathic pain. Gabapentin and pregabalin (anti-convulsants) are second-line agents licensed for this purpose. | ■ Chronic sciatica<br>■ Chronic brachialgia<br>■ Chronic back or neck pain with sleep disturbance<br>■ Chronic muscle tension |
| Injections (includes steroids and sclerosant delivered by injection) | Provide an accurate and effective way of delivering treatment to the specific source of pain (»pp.86–87). Steroids are synthetic drugs that are very similar to the body's natural steroid hormone. They work by a powerful anti-inflammatory action. Sclerosant injections stimulate the regrowth of ligaments. | ■ Localized back pain<br>■ Sprained and strained ligaments<br>■ Severe sciatica with symptoms of an inflamed nerve<br>■ Disc protrusion pain<br>■ Dural sheath irritation<br>■ Painful joints, including the spinal facet joints and sacroiliac joint |
| Surgery | Involves an operation carried out by a surgeon. Surgery is generally offered only after all other treatments have failed, or in severe cases of spinal disease (»pp.88–89). | ■ Disc prolapse (usually if it causes sciatica)<br>■ Central or lateral canal stenosis<br>■ Severe lower-back instability<br>■ Severe discogenic pain<br>■ Severe spondylolisthesis<br>■ Tumours of the vertebrae<br>■ Infections in the disc space and around the spinal column |
| Neuro-stimulation | Uses a small device similar to a pacemaker that is either placed over, or surgically inserted into, the spinal canal. The device sends mild electrical impulses to the nervous system which block the pain signals from reaching the brain and, in doing so, alleviate pain (»pp.104–05). Used when other forms of pain treatment are no longer effective. | ■ Chronic back pain |

# PERCEPTION OF PAIN

**We are only just beginning** to understand the psychology of pain perception. The amount of pain you feel depends not only on the physical damage sustained, but also on your mental state: if your mind is otherwise occupied, you can be unaware of some slight injury; or, at the other extreme, you can be so fixated with your condition that you become consumed with pain.

Pain is difficult to quantify: it is invisible and as such cannot be measured easily. There is no "instrument" that measures pain; instead your doctor relies on the information you give him to assess the type and level of pain you are experiencing. In turn, it is how you interpret your doctor's findings and how you choose to deal with them that influence the effectiveness of the treatment.

## TYPES OF PAIN

There are two main types of pain: nociceptive (where pain nerve receptors are directly stimulated) and neuropathic (where pain signals are generated spontaneously and perpetuated within the nervous system).

Acute pain caused by an initial injury usually settles within a few days or weeks, following the natural healing process. Sometimes, however, the pain becomes chronic (exceeding three months), and leads to changes within the nerves, spinal cord, and brain, which perpetuate the pain as if there were still an injury that has not healed. The reasons for this are numerous, but the psychological state you were in at the time of the initial injury, and your thoughts, reactions, and associations subsequent to the initial shock are very likely to set up this chronic neuropathic state. Chronic pain is difficult to diagnose and treat, and can leave you feeling anxious, helpless, and depressed. It is likely that the uncertainty of the diagnosis and its cure will have a far greater psychological impact on how you perceive pain.

## MIND OVER MATTER

Pain messages can be muted between the centre of your brain and the outer cortex. Your general state of mind, including your will to recover, expectations, anxieties, mood, and ability to concentrate on something else are the decisive factors in how you feel pain and deal with it. Both your conscious and subconscious mind work together either to subdue or increase the level of pain you are feeling, with the result that different people have different experiences of how they sense pain. For instance, some people seem not to be overly affected by considerable injury and pain, whereas others react with marked disability to what is deemed superficial damage and pain.

Research suggests that, to a certain extent, you can control and reduce the level of pain and disability you experience by adopting a positive attitude. Positive thinking reduces activity in the parts of your brain that process pain information and,

## FACTORS AFFECTING PAIN PERCEPTION

Susceptibility to pain is greater when your brain is aroused with fear and anxiety, and when the focus is on your pain and bodily symptoms. The mental and physical states listed here greatly influence your perception of pain: some of these states exaggerate or increase the intensity of the pain, while others dull or decrease it.

| FACTORS THAT INCREASE PAIN | FACTORS THAT DECREASE PAIN |
| --- | --- |
| ■ Anxiety and uncertainty | ■ Emotional tranquillity |
| ■ Negative beliefs and expectations | ■ Positive attitude |
| ■ Depression | ■ Sleep |
| ■ Prolonged stress | ■ Relaxation |
| ■ Fear | ■ Hypnosis |
| ■ Genetic factors | ■ Deep breathing |
| ■ Consuming excessive amounts of caffeine | ■ Consuming moderate amounts of alcohol |
| ■ Concentrating attention on pain | ■ Distracting the mind |
| ■ Drugs such as amphetamines | ■ Drugs such as diazepam and morphine |

as a consequence, pain is alleviated: if you expect pain to be less, it will be less. Conversely, if it is in your nature to worry and feel helpless in the face of pain, you will be more likely to experience greater levels of pain.

Your expectations also play a part in your perception of pain: if you have low expectations about pain (for instance, if you are told a moderately painful procedure will not hurt much), then your perception and processing of it will be influenced, compared to if you'd been warned to expect pain. Positive expectation actually reduces the amount of pain your brain processes.

In fact, it is only in the last few years that physicians have begun to unlock the mysteries of the mind–body connection. The more we understand about this complex association, the greater the benefits to patients and healthcare professionals alike.

## GATE CONTROL THEORY

In the mid-1960s the renowned neurologists Ronald Melzack and Patrick Wall developed the "gate control" theory of pain perception. They visualized a number of mental and physical factors working against each other, opening or closing a metaphorical "gate" and controlling the amount of pain a person experiences. This theory informs the current framework for conceptualizing chronic pain.

What causes pain? Stimuli such as a fall or a burn induce pain when they threaten to, or actually, cause tissue damage. These painful stimuli activate the nervous system through "nociceptors", receptors in the skin and internal organs that are sensitive to pain. These receptors are connected to small nerve fibres, and when they detect pain they relay pain messages from the site of the injury or inflammation to the spinal cord.

The gate control theory states that these small nerve fibres push open a "pain gate". On a normal basis the "pain gate" is closed and no pain is felt. However, when an injury occurs, various factors converge to push the gate open or to close it again. The intensity of the pain depends on how wide the gate is open.

To counteract this pain, massage, rubs, and other techniques are used to stimulate larger nerve fibres, which carry non-nociceptive information and help to close the gate again by reducing the intensity of the pain.

However, if small-fibre messages swamp those from large fibres, the gate reopens and a T-cell (pain transmission cell) is triggered, which starts a chain reaction through the spinal cord to the mid-brain (the emotional centre of the brain) and to the outer cortex of the brain, where it is registered as a conscious perception of pain.

As well as the pain-relieving aids mentioned above, the brain itself can also reduce the flow of pain through the gate. If you are in the right mental state, the brain stimulates the production of noradrenaline hormones, the body's natural pain relievers, which help to reduce your perception of pain. Acupuncture controls pain in a similar way by encouraging the production of endorphins in the spinal cord, and drugs such as morphine act like endorphins.

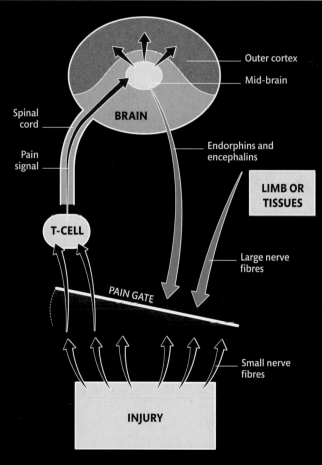

**The pain gate**
The diagram above shows how the pain gate is opened and closed, and how pain messages can be blocked even after the T-cell, which starts a chain reaction, has been triggered.

# PSYCHOLOGICAL FACTORS IN BACK PAIN

**It is unclear why some people** are prone to back pain, while others, who have a similar physique and live in similar circumstances, are not. But the answer seems to lie partly in emotional or psychological factors, which can play just as big a part in back pain as clearly diagnosed physical disorders.

Sufferers of chronic back pain often complain of high stress levels; indeed, medical professionals have found a strong connection between physical and emotional stress and chronic back pain. Continuous physical and emotional stress can cause various changes in your body and your bodily movements that influence the way you use your muscles and spine. Tightness or tension in your muscles is a common result, which can lead to neck and back pain, as well as headaches.

The constant discomfort of chronic back pain can then lead to depression: the pain makes sleeping difficult, leading to fatigue and irritability; participating in everyday activities becomes a struggle, which can cause feelings of isolation, hopelessness, despair, and, ultimately, depression. This vicious circle can be hard to break out of: you may feel trapped by your condition and believe that you are alone in your experience of pain. However, there are ways of dealing with stress-related pain, and with time you will find that the pain should gradually subside.

## MIND-BODY THERAPIES

The mind and body work in tandem and this is why psychological factors such as stress, anxiety, trauma, and depression, along with a lack of effective coping skills, can manifest themselves in the form of physical discomfort, including chronic back pain. Research studies have shown that a positive mental attitude in coping with pain, good self-esteem, and the ability to believe that pain can be overcome and a return to health possible, all lead to a speedier recovery. There are a number of mind-body therapies available, such as Cognitive Behavioural Therapy (where the objective is to modify the thoughts and feelings of the individual so their ability to cope with pain is more effective), imagery therapy (involving the use of the individual's imagination for healing), relaxation methods (》》pp.148–49), and hypnosis and meditation (》》pp.102–03).

## COPING STRATEGIES

There are two ways of coping with pain: you can either choose to be passive, and "grin and bear it" without taking any action to redress the problem; or you can take control of your pain and work towards a solution. If you choose the latter option, the first step is to realize that you are an active participant in the successful treatment of your condition. Once you take control, you will feel more positive, which will help in your pain management, and you will experience a sense of power that will spur you on even further. Don't be afraid to seek help: there are a range of medical and holistic approaches available, so find what works best for you.

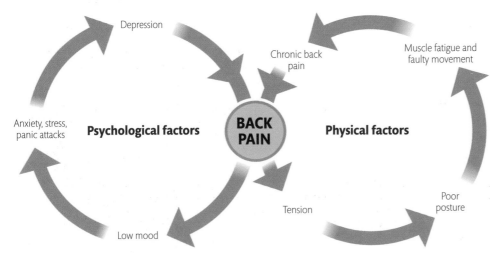

**Psychological factors**

Depression

Chronic back pain

Anxiety, stress, panic attacks

BACK PAIN

Low mood

Tension

**Physical factors**

Muscle fatigue and faulty movement

Poor posture

**Pain factors**
Try to become more aware of your moods and emotional state. Negative thoughts and feelings often lead to depression, which in turn can lead to chronic back pain. You may initially believe that an awkward movement has aggravated your back pain, but it is also possible that emotional tension is actually the causal factor.

# FACTORS AND COPING STRATEGIES

| FACTOR | STATE OF MIND | COPING STRATEGY |
|---|---|---|
| **Anxiety** | ■ This may be a general problem for you, or it may be specific to your pain and the uncertainty and fear of what might be wrong. Being overanxious makes you focus on your pain and bodily symptoms, and fear of pain can lead to fear of movement, which is disabling in itself. | ■ Adopt calming strategies. These include slow, diaphragmatic breathing, progressive muscle relaxation, mindfulness, and meditation.<br>■ Give yourself time to adapt to your pain and accept the occasional disruption it may cause in your life.<br>■ Seek reassurance from your doctor or therapist. Most back pain is benign. |
| **Thoughts and beliefs** | ■ Your preconceptions about pain, along with your previous experiences of pain and back trouble in yourself or significant others all influence your reactions and behaviour. | ■ Observe your thought process about your pain. Be aware of how it influences your body tension and pain experience. Negative thoughts, such as visualizing the worst outcome, are harmful to your recovery.<br>■ Believe that with the right help you have the resources to cope. |
| **Mood** | ■ This colours your view of your back trouble and how you cope with it. Low mood can affect your recovery and reduce your motivation and tolerance of pain. Chronic pain can have a depressing effect. | ■ An alteration in mood is possible if you attend to your thoughts and beliefs first (**》above**). If you are generally low or depressed, seek help from your doctor: they may prescribe medication or recommend counselling and psychotherapy. |
| **Stress** | ■ High stress levels, major life events such as bereavement or divorce, or just everyday hassles make you more prone to react unfavourably to back or neck pain. | ■ Reduce as many stresses as possible. There may be some that feel outside your control, which you may have to accept. Learn to prioritize so that only really essential matters are attended to. |
| **Coping skills** | ■ People's reactions vary in response to adversity: some see it as a challenge to overcome and a learning experience to avoid future attacks, while others struggle to cope and find it difficult to adapt to their changed circumstances. | ■ How well do you cope with adverse life events? You may be either too hard or too soft on yourself, so try to get the balance right.<br>■ Do you take responsibility and try to help yourself, or do you depend on others? Much of this is down to personality or learned behaviours, but this can be changed. Being proactive in the way you deal with pain will help you overcome it more easily. |
| **Environment** | ■ All pain is experienced within the context of your body, family and home life, social life, and interests. Pain and disability interrupt your normal rhythm and balance. Some of these factors may be part of the problem too. | ■ Make sure you take regular exercise such as walking, and stretch regularly throughout the day.<br>■ Don't let chronic back pain take over your life and intrude upon time with your family and friends. |
| **Occupation** | ■ If you are the sole breadwinner and your ability to function or hold down a job is under threat, this will have a huge influence on how you react to pain. The type of work you do may determine how quickly you can get back into action. | ■ Discuss the implications with your doctor. Ask him to liaise with your employer to find ways of alleviating your workload. Perhaps you could work part-time or take on lighter duties. If you are on sick leave, maybe they would consider a phased return to work. |
| **Sleep** | ■ Too little sleep, or sleep broken by feelings of pain and restlessness, makes nerves more sensitive and muscles more tense. Lack of sleep gets you down, lowers your pain threshold, reduces your body's ability to heal, and impacts on your ability to cope. | ■ Seek advice on sleeping posture and support. Night sedation with a low dose of amitriptyline (an antidepressant) can be very helpful. |

# PAIN RELIEF THROUGH RELAXATION

**Taking the time to relax properly** allows your body to unwind and can help to ease any physical, mental, and emotional stress you may be feeling. Relaxation can ease muscular tension in your neck and back and help to improve your breathing, which in turn has a calming effect on your entire body. It can therefore be a very useful element of your pain management.

Muscle tension brought on by emotional or physical stress can cause stiffness in the muscles of your back and neck. If this tension persists for too long it can lead to chronic pain. To help with your pain management, or prevent the onset of back and neck pain in the first place, you should try a range of relaxation techniques, find out which ones work best for you, and then build them into your routine. There are numerous options you can choose from, including relaxation positions, deep breathing exercises, and positive visualization techniques.

### RELAXATION POSITIONS

Relaxation positions (»below) can help you to relieve stress, and are important in maintaining a healthy back and neck as they help you to ease tension in your muscles, reduce your blood pressure, and slow your heart rate. If practised regularly they can help to increase your energy levels and focus your mind. You may want to use these positions in conjunction with meditation and self-hypnosis techniques (»pp.102–03).

### BREATHING METHODS

Deep breathing is a simple, yet very effective, relaxation method that can help to ease pain, especially as most people tend to take short, shallow breaths. Your therapist may teach you diaphragmatic, or abdominal, breathing (»pp.102–03); however, you can practise the following technique on your own:

■ Begin by breathing in through your nose and out through your mouth, allowing your mouth to stay open in a relaxed way. Concentrate on breathing in deeply, so that you feel

---

## CROSS-LEGGED SITTING POSITION

This basic yoga sitting posture is often used for meditation. It is a perfect relaxation position as it is versatile and easy to perform.

Keep your shoulders down and relaxed

Straighten your torso

1 Sit on a cushion or on the floor with your legs crossed at the ankles and your back straight. Rest your hands on your knees or upper thighs, relax your shoulders and back, and breathe in and out deeply for a few minutes, using your abdomen to control each breath.

## PSOAS AND BACK RELAXATION

This position helps to relax your psoas muscles, which are located deep in your lower back and help to keep your spine and legs mobile. When they tighten, they cause lower-back pain, so it is important to keep them supple.

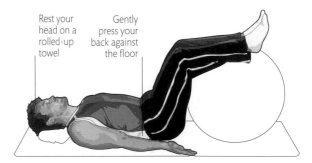

Rest your head on a rolled-up towel

Gently press your back against the floor

1 Lie on your back with your arms by your sides, palms up, your hips and knees bent at right angles, and your calves resting on a Swiss ball or chair. Relax your shoulders and back, and take deep breaths in and out for several minutes, using your abdomen to control each breath.

your abdomen rising as your diaphragm descends. Avoid breathing in too quickly or taking short, shallow breaths. Your chest hardly needs to rise at all – it is your diaphragm that should provide the automatic rhythm.

■ Next, concentrate on breathing out properly. Keep your jaw relaxed, your mouth open, and allow your abdomen to sink when you breathe out. It can help to let go with a prolonged and audible sigh.

■ Once you have taken a few deep breaths in and out, focus on your breathing as a whole, and be aware of your diaphragm rising and falling. While you will be very aware of your breathing at first, it will come more naturally with practice and, with a regular breathing rhythm, your muscles will start to relax.

## VISUALIZATION TECHNIQUES

You may find that practising visualization techniques can help you to relax. While such techniques vary in approach and scope, most involve using positive thinking to promote rest, calm, and well-being. One particular form, known as autogenic training, is sometimes used by physiotherapists as part of pain management treatment (**»pp.102–03**).

### PROGRESSIVE MUSCLE RELAXATION

One of the most simple relaxation techniques, Progressive Muscle Relaxation is often used by therapists as a pain management treatment. The technique works through the deliberate tensing and relaxing of different muscle groups, focusing on one at a time, to increase your awareness of what tension and relaxation feel like. This way you can identify and counteract signs of muscular tension at an early stage. Start with your feet, and work your way up your body:

■ **Breathe in deeply** and tense the muscles in your left foot as hard as you can.
■ **Keep the muscles** in your foot tense for about 10 seconds, then breathe out, releasing the tension and feeling it flow out of your body as you exhale.
■ **Repeat** with the other parts of your body: your right foot, then your calves, thighs, hips and buttocks, stomach, chest, back, arms and hands, neck and shoulders, and, finally, your face. At each stage concentrate on the left side of your body first, then your right.

### RELAXATION CDS

You may find the soothing music of relaxation CDs a useful relaxation aid, helping you to empty your mind of stressful thoughts, especially when you are practising other relaxation techniques.

## CORPSE POSE

This position is widely used in yoga at the beginning and end of a session. While it is relatively straightforward, it can take a certain amount of practice to master because the movements involved are quite subtle. When done correctly it is a pose that enables deep relaxation, both of your body and your mind.

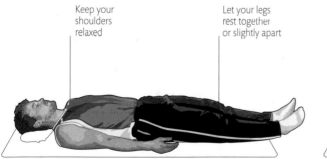

Keep your shoulders relaxed

Let your legs rest together or slightly apart

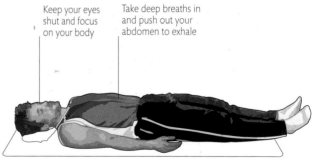

Keep your eyes shut and focus on your body

Take deep breaths in and push out your abdomen to exhale

1 Lie face-up on a mat with a rolled-up towel or a small pillow under your head, and close your eyes. Rest your arms by your sides with your palms facing in towards your body, and relax completely, shaking out your limbs and allowing them to loosen.

2 Turn your head from side to side to mobilize your spine, then stretch your body to its full length from head to toe. Feel the stretch between your head and shoulders, and your legs and pelvis. Breathe deeply in and out for several minutes, using your abdomen.

# LYING DOWN AND SLEEPING

**You may find that** you are most comfortable when you are lying down. This is because a lying position relieves most of the pressure that your body weight puts on your spine. You don't have to lie flat on your back, however: try out the positions shown below until you find one that works best for you.

## YOUR BED

If you find that your back pain is at its worst in the morning or that this is the only time your back aches, you may need a new mattress. Likewise, if you have only developed pain since you bought a new mattress, you should consider replacing it. Bear in mind that aching and stiffness can also result from inactivity, so it may not matter which surface you lie on.

When purchasing a mattress, make sure you choose one that is firm, finely sprung, and provides sufficient support, and is at least 15cm (6in) longer than you are to allow freedom of movement. No matter how good your mattress is, a sagging bed base can harm your back, so make sure that the base is firm and strong enough to support your mattress.

Adjustable beds are now widely available and affordable, and offer positional comfort. They allow you to raise your legs or head to any angle at the touch of a button, meaning that you can even set them for the Fowler position (**»below**).

## POSITIONS TO LIE IN

Lying on your front increases the curve in your lower back, which aggravates backache caused by facet joint problems (**»p.68**). However, such a position will probably not hurt your back if your pain is caused by a herniated disc (**»p.70**).

## SLEEPING POSITIONS

If you suffer from back pain there are a number of positions you can adopt to help you sleep. Different types of pillows or a folded towel can alleviate back pain. Try these positions and see what works for you.

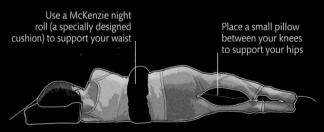

Use a McKenzie night roll (a specially designed cushion) to support your waist

Place a small pillow between your knees to support your hips

**Lying on your side I**
Lie on your side, with a pillow supporting your head and a McKenzie night roll supporting your waist so your spine is straight. Place a pillow between your knees to help with your alignment.

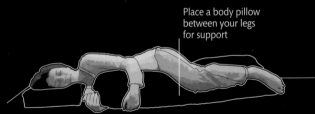

Place a body pillow between your legs for support

**Lying on your side II**
Rest your head on a support pillow (**»opposite**) so that your head is in line with your spine, and use a body pillow to support your entire body. Pregnant women will find this type of pillow particularly comfortable.

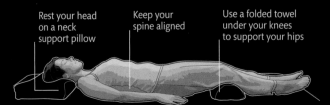

Rest your head on a neck support pillow

Keep your spine aligned

Use a folded towel under your knees to support your hips

**Lying on your back**
Lie on your back and rest your head on a neck support pillow to prevent your head flopping from side to side. Place a rolled-up towel under your knees to help with lower-back pain.

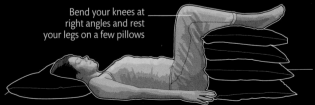

Bend your knees at right angles and rest your legs on a few pillows

**The Fowler position**
If lying flat on your back causes you pain, lie with your knees bent at right angles and your calves supported on a stack of pillows. This reduces the curve in your lower back and minimizes the pressure on your discs.

Lying flat on your back with your legs straight may also increase the curve in your lower back and cause backache. The Fowler position (**»opposite**) helps to flatten out this excessive curve and relaxes the psoas muscles, which run from your lower back to your thighs. If you have acute back pain (**»pp.36–39**), you should place several pillows under your knees, but for most other conditions, a rolled-up towel may be enough.

With an adjustable bed (**»opposite**), you can raise or lower your head and legs to relieve aching limbs, or lie in a semi-recumbent position if you have breathing or cardiac problems. The bed may also have a vibration mode to micro-massage your joints.

To avoid neck pain, make sure your head rests fairly square on your shoulders to minimize the strain. You should only use one pillow if you lie on your back; if you sleep on your side, the width of your shoulders will determine whether you need one or two pillows to support your head.

## PILLOW SUPPORT

It is important to ensure you get the correct support from your pillow. To test a pillow, lift it horizontally, with the edge of your hand running across the centre: if it stays more or less level, it is fine; if it sags, you should replace it. If you wake with a stiff neck, try twisting the pillow into a butterfly shape or use a rolled towel placed around your neck to act as a soft collar. Alternatively, try a neck support pillow, which prevents your head lolling from side to side.

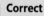

**Correct**

Neck support pillows are made from a foam material that moulds itself to the shape of your neck. They are ridged at the front to hold your neck and head firmly.

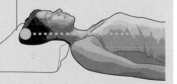

A neck support pillow ensures your head and neck are correctly positioned

The raised position of your head will put pressure on your spine

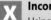

**Incorrect**

Using more than one pillow can cause excessive flexion of your head and neck, which can put pressure on your spine and cause or exacerbate pain.

## SEX AND BACK PAIN Q&A

**Q** | **Can I still have sex if I have back pain?**

**A** | Yes, but you may have to modify your favourite positions to accommodate your pain (**»below**). Depending on the type of back pain you have, you should try placing a pillow or rolled-up towel under your pelvis for extra support and comfort. You may also find that a hot bath or gentle massage before sex can help to relax your muscles and ease pain.

**Q** | **What do I do if my partner has back pain?**

**A** | If either one of you has back or neck problems, it is likely to affect both of you. Sex can be difficult or painful, causing frustration and distress to both parties. Try to open up the channels of communication so that you can discuss how you feel. Reassure your partner and make it clear that you want to work together to find a way to restore a fulfilling sex life that gives both of you pleasure.

**Q** | **How can I tell my partner I'm in pain?**

**A** | Back pain can be stressful as well as debilitating. Because back pain is invisible, it can be hard for your partner to fully understand your pain. Talking to your partner about your discomfort is very important: describe your pain as clearly as possible and explain that you are still attracted to him or her but that the pain in your back is causing you distress.

**Q** | **How can we make sure sex is still special?**

**A** | Set aside some time when you know that neither of you will be interrupted and find a comfortable environment. Be gentle and tune into each other's feelings and reactions: honesty, support, and reassurance will go a long way to restoring your sexual relationship. Explore other forms of sensuality as part of your sex life, and spend more time on kissing and stroking. There are many ways to enjoy a fulfilling physical relationship, so it is up to you and your partner to use your creativity and imagination and explore other avenues to find activities that will not put undue stress on areas of pain.

**Q** | **What are the least painful positions for intercourse?**

**A** | One of the most gentle positions is known as "spoons". For this, the female partner lies on her side with the male partner directly behind her in the same position, so that their bodies fit together like spoons. The "doggie" position can work well for women who have back pain. For this, she kneels on all fours with her partner positioned behind her. For men who find it painful to straighten their backs, the seated position works well, in which he sits on a chair or the edge of the bed with his partner straddling him, face to face.

# TURNING IN BED

If you need to turn in bed from one side to the other, start by turning your upper arm and head – this is the natural way that babies and toddlers turn over. Your arm will initiate the movement of your upper trunk.

As you begin to roll onto your back, move your other arm in the same direction. Your pelvis will follow the movements of your arms and trunk without putting any strain on your back.

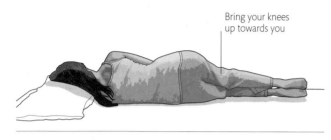

Bring your knees up towards you

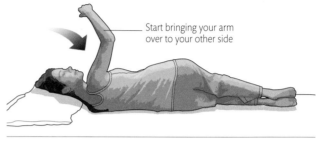

Start bringing your arm over to your other side

1 If you are lying on your side and want to roll over onto your back or your other side, start by bringing your knees up towards you until they are at right angles.

2 To roll over onto your back, bring your top arm over while turning your head at the same time.

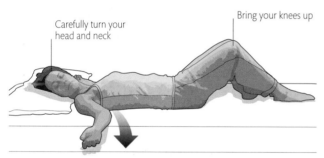

Carefully turn your head and neck

Bring your knees up

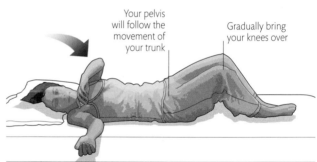

Your pelvis will follow the movement of your trunk

Gradually bring your knees over

3 Bring your legs over so that your feet and back are flat on the mattress. Your leading arm should lie out to the side you are turning towards.

4 Now bring your other arm over and drop your legs towards the mattress. As you do this, your head and torso will turn too.

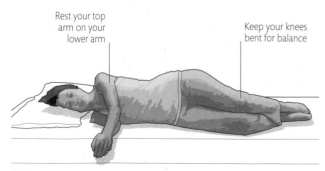

Rest your top arm on your lower arm

Keep your knees bent for balance

5 Bring your arm over until it rests on your other arm, and rest your legs on the mattress. Practise this during the day so that it becomes your habit during the night time.

## SLEEPING PROBLEMS

You may find that back pain interrupts your sleeping patterns and leads to insomnia. Follow these steps to readjust your sleeping habits:

- Lie down to sleep only when you feel sleepy.
- Do not do anything in bed (apart from sexual activity) except sleep.
- If you do not fall asleep within 15 minutes of getting into bed, get up and leave the room. Do not return to bed until you are sleepy.
- Set the alarm for the same time every morning. When it goes off, get up, regardless of how much sleep you've had.
- Avoid naps during the day.
- Cut down on tea, coffee, and other stimulants.
- If you and your partner prefer different types of mattress, buy two separate mattresses and place them next to each other.

# GETTING IN AND OUT OF BED

To get into bed, sit on the bed with your arms either side of you. Lower yourself down on one side by leaning on your elbow and then putting your head down onto the pillow, while at the same time raising your legs up onto the bed. To get out of bed, try the sequence in reverse: lie on your side and raise your head from the pillow, put your legs down onto the floor and use your arm to lift yourself up into a sitting position.

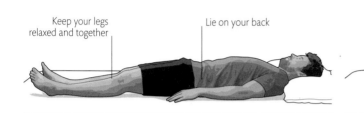

Keep your legs relaxed and together

Lie on your back

1 If you usually sleep on your front or side, turn over so that you are lying on your back, with your arms resting on either side of your body and your legs together.

Keep your knees and feet together

2 Bring your feet towards you so that your knees are at right angles.

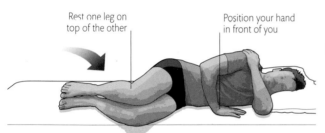

Rest one leg on top of the other

Position your hand in front of you

3 Lower your bended knees towards the edge of the bed. Rest the hand of your top arm in front of you and position your other arm so that your elbow is on the mattress and your hand is resting on your top shoulder.

Keep your shoulders relaxed

Swing your legs down as you push up on your arms

4 Lift your head off the pillow, pushing down on your elbow and supporting hand at the same time, while bringing your feet over the edge of the bed.

5 To take the extra weight, rest your forearm against the mattress and continue pushing yourself up until you are sitting upright.

Keep your head in line with your back

6 Place your arms either side of your body. With your feet firmly on the floor, stand up as you would from a chair.

Shift your body to the edge of the bed before you try to get up

# WASHING AND DRESSING

**You can make washing** and dressing easier by incorporating simple coping strategies into your daily routine. For instance, when you are standing at the sink to wash, shave, or brush your teeth, avoid bending or leaning over it; as always, it is best to try to stand up straight.

If you have to stand at the sink for any length of time, try putting one hand on the basin to support your weight, and bend from your hips, not at your waist. Keep your head up and your back straight throughout. You might prefer to wash with a face cloth.

## USING THE SHOWER AND BATH

You may find it easier to stand in the shower than sit in a bath. Put a rubber nonslip mat in the shower to stop you from slipping. Keep your toiletries in a wall rack to avoid having to bend or reach for them. Use a sponge or long-handled brush to wash with; the latter is particularly useful for washing hard-to-reach areas, such as your back and feet. If you would rather have a bath, avoid lying with your back in a rounded position for too long, as getting out may be difficult. You may find a hand-held shower head useful when washing your hair. Fit a handrail to the bath if you have chronic back trouble to help you get out of the bath more easily. It may be easier to dry yourself by wearing a towelling bath robe rather than by using a towel.

## USING THE TOILET

A raised seat can make it easier for you to sit on the toilet, especially if you are tall. Lower yourself down onto the seat carefully by bending your knees and steadying yourself with a hand placed against a wall or holding onto a door in front of you. Be careful not to twist or reach round behind while you are sitting on the toilet.

## YOUR MORNING ROUTINE

Washing your face and brushing your teeth are part of your daily washing routine. If you suffer from back pain, it is important you do not hunch over the sink. Stay upright, and, if you do need to bend, bend from your hips and knees. Your toiletries should be within easy reach to avoid unnecessary reaching or bending.

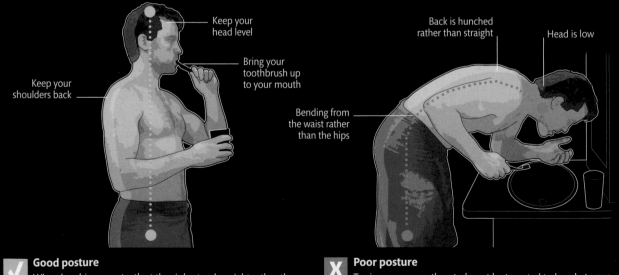

Keep your head level

Bring your toothbrush up to your mouth

Keep your shoulders back

Back is hunched rather than straight

Head is low

Bending from the waist rather than the hips

**✔ Good posture**
When brushing your teeth at the sink, stand upright rather than crouched over the sink. You may find it easier to use a cup filled with water to rinse out your mouth. If you shave, the mirror should be directly in front of you. An extendable mirror to the side of the basin may also be handy.

**✗ Poor posture**
To rinse your mouth out, do not be tempted to bend at your waist as this could aggravate a back injury. Instead, bend from your hips and bend your knees, keeping your back in a neutral position to take the stress off your spine.

## WASHING AND DRESSING Q&A

**Q | Should I shower, or bathe?**

**A |** If you are experiencing acute pain, and/or suffering from disc problems, you should shower instead of taking a bath. This will stop you from bending your back for a prolonged period and aggravating the condition. Take care when stepping in and out of the shower – a nonslip mat will help prevent accidents.

**Q | How can I wash my back properly?**

**A |** It can be tricky reaching all parts of your body, your back in particular. A long-handled body brush will reach areas that would otherwise be hard to get to.

**Q | How do I wash my feet?**

**A |** Stand on a mat next to the shower or bath, and place one foot on the side of the tub. If you are able to bathe, bring your foot up towards you while lying in the bath.

**Q | What sort of clothing should I wear?**

**A |** Loose clothing that is easy to put on and take off and that does not restrict your movement is always a good option. Tops with a zip or buttons are good for the same reasons.

**Q | What type of shoes should I wear?**

**A |** Shoes without laces are easy to slip on and off. Women should avoid wearing high heels as these can cause lower-back pain. If in doubt, choose comfortable footwear that requires the least possible amount of effort.

**Q | Can I wear boots?**

**A |** You should avoid wearing boots or any other kind of heavy or stiff footwear that requires you to apply unnecessary force to put them on or take them off (»above).

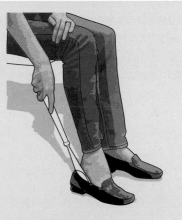

**Putting on shoes**
A long-handled shoe horn is a useful tool when bending over is painful. Simply sit on a chair and use the shoe horn to ease your foot into the shoe.

## GETTING DRESSED

You should try to avoid having to bend your back while dressing – instead, lie flat or stand up straight. In general, it is best to avoid wearing tight clothing that restricts your movement. You will also find slip-on shoes much easier to put on and take off.

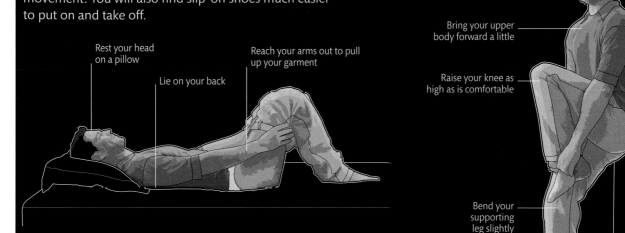

Rest your head on a pillow

Lie on your back

Reach your arms out to pull up your garment

Keep your head in line with your spine

Bring your upper body forward a little

Raise your knee as high as is comfortable

Bend your supporting leg slightly

**Putting on underwear and trousers**
You may find putting on underwear or trousers more comfortable when performed lying down. Step into your trousers and carefully move onto the bed, taking care not to bend, and lie down on your back. Raise your hips off the bed slightly to pull your garment all the way up. To remove the garment, reverse the sequence.

**Putting on socks**
Don't sit down to put on your socks; instead, lean your buttocks against a wall with your feet about 30cm (12in) from the wall. Raise one leg and slip on your sock. Repeat for the other sock.

# MOVING AROUND

**When performing everyday tasks** such as household chores, personal care, or social activities, it is important to maintain good neck and back posture so you can carry on with daily life without putting undue stress on your back.

Additionally, it is a good idea to help yourself by making use of the many mobility aids available to simplify routine tasks, whether in the home or outside (**»opposite**).

## HOME AND GARDEN
Nobody knows your home as well as you do. There may be areas that you know could be made more accessible: make a note of these and aim to make the necessary changes. For instance, you may find you have to reach beyond your comfortable range to access an everyday item in the kitchen; or you may need to crouch down to get to the cleaning

products in the bathroom. As a general rule, put objects that you use more frequently at an easily accessible height so that you do not have to bend, stretch, twist, or lift unnecessarily.

In the garden, use long-handled tools, and if you need to do labour-intensive work such as digging or shovelling, take the necessary precautions (**»pp.132–33**).

If you find that you are struggling to make your home more user-friendly, an occupational therapist will be able to assess your home in relation to your needs and advise you on how best to adapt it. They will also be able to teach you new ways of doing things.

## SOCIAL ACTIVITIES
Some social activities may require you to stand on your feet for hours on end, leading to back pain and aching joints. Wear flat, comfortable shoes, take regular rests, and, if you are attending an event where seating will not always be available, take your own portable stool with you (**»opposite**).

## GETTING OUT OF AN ARMCHAIR

It is important to learn how to get out of an armchair safely to avoid potential back injuries and falls. If you suffer from back pain, using your arms to help raise yourself up will relieve stress on your lower back.

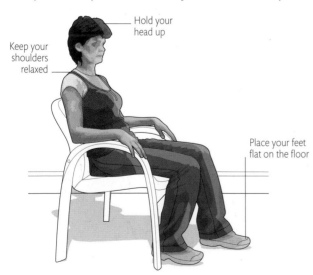

Keep your shoulders relaxed

Hold your head up

Place your feet flat on the floor

1 When you are ready to stand up, place your arms and hands on the arm rests. Make sure your feet are flat on the floor about hip-distance apart, with one foot positioned slightly in front of the other for balance.

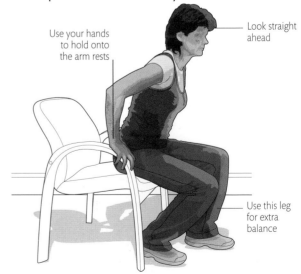

Use your hands to hold onto the arm rests

Look straight ahead

Use this leg for extra balance

2 Move your buttocks towards the edge of the chair. Lean forwards until your nose is above your knees and use your arms to help push yourself up. Keep your head, shoulders, and back aligned.

## MOBILITY AIDS

A range of mobility aids can reduce the strain of everyday activities and ease chronic back pain and knee joint stress. For instance, if you struggle to reach high or low objects, a compact reaching aid will extend your reach so that you can pick up items easily without straining your back. Collapsible walking sticks are lightweight, compact, and can be stored away when not in use. Portable folding stools are ideal for when you are working in low, uncomfortable positions, such as tending the garden, where you would otherwise be on your knees, bending, or crouching in awkward positions.

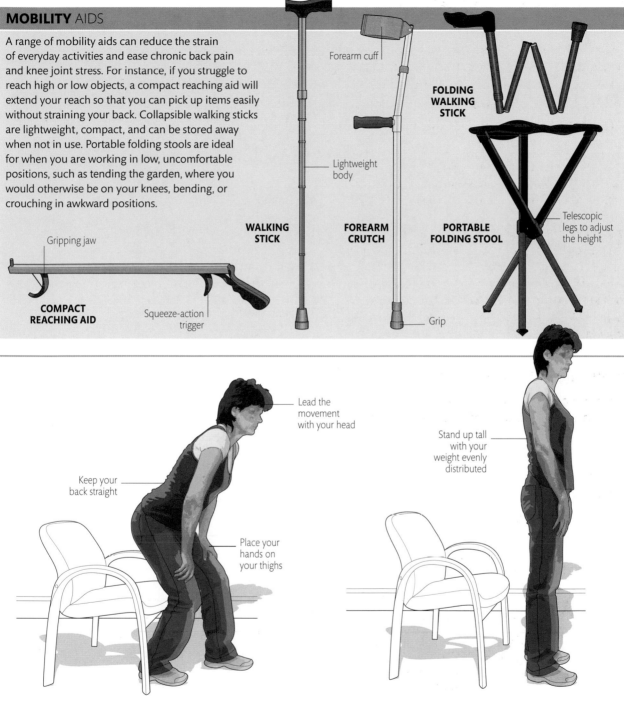

Forearm cuff

**FOLDING WALKING STICK**

Lightweight body

Gripping jaw

**WALKING STICK**

**FOREARM CRUTCH**

**PORTABLE FOLDING STOOL**

Telescopic legs to adjust the height

**COMPACT REACHING AID**

Squeeze-action trigger

Grip

Lead the movement with your head

Stand up tall with your weight evenly distributed

Keep your back straight

Place your hands on your thighs

3 As you push yourself up, gradually straighten your legs and let go of the arm rests. Place your hands on your thighs to support your weight and keep your head in line with your back throughout the move.

4 Continue straightening your legs until you are fully upright, and move your back leg forwards so that your feet are together.

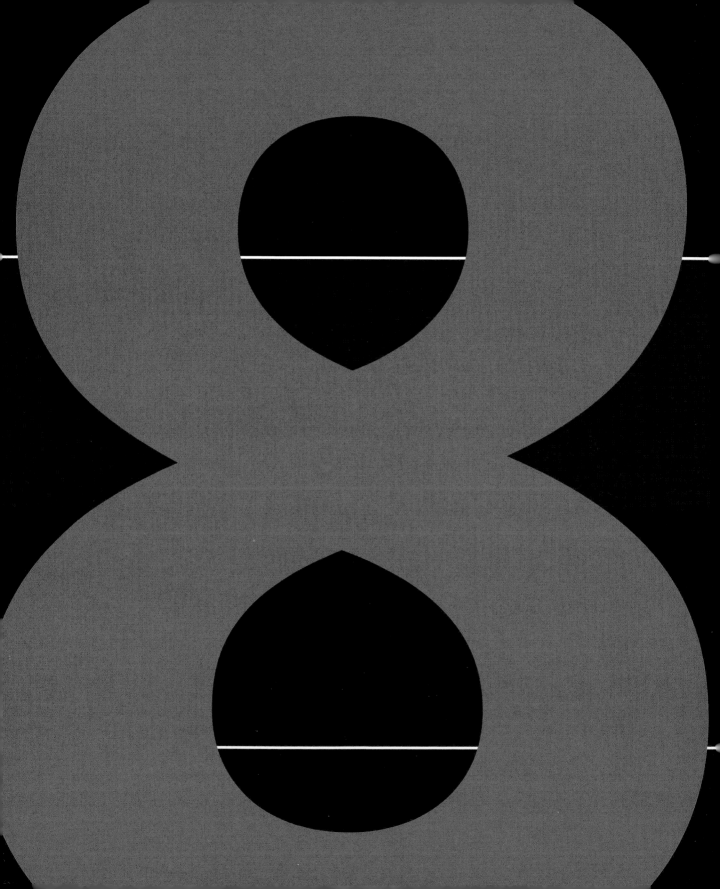

# REHABILITATION EXERCISES

**This chapter guides you step by step** through a wide range of exercises that your physiotherapist may recommend as part of your recovery programme. Most of them can also be used as part of a general fitness regimen to increase your overall flexibility, mobility, and strength, reduce your body fat and improve your posture, all of which can help to reduce your chances of back and neck trouble. Ensure you consult your doctor and physiotherapist before beginning any exercise programme, and follow the general safety guidelines in this book (»p.224).

# NECK AND BACK

**Improving the mobility and strength in your back and neck is one of the best ways to help prevent problems occurring in the first place, because this improves your posture and** **reduces muscular tension. Performed as part of a rehabilitation programme, exercises can help with recovery from acute conditions and may help if you have chronic pain.**

## NECK ROTATION

This simple movement helps to ease neck ache, maintain neck flexibility, and delay or prevent age-related stiffness.

You should be able to rotate your neck through 70–90 degrees on either side without straining.

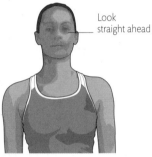

Look straight ahead

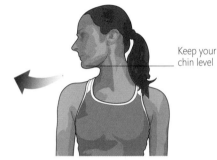

Keep your chin level

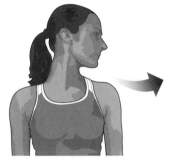

1 Look straight ahead, keeping your spine in a neutral position. Keep your upper body relaxed and your arms loose by your sides.

2 Move your head slowly to the side to look over your right shoulder. Turn it as far as is comfortable and hold for a few seconds.

3 Move your head back through the starting position, until you are looking over your left shoulder, without straining. Return to the start position.

## NECK SIDE FLEXION

This useful mobility exercise is ideal if you suffer from aching muscles in your upper back and neck. Poor posture or an awkward sleeping position can result

in imbalances in the muscles of your neck and shoulders. This may cause pain or even headaches, and is a common condition in desk workers.

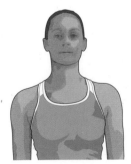

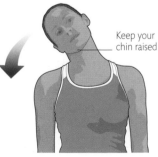

Keep your chin raised

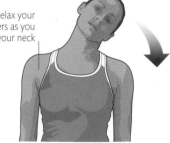

Relax your shoulders as you flex your neck

1 Stand upright, holding your body in a relaxed posture, with your shoulders loose and your eyes looking straight ahead.

2 Tilt your head so that your right ear moves towards your right shoulder as far as is comfortable. Hold for a few seconds.

3 Flex your neck in the opposite direction as far as you can go. Hold for a few seconds and return to the start position.

## 3 ▪ **NECK EXTENSION** AND FLEXION

This easy movement, which can be carried out either standing or seated, will help prevent a build-up of tension in your neck and upper-back muscles, and mobilizes the joints and nerves in your neck.

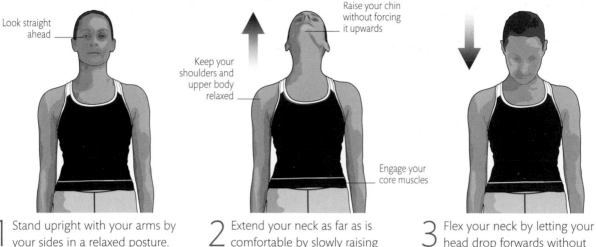

Look straight ahead

Raise your chin without forcing it upwards

Keep your shoulders and upper body relaxed

Engage your core muscles

1 Stand upright with your arms by your sides in a relaxed posture. Look straight ahead and keep your spine in a neutral position.

2 Extend your neck as far as is comfortable by slowly raising your chin so you are looking directly upwards. Hold for a few seconds.

3 Flex your neck by letting your head drop forwards without straining. Hold for a few seconds and return to the start position.

## 4 ▪ **SHOULDER** ROTATION

If you have a stiff neck, you will benefit from this exercise, which loosens the muscles in the head, neck, and shoulder areas. It also helps to increase mobility in your neck and shoulders.

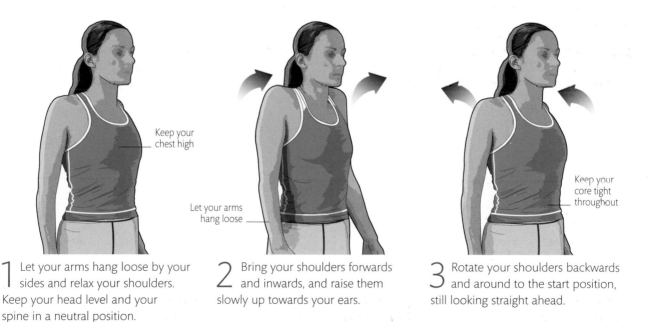

Keep your chest high

Let your arms hang loose

Keep your core tight throughout

1 Let your arms hang loose by your sides and relax your shoulders. Keep your head level and your spine in a neutral position.

2 Bring your shoulders forwards and inwards, and raise them slowly up towards your ears.

3 Rotate your shoulders backwards and around to the start position, still looking straight ahead.

## 5 NEURAL GLIDE

Also known as "flossing", this exercise is great for helping with neural tension in your spine and legs. When you are starting off, be gentle and don't push yourself too hard – you will develop the range of movement eventually.

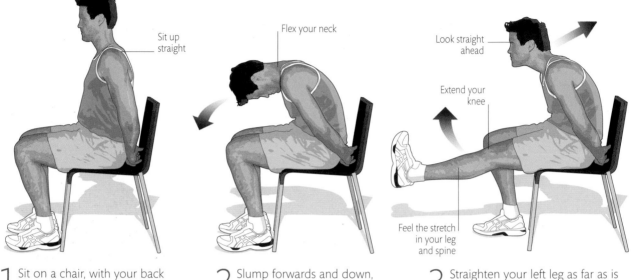

Sit up straight

Flex your neck

Look straight ahead

Extend your knee

Feel the stretch in your leg and spine

1 Sit on a chair, with your back straight, your spine lengthened, and your arms tucked behind your back, with your hands resting on the chair.

2 Slump forwards and down, so that your spine is rounded and your neck is flexed.

3 Straighten your left leg as far as is comfortable and, at the same time, lift your head. Hold the position for 5 seconds. Return to the position in Step 2 and repeat with your right leg.

## 6 UPPER-BACK STRETCH

This easy stretch specifically mobilizes the muscles in your upper back, making it a useful rehabilitation movement for those recovering from injuries to that area (»pp.34–35), as well as a good warm-up for any activity involving your shoulders.

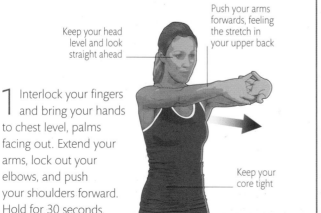

Keep your head level and look straight ahead

Push your arms forwards, feeling the stretch in your upper back

Keep your core tight

1 Interlock your fingers and bring your hands to chest level, palms facing out. Extend your arms, lock out your elbows, and push your shoulders forward. Hold for 30 seconds.

## 7 PEC STRETCH

This stretch targets the pectoral muscles of your upper chest, easing any tightness to help increase flexibility and movement in your shoulders and upper back.

Push your chest out

Feel the stretch here

Rest your free hand on your hip

1 Stand sideways close to a solid vertical support. Rest one arm behind the upright support, keeping your upper arm in line with your shoulder. Rock your body gently forwards until you can feel the stretch in your chest.

## 8 **MANUAL** ISOMETRICS

These neck-strengthening exercises use your hands for resistance and can be performed either standing or sitting down. These are essential exercises if you have suffered a neck injury (**》pp.26-33**) or are starting to strengthen your neck. As you progress, you can use bands or a pulley machine to provide the required resistance.

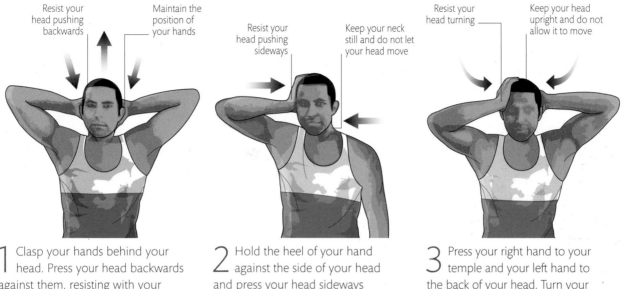

Resist your head pushing backwards

Maintain the position of your hands

Resist your head pushing sideways

Keep your neck still and do not let your head move

Resist your head turning

Keep your head upright and do not allow it to move

1 Clasp your hands behind your head. Press your head backwards against them, resisting with your hands and ensuring that your head doesn't move. Hold for 6 seconds, then relax.

2 Hold the heel of your hand against the side of your head and press your head sideways against it, while resisting with your arm. Hold for 6 seconds, relax, then switch sides.

3 Press your right hand to your temple and your left hand to the back of your head. Turn your head to the right, resisting with both arms. Hold for 6 seconds, relax, then switch hands and direction.

## 9 **TRUNK** ROTATION

Rotating the trunk of your body to each side will gently work the muscles around your spine. You should be able to feel the stretch in your upper back as you turn in either direction, but do not push the movement too hard.

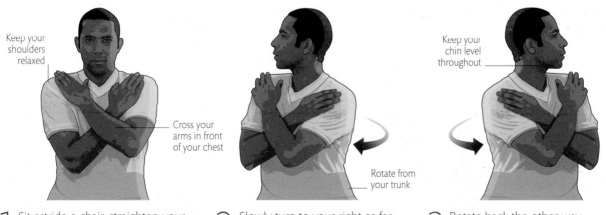

Keep your shoulders relaxed

Cross your arms in front of your chest

Rotate from your trunk

Keep your chin level throughout

1 Sit astride a chair, straighten your spine, cross your arms in front of your chest, and breathe in deeply.

2 Slowly turn to your right as far as you can, breathing out as you do so, and holding the position briefly.

3 Rotate back the other way, as far as you can. Hold briefly and return to the start position.

## 10 LYING TRUNK ROTATION

This exercise helps to improve the rotational mobility of your upper-back muscles and your thoracic spine, while stretching the muscles of your chest.

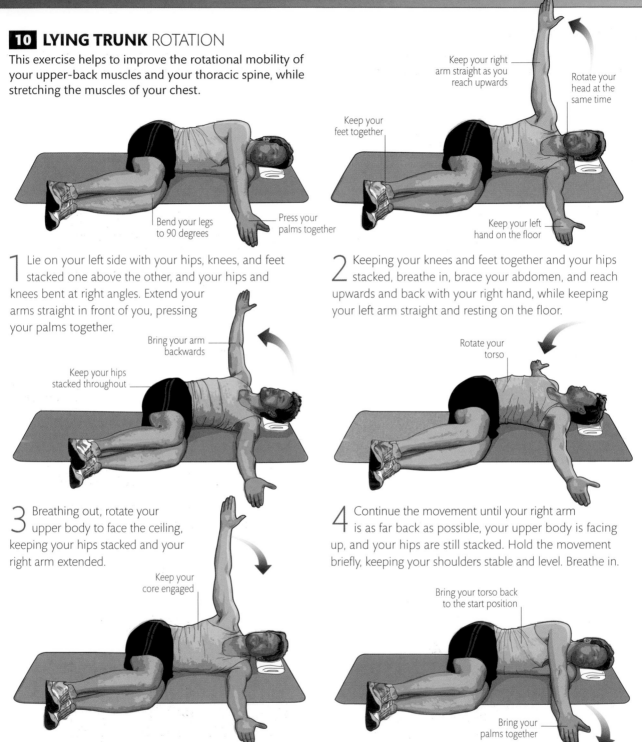

Bend your legs to 90 degrees

Press your palms together

**1** Lie on your left side with your hips, knees, and feet stacked one above the other, and your hips and knees bent at right angles. Extend your arms straight in front of you, pressing your palms together.

Keep your right arm straight as you reach upwards

Rotate your head at the same time

Keep your feet together

Keep your left hand on the floor

**2** Keeping your knees and feet together and your hips stacked, breathe in, brace your abdomen, and reach upwards and back with your right hand, while keeping your left arm straight and resting on the floor.

Bring your arm backwards

Keep your hips stacked throughout

**3** Breathing out, rotate your upper body to face the ceiling, keeping your hips stacked and your right arm extended.

Rotate your torso

**4** Continue the movement until your right arm is as far back as possible, your upper body is facing up, and your hips are still stacked. Hold the movement briefly, keeping your shoulders stable and level. Breathe in.

Keep your core engaged

**5** Breathing out, reach back towards the ceiling with your right arm, while rotating your torso back towards the start position slowly and under control.

Bring your torso back to the start position

Bring your palms together

**6** Continue the movement towards the start position and touch the palms of your hands together. Repeat the movement as required, then switch sides.

## 11 CAT STRETCH

This dynamic exercise works really well as a lower-back stretch that also works your upper back and shoulders.

It promotes spinal flexibility and increases abdominal strength. Move slowly, breathing deeply as you perform it.

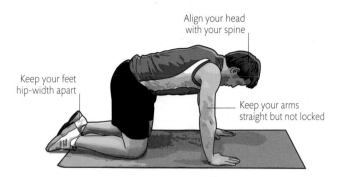

Align your head with your spine

Keep your feet hip-width apart

Keep your arms straight but not locked

1 Kneel on all fours, with your hands in line with your shoulders, your fingers pointing forward, and your knees below your hips. Keep your feet hip-width apart.

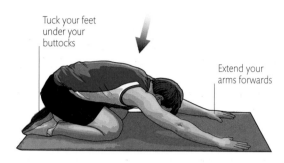

Tuck your feet under your buttocks

Extend your arms forwards

2 Sit back onto your heels and stretch your arms out in front of you, keeping your palms flat on the floor.

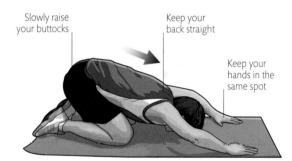

Slowly raise your buttocks

Keep your back straight

Keep your hands in the same spot

3 Slowly start to raise your buttocks, sliding your body forward while lowering your forehead towards the mat. Keep your hands in position and flat on the floor.

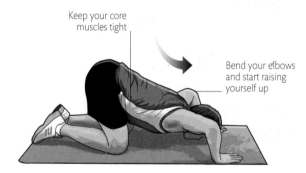

Keep your core muscles tight

Bend your elbows and start raising yourself up

4 As you continue to raise your buttocks, bend your elbows and start raising your upper body.

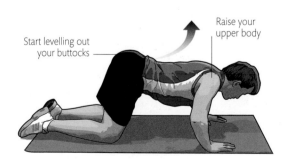

Start levelling out your buttocks

Raise your upper body

5 Continue lifting yourself up, gradually straightening your elbows and back. Keep your head level with your back.

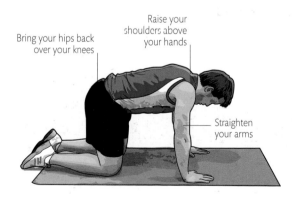

Raise your shoulders above your hands

Bring your hips back over your knees

Straighten your arms

6 Continue the movement until you return to the start position. Repeat the exercise for the required number of reps.

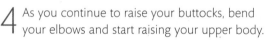

## 12 SHOULDER SHRUG

If you have a stiff and painful neck, this exercise is helpful for releasing tension in those muscles closest to your head.

Raise your shoulders as high as you can: you will really feel the stretch in your neck when you lower them.

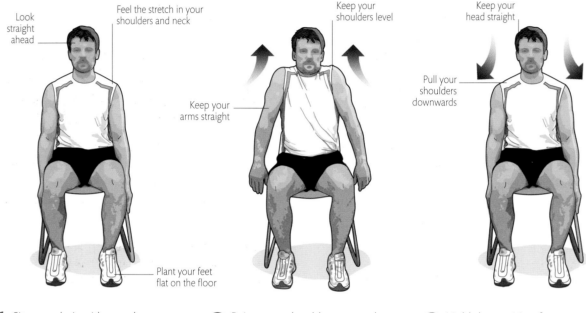

Look straight ahead

Feel the stretch in your shoulders and neck

Keep your arms straight

Plant your feet flat on the floor

Keep your shoulders level

Keep your head straight

Pull your shoulders downwards

1 Sit on a chair with your knees at right angles and your feet hip-width apart. Let your shoulders drop, and your arms hang by your sides.

2 Raise your shoulders upwards as high as you can, keeping your elbows as straight as possible.

3 Hold the position for around 5 seconds, then relax to return to the start position. Repeat for the required number of reps.

## 13 PRONE BREASTSTROKE

This exercise strengthens the muscles of your upper back and is recommended for scoliosis (**»pp.58**; **74**), hypermobility (**»pp.56**; **66**), and postural upper-back pain (**»pp.34–35**).

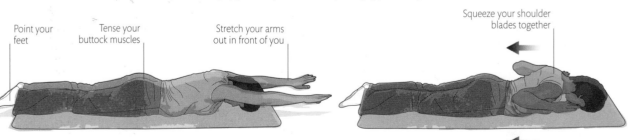

Point your feet

Tense your buttock muscles

Stretch your arms out in front of you

Squeeze your shoulder blades together

1 Lie face-down on a mat with your feet touching and your buttocks contracted. Hold your neck in a neutral position off the mat and stretch your arms forwards past your head, keeping them raised off the floor and parallel. Take a deep breath in.

2 With your arms still raised, bring them back close to your chest, slowly and under control, bending your elbows and keeping them at the same level as your hands, squeezing your shoulder blades together. Breathe out. Repeat for the required number of reps, then relax.

## 4 PRONE SHOULDER SQUEEZE

This exercise strengthens your upper back and the back of your shoulders, and helps to improve your posture. It is a useful movement for people with rounded back and shoulders, which is common in desk workers.

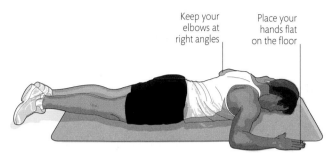

Keep your elbows at right angles

Place your hands flat on the floor

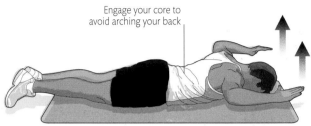

Engage your core to avoid arching your back

1 Lie face-down with your forehead resting on a mat and your elbows at right angles, palms facing down and on the floor. Point your feet back, with your toes on the floor.

2 Raise your arms off the floor to head height and squeeze your shoulder blades together. Return to the start position and repeat for the required number of reps.

## 5 SEATED SHOULDER SQUEEZE

This exercise mobilizes the muscles and nerves of your upper back and shoulders, and is ideal for people in sedentary or desk-based jobs. It can also help prevent repetitive strain injury (RSI), and can ease cases of pain in your hands and forearms. Aim to perform 10 reps 5 or 6 times per day.

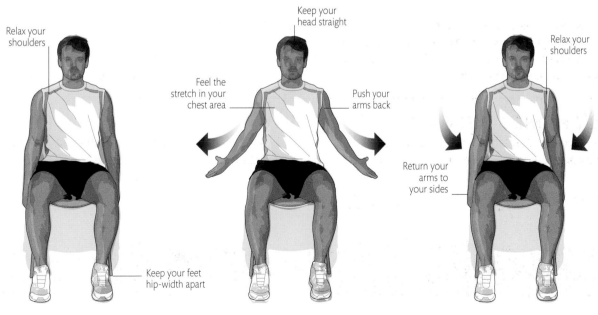

Relax your shoulders

Keep your head straight

Feel the stretch in your chest area

Push your arms back

Relax your shoulders

Return your arms to your sides

Keep your feet hip-width apart

1 Sit on a backless seat with your back straight, your arms hanging loosely by your sides, and your feet hip-width apart and flat on the floor.

2 With your palms facing out, push your arms backwards and away from your body as far as you can go without straining.

3 Hold for a few seconds then return to the start position, slowly and under control. Repeat for the required number of reps.

## 16 LEVATOR SCAPULAE STRETCH

This simple stretch involves using the weight of your head to stretch your neck muscles. It offers instant relief from tense neck and shoulder muscles and can be a useful exercise for office workers.

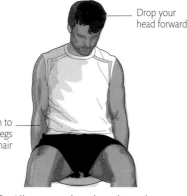

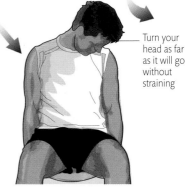

Look straight ahead

Relax your shoulders

Hold on to the back legs of the chair

Drop your head forward

Turn your head as far as it will go without straining

1 Sit unsupported on a chair with your shoulders aligned and your arms straight. Grip the underside or the back legs of the chair with your hands.

2 Allow your head to drop down as far as it can without bending your upper back, then slowly turn your head towards your left shoulder.

3 Hold the position for around 5 seconds, until you feel the stretch in the muscles to the right of your neck. Return to the start position and swap sides.

## 17 DOORWAY CHEST STRETCH

Similar to the corner chest stretch (》p.176), this exercise mobilizes the muscles and nerves in your arms and improves mobility in your shoulder blades. Perform this movement slowly and fluidly.

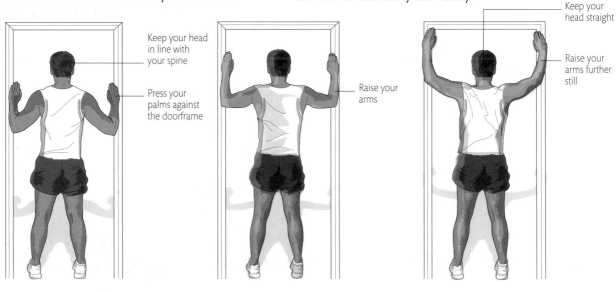

Keep your head in line with your spine

Press your palms against the doorframe

Raise your arms

Keep your head straight

Raise your arms further still

1 Stand in a doorway, with your feet hip-width apart, and your hands at shoulder height and resting flat against the doorframe.

2 Slowly and with control, slide your hands up the doorframe, until your elbows are bent at right angles.

3 Continue the movement until your elbows are at shoulder height. Reverse the movement to return to the start position.

## 18 SUPINE NECK FLEXION

This is a mobilizing exercise, which activates the deep muscles of your neck along with the upper and lower joints of your neck. It is often used in the rehabilitation of whiplash injuries (»pp.29; 72) and tension headaches.

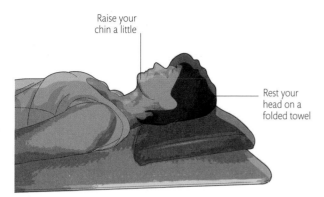

Raise your chin a little

Rest your head on a folded towel

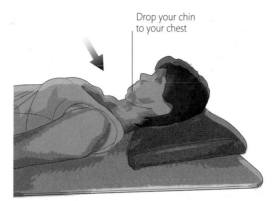

Drop your chin to your chest

1 Lie on your back with your head supported by a folded towel, your pelvis and upper back relaxed, and your arms resting either side of your body. Lift your chin a little so that your face points slightly upwards.

2 Slowly slide the back of your head up the towel until the plane of your face tilts forwards as far as it will go and your chin drops all the way towards your throat. Hold for a few seconds then return to the start position.

## 19 NECK EXTENSION WITH OVERPRESSURE

This is a mobilizing exercise for your neck that is used in the rehabilitation of most neck conditions (»pp.26-33). You should perform it in one fluid movement for no more than 10 reps 5 or 6 times per day. If you experience pain or pins and needles in your arm while doing the exercise, you should stop immediately and consult your therapist.

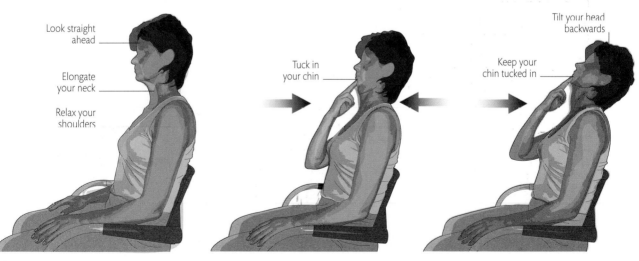

Look straight ahead

Elongate your neck

Relax your shoulders

Tuck in your chin

Tilt your head backwards

Keep your chin tucked in

1 Sit in a chair and rest your arms on your thighs. Keeping your head straight, drop your shoulders and elongate your neck.

2 Applying gentle pressure with your hand, tuck your chin in. Your neck and head will shift backwards automatically.

3 Keeping your chin tucked in, extend your neck by bending it backwards in one fluid movement. Hold this position for no more than 2 seconds, then return to the start position.

## 20 UPPER-BACK EXTENSION

This stretching movement works the muscles of your upper back and shoulders. It helps to support your spine and improve your posture, and is a good exercise for desk workers.

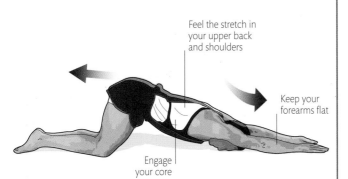

Feel the stretch in your upper back and shoulders

Keep your forearms flat

Engage your core

1 Kneel on an exercise mat and lower your body forwards slowly and carefully, extending your arms forwards so that your forehead touches the mat. Press down against the floor with your hands and forearms, and ease your buttocks backwards as far as you can. Pause at the edge of the movement, then relax to return to the start position.

## 21 SWISS BALL BACK STRETCH

This exercise stretches the joints of your upper and lower back, and helps to improve the alignment of your spinal joints.

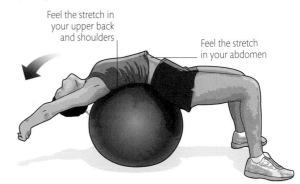

Feel the stretch in your upper back and shoulders

Feel the stretch in your abdomen

1 With your feet shoulder-width apart and flat on the floor, squat down onto a Swiss ball, and lean back over it so that both your shoulders and buttocks are resting on it. Stretch both arms over your head and allow your arms to fall as far as they will go. Hold the position for a few seconds, breathing in and out, then return to the start position.

## 22 SEATED BACK EXTENSION

This stretch helps to loosen tight muscles in your upper back, while working those that support your spine, improving your posture and helping to ease the muscle tension that can result from working at a desk or long periods of sitting. The exercise can be performed in most chairs, making it a versatile and easy movement, and is especially recommended to those in sedentary jobs, or who suffer from a stiff neck and upper back.

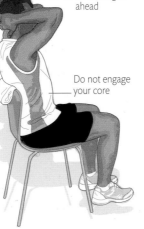

Look straight ahead

Rest your hands behind your head

Press your back against the chair

Do not engage your core

1 Sit on a chair with your knees at right angles and your feet flat on the floor. Bring your arms up and clasp your hands behind your head with your elbows facing forwards. Relax your body and let your shoulders drop.

Keep your elbows in line

Push your chest out

2 Lean back as far as you can within a painless range of movement. Breathe in and out slowly and enjoy the stretch. Hold for a few seconds and return to the start position.

NECK AND BACK

## 23 **UPPER-BACK** BAND ROW

This exercise works the muscles of your shoulders and upper back, and is recommended to those who suffer from postural strain or scoliosis (»p.58; 74). Loop the resistance band safely through a door handle or similar.

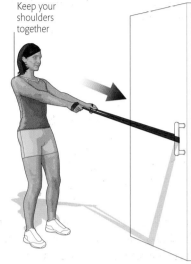

Keep your palms down

Plant your feet firmly on the floor

Engage your core

Keep your knees slightly bent

Keep your shoulders together

1 Hold the ends of the band with your arms extended. Squeeze your shoulder blades down and together, and inhale.

2 Exhale as you pull the band to shoulder height, bending your elbows out to the sides.

3 Inhale as you release the band and return to the start position. Repeat several times.

## 24 **LAT BAND** ROW

This exercise works the large muscles of your upper back and the back of your shoulders. It is particularly effective for sufferers of postural pain (»p.57) or scoliosis (»pp.58; 74). Keep your feet in the same spot throughout.

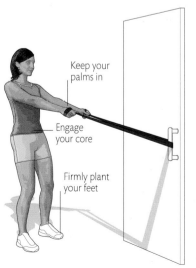
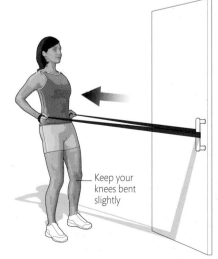
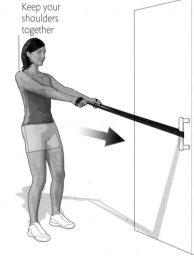

Keep your palms in

Engage your core

Firmly plant your feet

Keep your knees bent slightly

Keep your shoulders together

1 Hold the ends of the band with your arms extended. Squeeze your shoulder blades down and together, and inhale.

2 Exhale as you pull the band into the sides of your waist. Keep your elbows parallel.

3 Inhale as you release the band and return to the start position.

## 25 PASSIVE NECK RETRACTION

This is a mobilizing exercise for your neck and is especially helpful if you have a facet joint problem (»pp.31; 42; 68), disc problem (»pp.27; 33), or nerve impingement in your neck. Start gently and perform no more than 10 reps 5 or 6 times a day. You may feel some discomfort, but you should stop immediately if the exercise becomes painful.

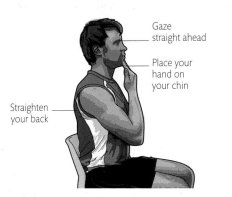

Gaze straight ahead

Place your hand on your chin

Straighten your back

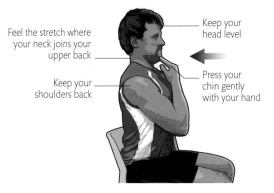

Feel the stretch where your neck joins your upper back

Keep your shoulders back

Keep your head level

Press your chin gently with your hand

1 Sit up straight with your shoulders relaxed. Look straight ahead and place your hand on your chin. Try to elongate your neck, increasing the distance between your shoulders and ears.

2 Keeping your shoulders relaxed, push your chin in with your hand, applying gentle pressure. Hold for 3 seconds, then ease the pressure and return to the start position for 3 seconds. Repeat as required.

## 26 ACTIVE NECK RETRACTION

Following on from the passive neck retraction exercises (»above), activating the deep muscles in your neck helps to increase the strength of the muscles responsible for good head and neck posture (»pp.112–15).

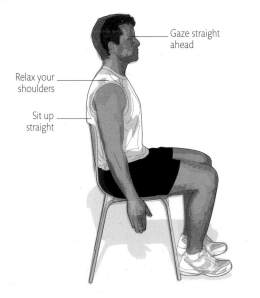

Gaze straight ahead

Relax your shoulders

Sit up straight

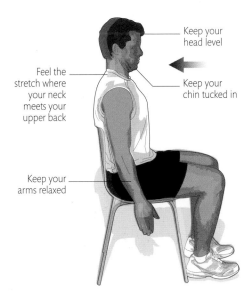

Feel the stretch where your neck meets your upper back

Keep your arms relaxed

Keep your head level

Keep your chin tucked in

1 Sit on a chair with your back straight and your shoulders and upper back relaxed. Look straight ahead, and allow your arms to rest at your sides with your palms towards you.

2 Tuck in your chin and elongate your neck, so that the top of your head moves upwards. Hold for 5 seconds and then relax to the start position. Repeat as required.

## 27 **SUPINE BACK** ROTATION

This more gentle version of the back rotation (»p.203) improves general mobility and is useful for relaxing the muscles of your back and around your pelvis.

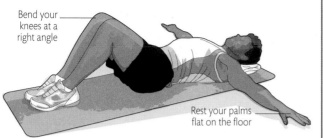

Bend your knees at a right angle

Rest your palms flat on the floor

1 Placing a folded towel under your head, if required, lie on your back with your knees together and your legs bent, your feet flat on the floor, and your arms extended with your palms facing downwards.

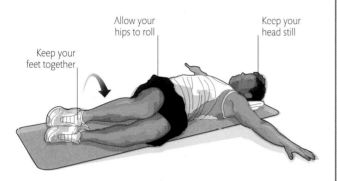

Keep your feet together

Allow your hips to roll

Keep your head still

2 Keeping your knees together, slowly roll them to your left and hold for a few seconds. Keep your upper body flat against the floor, bracing yourself with your arms.

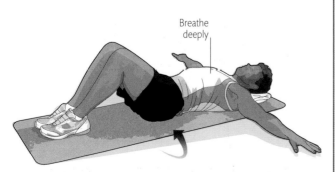

Breathe deeply

3 Slowly return to the start position. Repeat for the required number of reps before switching sides.

## 28 **TOWEL** ROCK

This can help a stiff or aching neck. If one side of your neck is tight, begin by rocking away from that side, then if it's not too painful, back towards the stiff side. Moving your head both ways can help to restore a full range of motion.

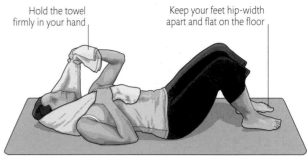

Hold the towel firmly in your hand

Keep your feet hip-width apart and flat on the floor

1 Fold a towel in three lengthways and place it behind your head. Lie on a mat with your knees bent and your lower back pressed into the mat. If the left side of your neck is stiff, hold the left end of the towel above your head with your left hand, and the right end by your chest with your right hand.

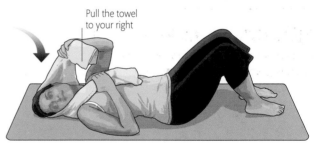

Pull the towel to your right

2 Grasping the right end firmly by your chest with your right hand, pull the left end with your left hand so that your head rocks gently to the right. Perform about 10 small rocking motions, and keep your neck muscles relaxed.

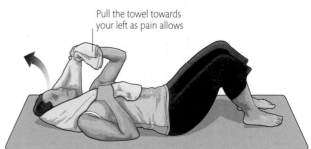

Pull the towel towards your left as pain allows

3 Return to the start position, and repeat the movements in the opposite direction if it is comfortable to do so, but don't force the movement if you feel any pain.

## 29 TOWEL NECK FLEXION

This self-mobilizing technique is ideal if you suffer from a stiff, painful neck, as it improves neck flexion. Let your arms do the work – your neck muscles should be fully relaxed, and the movements controlled and slow.

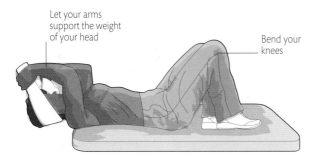

Let your arms support the weight of your head

Bend your knees

1 Lie on your back with your shoulders off the edge of a thick exercise mat or mattress. Fold a towel lengthways and place it behind your head, gripping either end to support your head and neck, which should be roughly level with your upper back. Inhale deeply.

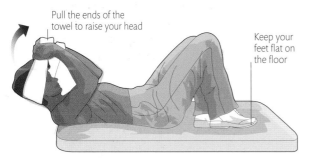

Pull the ends of the towel to raise your head

Keep your feet flat on the floor

2 Gently pull the towel forwards and up. Carry the weight of your head with your arms so that your neck flexes without you using your neck muscles. Hold for 3–5 seconds and breathe out through your mouth.

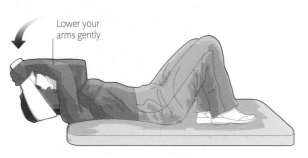

Lower your arms gently

3 Still gripping the towel, lower your arms to return to the start position slowly and under control.

## 30 TOWEL NECK EXTENSION

This neck exercise improves neck extension and can be done alongside the towel neck flexion exercise (»left). Remember to relax the muscles in your neck and to keep the movements slow and controlled.

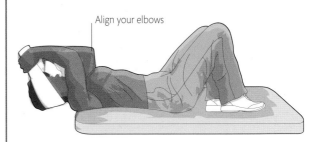

Align your elbows

1 Lie on your back with your shoulders off the edge of a thick exercise mat or mattress. Fold a towel lengthways and place it behind your head. Tightly hold the ends of the towel to support your head and neck, which should be level with your upper back. Breathe in deeply.

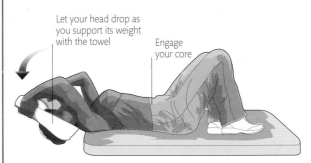

Let your head drop as you support its weight with the towel

Engage your core

2 Gripping the towel, move your arms back and down, allowing your head to drop gently. Take the weight of your head in your arms, rather than using your neck muscles. Hold for 3–5 seconds and exhale through your mouth.

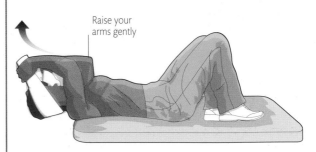

Raise your arms gently

3 Maintaining a firm grip on the towel, raise your arms slowly and under control to return to the start position.

## 31 OVAL SHOULDER STRETCH

This versatile exercise mobilizes your shoulders and upper back, which will improve the function of your shoulder girdle, which in turn will increase the range of motion in your upper back and prevent injuries to this area. To do this exercise correctly, perform the stretch in a slow, controlled manner, and bend from your hips, not at your waist. You may also want to bend your knees slightly to take the strain from your lower back.

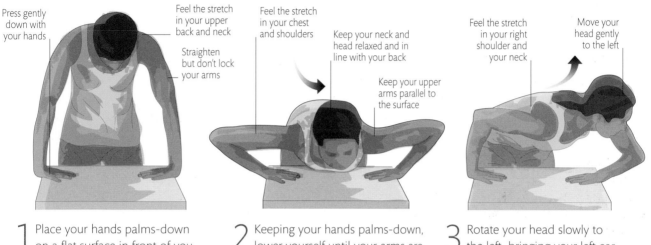

Press gently down with your hands

Feel the stretch in your upper back and neck

Straighten but don't lock your arms

Feel the stretch in your chest and shoulders

Keep your neck and head relaxed and in line with your back

Keep your upper arms parallel to the surface

Feel the stretch in your right shoulder and your neck

Move your head gently to the left

1 Place your hands palms-down on a flat surface in front of you with your fingers slightly splayed and pointing inwards. Round your upper back and tilt your head downwards.

2 Keeping your hands palms-down, lower yourself until your arms are parallel to the surface and your upper body is 5cm (2in) above it. Slide your body left, keeping your back straight.

3 Rotate your head slowly to the left, bringing your left ear around towards your shoulder, and raise your upper body up and around towards the start position.

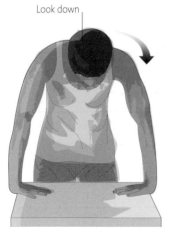

Look down

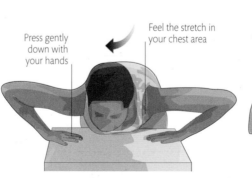

Press gently down with your hands

Feel the stretch in your chest area

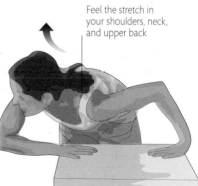

Feel the stretch in your shoulders, neck, and upper back

4 Once back in the start position, repeat the movement, but this time in the opposite direction, aiming for a slow and continuous fluid motion.

5 Lower yourself down again until your arms are parallel to the surface and your upper body is 5cm (2in) away from the surface. Slide your body right, keeping your back straight and your upper arms parallel to the surface.

6 Rotate your head slowly to the right and up, bringing your right ear around towards your shoulder, while lifting your upper body back to the start position. Repeat for the required number of reps in either direction, then relax.

## 32 ROLL-DOWN STRETCH

This exercise is an excellent stretch for your neck, but it is important to keep your head back and your chin tucked in as you roll your head down. This ensures that you stretch your entire neck, not just the lower part of it, and your upper back. It is recommended if you suffer from postural pain (»p.57) and tension headaches.

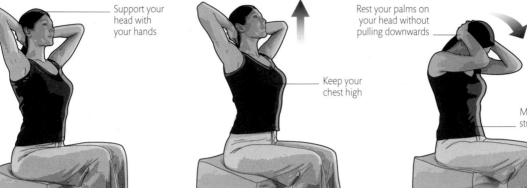

Support your head with your hands

Keep your chest high

Rest your palms on your head without pulling downwards

Maintain a strong core

1 Sit slightly forwards on a box or a chair with your feet flat on the floor. Clasp your hands behind your head and press your head back into them.

2 Gently lift your gaze and look diagonally upwards. Pull your elbows up and out as you stretch up, lifting your chest.

3 Tuck your chin into your neck and roll your head downwards to look at your chest. Hold briefly, then roll back up to the start position.

## 33 CORNER CHEST STRETCH

This exercise is ideal for improving your posture, especially if the muscles of your chest and shoulders are feeling tight. To perform the stretch correctly and safely, make sure your feet are well grounded so that you can push yourself away from the wall.

### VARIATION

You can vary this exercise by raising or lowering the position of your arms. By doing this you alter the stretch to focus on different parts of your chest.

Keep your back straight

Keep your palms flat against the wall

Support your body weight with your arms

Engage your core

Keep your feet flat

1 Stand facing a corner, hands raised at your sides and facing up, elbows bent. Place your palms on the walls at shoulder height.

2 Lean forwards and feel the stretch in your chest and upper back between your shoulder blades. Hold this position for 15 seconds, then relax. Repeat 3 times.

## 34 SEATED TWIST STRETCH

This is a good exercise for the muscles around your spine. It is important to push with one arm to leverage the twist and stretch your upper back without stretching your lower back. This exercise improves the rotational mobility of your upper back, but you should go only as far as is comfortable.

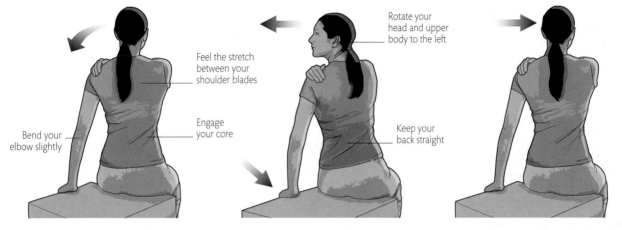

Feel the stretch between your shoulder blades

Rotate your head and upper body to the left

Bend your elbow slightly

Engage your core

Keep your back straight

1 Sit on the edge of a box or chair, your feet flat on the floor. Hold the edge of the box with your left hand, and place your right hand on your left shoulder.

2 Twist to the left, pulling your left shoulder back and pushing against the edge of the box with your left hand. Pause at the edge of the movement.

3 Relax to return to the start position. Repeat for the required number of reps, then swap sides.

## 35 SEATED WAIST STRETCH

This is a great stretch for the muscles of your upper back. To get the full benefit of the movement, elongate both sides of your torso as you reach up. Look straight ahead and try to hold yourself back to avoid leaning forwards. Holding onto the side of the seat will prevent movement in your lower back, allowing your upper body to feel the full effect of the stretch.

1 Sit slightly forwards on a box or chair, with your feet flat on the floor. Reach up with your left hand, palm facing inwards, holding onto the edge of the box with your right hand.

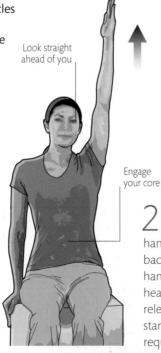

Look straight ahead of you

Engage your core

Keep your elbow slightly bent

Feel the stretch in your left arm and left side

Keep your shoulders aligned

2 Pressing down on the seat with your right hand, and with a straight back, stretch your left hand up and over your head. Hold briefly, then release to return to the start position. Repeat as required, then switch arms.

# BACK AND BUTTOCKS

**Weakness or tension in the muscles of your thighs, buttocks, and hips can cause lower-back pain, so it is important to keep them strong and mobile. Likewise, strengthening the muscles of your core improves your posture, reducing your chance of back problems. Such exercises are useful in both maintenance and the process of recovery.**

## 36 SEATED HIP TILT

This exercise works your whole spine, from neck to pelvis, gently mobilizing your joints, muscles, and nerves. It is a good exercise for easing postural pain (»p.57).

1 Sit towards the front of your seat so that your thighs slope downwards a little. Rest your hands on the seat on either side of your body, with your head level. Keep your feet slightly apart and flat on the floor.

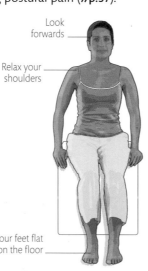

Look forwards

Relax your shoulders

Keep your feet flat on the floor

2 Tilt your head to the right, while leaning your body to the left, taking the weight off your right hip bone. Hold briefly, then return to the start position. Repeat with your right side if required, this time leaning to the right and tilting your head to the left.

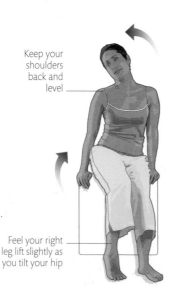

Keep your shoulders back and level

Feel your right leg lift slightly as you tilt your hip

## 37 SEATED HIP WALK

As with the seated hip tilt (»left), this exercise works your entire spine in multiple directions and is recommended for alleviating postural pain (»p.57).

1 Sit towards the front of the seat with your thighs sloping slightly downwards. Make sure you are sitting up straight with your feet flat on the floor. Line up your knees and look straight ahead.

Look straight ahead

Keep your back straight

Keep your feet slightly apart

2 Press your right hip back into the seat and turn your head to the left. Hold briefly then return to the start position. Switch sides, and repeat the movement, pressing your left hip back and turning your head to the right.

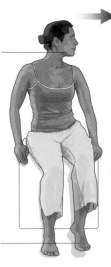

Turn your head back and keep your chin level

Feel your left foot rise as you tilt your hip

## 38 SQUAT

This is a key mobilizing movement for your lower body and core, and can help to improve flexibility and strength in your hips, reducing the chances of back problems occurring. Good form is crucial: go as low as possible to improve your range of motion and do not "bounce" at the bottom.

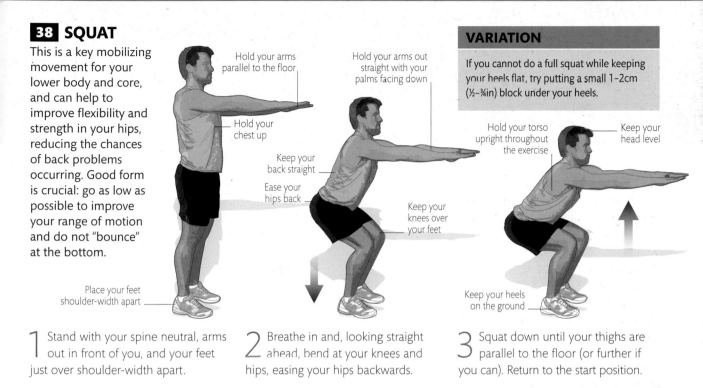

Hold your arms parallel to the floor

Hold your chest up

Place your feet shoulder-width apart

Hold your arms out straight with your palms facing down

Keep your back straight

Ease your hips back

Keep your knees over your feet

**VARIATION**

If you cannot do a full squat while keeping your heels flat, try putting a small 1–2cm (½–¾in) block under your heels.

Hold your torso upright throughout the exercise

Keep your head level

Keep your heels on the ground

1 Stand with your spine neutral, arms out in front of you, and your feet just over shoulder-width apart.

2 Breathe in and, looking straight ahead, bend at your knees and hips, easing your hips backwards.

3 Squat down until your thighs are parallel to the floor (or further if you can). Return to the start position.

## 39 WALKING LUNGE

This is an excellent way to strengthen your hips and thighs, reducing the chances of straining your back. The walking lunge tests both your balance and coordination. You can also perform it from a fixed position.

1 Stand with your feet hip-width apart and your shoulders, hips, and feet in line.

2 Take a long step forwards with your right leg. Drop down and bend at your knees.

3 Push off with your left leg back to an upright position, keeping your core engaged and your head up.

4 Step forwards with your left leg and drop down again. Return to the start position, repeat as required, then switch legs.

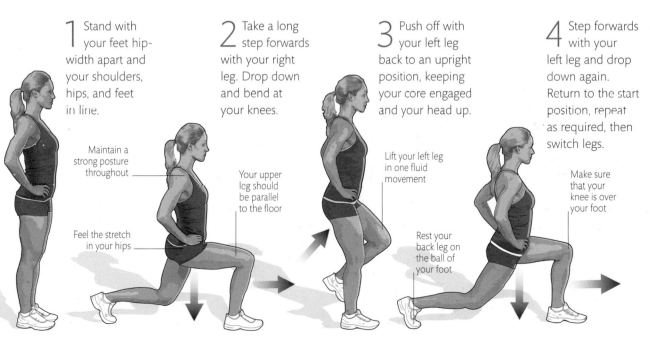

Maintain a strong posture throughout

Feel the stretch in your hips

Your upper leg should be parallel to the floor

Lift your left leg in one fluid movement

Rest your back leg on the ball of your foot

Make sure that your knee is over your foot

## 40 PRESS-UP

This simple exercise is a useful form of self-traction for your upper and lower back that helps to elongate your spine. It can help with a range of back conditions and is a good general maintenance stretch for desk workers.

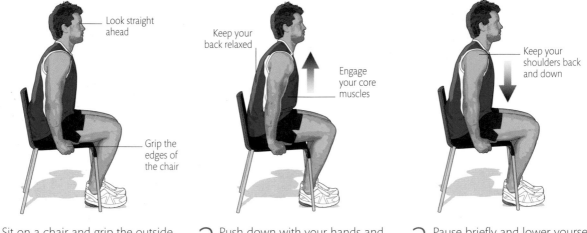

1 Sit on a chair and grip the outside edges of the seat with your hands, placing them roughly in line with your shoulders.

2 Push down with your hands and relax your back, breathing in and out slowly, and allowing your pelvis to drop so that your back elongates.

3 Pause briefly and lower yourself to the start position, repeating the movement as required, slowly and gently.

## 41 HIP-HITCHER

This exercise works the muscles around your hip joint. It is a very useful movement if you are suffering from facet joint dysfunction (»p.68), and is also good for improving hip and sacroiliac joint mobility (»p.39; 69).

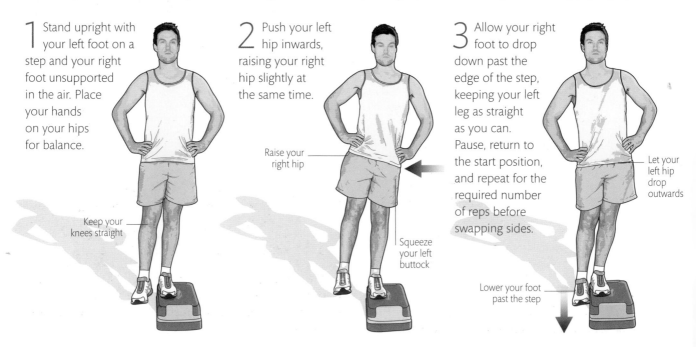

1 Stand upright with your left foot on a step and your right foot unsupported in the air. Place your hands on your hips for balance.

2 Push your left hip inwards, raising your right hip slightly at the same time.

3 Allow your right foot to drop down past the edge of the step, keeping your left leg as straight as you can. Pause, return to the start position, and repeat for the required number of reps before swapping sides.

## 42 WALL SIT PRESS

This exercise is great for releasing tension in your thoracic spine, and opening up your shoulders and the muscles of your upper body.

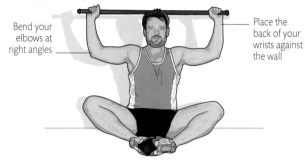

Bend your elbows at right angles

Place the back of your wrists against the wall

1 Sit with your hips, back, shoulders, elbows, wrists, and head against a wall, and the soles of your feet together. Hold a bar above your head with your elbows at 90 degrees.

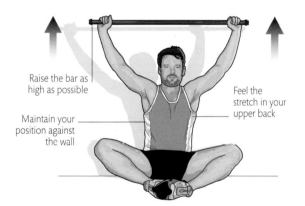

Raise the bar as high as possible

Maintain your position against the wall

Feel the stretch in your upper back

2 Slowly push the bar above your head, maintaining full contact with the wall throughout the movement.

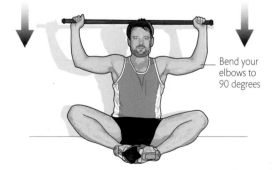

Bend your elbows to 90 degrees

3 Once you have raised the bar as far as you can, lower it back to the start position. Repeat as required.

## 43 CLAM

This straightforward exercise works your hip flexors and the muscles of your buttocks, while also improving overall stability in your pelvis and core.

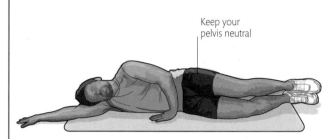

Keep your pelvis neutral

1 Lie on your right side, bending about 45 degrees at your hips and knees. Extend your right arm so that it is in line with your body, and rest your head on it. Bend your left arm at the elbow and place your left hand on the floor in front of you.

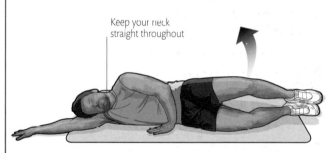

Keep your neck straight throughout

2 Keeping your neck straight, your hips and shoulders in line, and your feet touching, engage your core and begin lifting the knee of your left leg, rotating it at your hip.

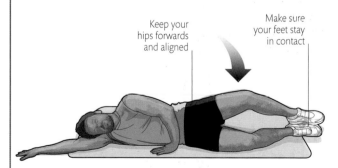

Keep your hips forwards and aligned

Make sure your feet stay in contact

3 Lift your left knee as far as it will go, while keeping your hips aligned. Slowly lower your knee back to the start position, and repeat for the required number of reps before swapping sides.

## 44 SINGLE ARM AND LEG RAISE

This exercise engages the muscles of your core, using them to stabilize your pelvis against the motion of your arms and legs. Your core acts as a natural girdle, flattening your abdomen and supporting your lower back.

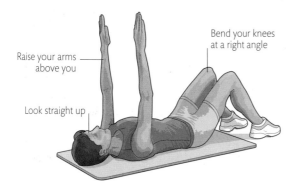

Raise your arms above you

Look straight up

Bend your knees at a right angle

1 Lie on your back with your knees bent, your feet flat on the ground, and your arms extended above you, palms facing forwards. Keep your back straight and pelvis neutral.

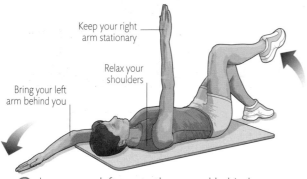

Keep your right arm stationary

Relax your shoulders

Bring your left arm behind you

2 Lower your left arm to the ground behind you as you lift your right knee above your hip, contracting your abdominals as you do so.

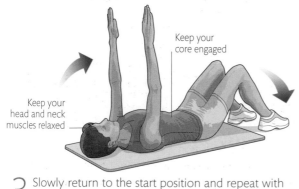

Keep your core engaged

Keep your head and neck muscles relaxed

3 Slowly return to the start position and repeat with your right arm and left leg.

## 45 DEAD BUG

This exercise works your lower back, pelvis, trunk, and shoulders. A moderate- to high-level Pilates exercise, you should only attempt it after mastering more basic Pilates exercises, such as the single arm and leg raise (»left). If you are recovering from a back injury, ensure that you keep your lower back pressed against the floor.

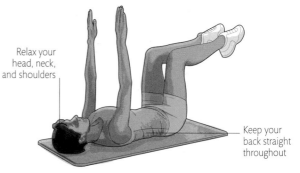

Relax your head, neck, and shoulders

Keep your back straight throughout

1 Lie on your back on a mat and contract your abdominals. Bend your hips and knees at 90 degrees, and position your feet roughly hip-width apart in the air. Point your arms up directly over your shoulders, palms facing forwards.

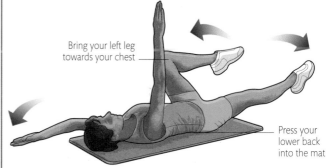

Bring your left leg towards your chest

Press your lower back into the mat

2 Lower your left arm behind you and extend your right leg, bringing it as close to the floor as possible without arching your back. Draw your left knee to your chest.

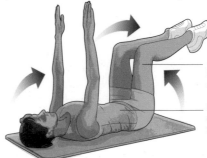

Make sure your knees and hips are at right angles

Keep your core engaged throughout

3 Briefly hold the position, ensuring you do not arch your back, then return to the start position and switch sides.

## 46 **SACRAL** CIRCLE

This exercise relaxes the muscles surrounding your sacroiliac joints, and provides a form of self-massage that helps to mobilize them. It can be used to help with sacroiliac strain (»p.69).

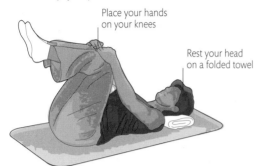

Place your hands on your knees

Rest your head on a folded towel

1 Lie on a mat, placing a folded towel under your head for support. Gently exhale as you slowly bring your knees back towards your chest and place your hands on them.

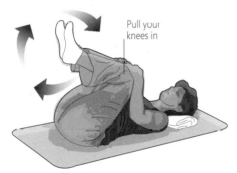

Pull your knees in

2 Circle your knees from right to left 5 times, using your hands to guide the movement. Breathe normally.

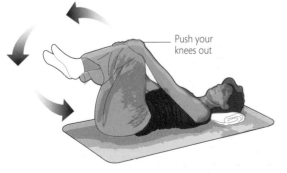

Push your knees out

3 Repeat the exercise 5 times in the opposite direction, from left to right, drawing your arms in and out as you perform the movement.

## 47 **ONE-LEG** CIRCLE

This exercise can be used as a mobilizing technique for your sciatic nerve, and can help with sciatica (»p.38). The movement should be fluid and gentle.

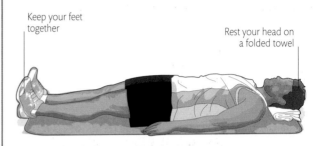

Keep your feet together

Rest your head on a folded towel

1 Lie on your back with a folded towel under your head for support. Rest your arms either side of your body.

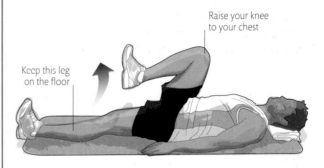

Raise your knee to your chest

Keep this leg on the floor

2 Bring your right knee to your chest, extending your foot upwards towards your body as you do so.

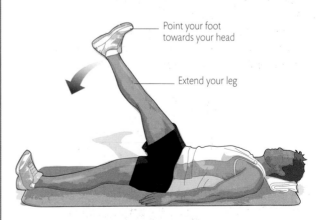

Point your foot towards your head

Extend your leg

3 Without pausing, stretch your right leg up towards the ceiling and then drop it towards the mat with control, in a circular motion. Repeat the circle for the required number of reps, then return to the start position and swap legs.

## 48 ALLIGATOR

This exercise mobilizes your whole spine with a side-to-side movement, and is a great exercise to increase your spinal flexibility. It should be performed in one fluid motion from one side to the other.

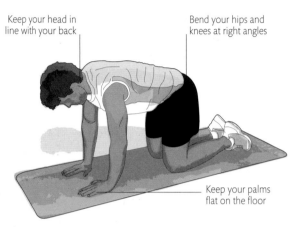

Keep your head in line with your back

Bend your hips and knees at right angles

Keep your palms flat on the floor

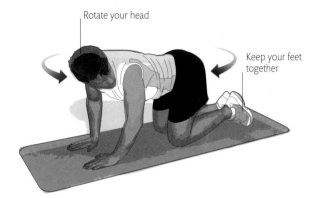

Rotate your head

Keep your feet together

1 Start on all fours with your back flat and your neck in a relaxed position. Position your arms directly under your shoulders, and bend your hips and knees at right angles. Keep your feet together. Take a deep breath in.

2 Breathing out, turn your head and pelvis to the left and towards each other, feeling the stretch along the right side of your body. Pause, then repeat the movement to your right. Complete the desired number of repetitions on either side, then relax to the start position.

## 49 LYING WAIST TWIST

This exercise increases the mobility of the joints and muscles in your lower and upper back. Perform the exercise 3 times on each side, holding the position for 15 seconds.

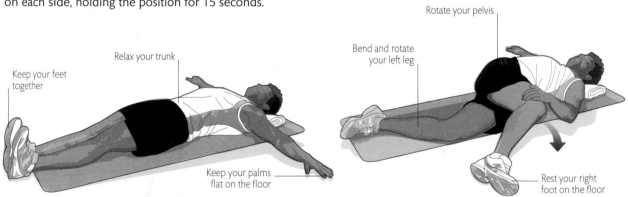

Keep your feet together

Relax your trunk

Keep your palms flat on the floor

Rotate your pelvis

Bend and rotate your left leg

Rest your right foot on the floor

1 Placing a folded towel under your head for extra support, lie on your back, with your body relaxed and your arms loose but extended at a 90-degree angle from your upper body. Keep your legs and feet together.

2 Keeping your upper body flat against the mat, bend your right leg at the knee and bring it across your body, using your left hand to increase the stretch, and allowing your left leg to turn and bend in the same direction. Hold the move, then return to the start position and switch sides.

## 50 GLUTEAL/PIRIFORMIS FOAM ROLLER

This exercise loosens up the gluteals at the outside of your buttocks and the piriformis towards the middle of them.

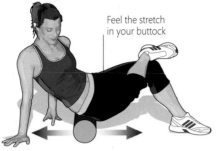

Feel the stretch in your buttock

1 Sit on the roller with your right buttock and cross your right leg over your left leg. Rolling backwards and forwards, work on the outside of your buttock before shifting your weight to the middle of your buttock. Repeat for at least 30 seconds before switching sides.

## 51 LAT FOAM ROLLER

This exercise helps to loosen up the large muscles of your middle and upper back, reducing tightness.

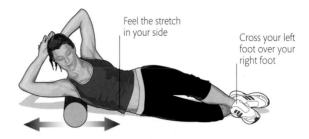

Feel the stretch in your side

Cross your left foot over your right foot

1 Lie on your right side over the roller, which should be placed under your armpit, and place your hands behind your head for stability. Use your back muscles to roll down from your armpit to the base of your shoulder blade. Roll back up and repeat for at least 30 seconds, then switch sides.

## 52 ITB FOAM ROLLER

This exercise loosens your iliotibial band (ITB), the band of muscular tissue on the outside of your upper leg, and can help to prevent piriformis syndrome (»pp.49; 76).

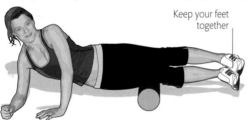

Keep your feet together

1 Lie on your right side with the foam roller beneath your outer thigh, just above your knee. Propping yourself up on your right forearm, bend your left arm slightly and place your left hand, palm-down, in front of you for support.

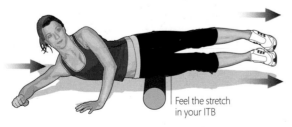

Feel the stretch in your ITB

2 Using your right forearm and left hand, push your body over the roller so that your outer thigh slides across the roller, up towards your hip bone. Slide back the opposite way and repeat for at least 30 seconds, then swap sides.

## 53 THORACIC FOAM ROLLER

Here, the foam roller acts as a hinge to help improve the range of motion in your middle and upper back. It is a good movement to help prevent neck and back pain.

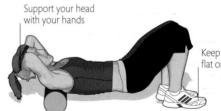

Support your head with your hands

Keep your feet flat on the floor

1 Sit with your heels planted on the floor and the roller beneath the middle of your back. Lie back onto the roller so that it is just below your shoulder blades. Clasp your hands together and lightly cradle your head.

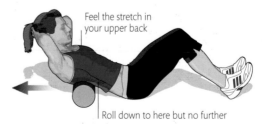

Feel the stretch in your upper back

Roll down to here but no further

2 With your chin tucked in, slide up and down the roller, from your neck down to the level of your lowest ribs. Do not go too low into your lumbar spine as this will cause some discomfort. Repeat for at least 30 seconds.

## 54 CURL-UP

A key part of most exercise programmes, this movement strengthens your abdominal muscles, which help to stabilize your pelvis. If it is recommended as part of your rehabilitation, you can increase the difficulty of the exercise through five levels as your strength and endurance gradually improve.

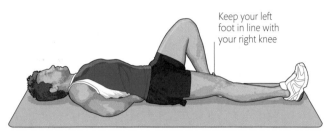

Keep your left foot in line with your right knee

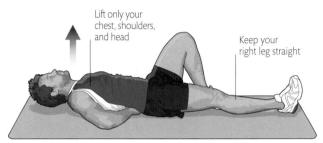

Lift only your chest, shoulders, and head

Keep your right leg straight

1 Lie on your back with one leg straight and the other bent at a 90-degree angle with your foot flat on the floor. Bend your elbows and place your hands palm-down under your lower back. Rest your elbows against the floor.

2 Use your stomach muscles to lift your chest, shoulders, and head off the floor, and breathe out. Hold for 8 seconds, then return to the start position for 2 seconds. Repeat as required, then switch leg positions.

### PROGRESSION – LEVEL 2

Perform the curl-up as in Level 1, with your hands under the small of your back, but this time with your elbows off the floor. As for Level 1, keep one leg straight along the floor and the other bent at a right angle with your foot flat on the floor. Hold for 8 seconds at the top of the movement, then return to the start position for 2 seconds. Repeat as required, then switch leg positions.

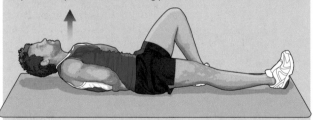

### PROGRESSION – LEVEL 3

Place your hands across your chest instead of behind your back, straightening one leg along the floor and bending the other at 90 degrees with your foot flat on the floor, and only lift your chest, shoulders, and head off the floor. Hold for 8 seconds at the top, then return to the start position for 2 seconds. Repeat for the required number of reps, then switch leg positions.

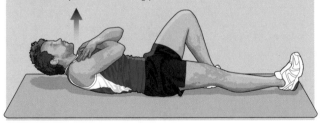

### PROGRESSION – LEVEL 4

Position yourself with a wobble-board under your lower back and your hands across your chest, with one leg straight along the floor and the other bent at a right angle with your foot flat on the floor. Lift your chest, shoulders, and head, hold at the top for 8 seconds, then return to the start position for 2 seconds. Repeat for the required number of reps, then switch leg positions.

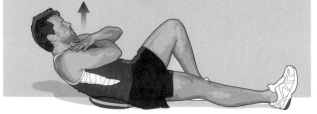

### PROGRESSION – LEVEL 5

Perform the exercise with your lower back positioned on a Swiss ball and your hands across your chest. Plant your feet firmly on the floor and bend your knees at 90 degrees. Hold for 8 seconds, then return to the start position for 2 seconds. Repeat for the required number of reps.

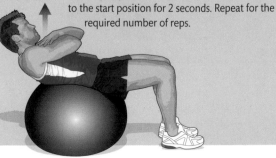

## 55 **CAT** AND CAMEL

A great muscle-releasing exercise, this stretch helps to lubricate your spine and get your spinal discs moving. It is one of the best exercises you can do as part of a general warm-up.

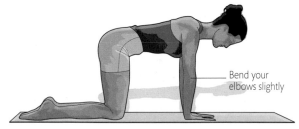

Bend your elbows slightly

1 Kneel on all fours with your hands in line with your shoulders, your fingers pointing forwards, and your knees below your hips.

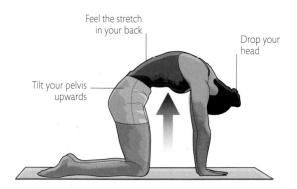

Feel the stretch in your back

Drop your head

Tilt your pelvis upwards

2 Round your back upwards and pull in your stomach, letting your head drop down. Pause at the top of the movement.

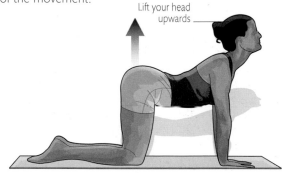

Lift your head upwards

3 In one fluid movement, raise your buttocks and curve your spine downwards while lifting your head so that you are looking straight ahead. Return to the start position and repeat as required.

## 56 **SWISS BALL** TWIST

This exercise not only helps to build your abdominal muscles, but also strengthens the rotational muscles of your torso, improving your core stability and balance.

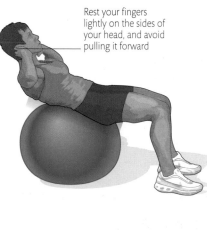

Rest your fingers lightly on the sides of your head, and avoid pulling it forward

1 Lie on a Swiss ball with your lower back supported, your feet flat on the floor, your knees at right angles, and your hands touching your head.

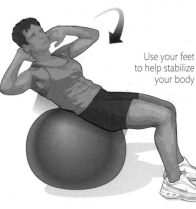

Use your feet to help stabilize your body

2 Once you feel steady, begin to crunch up. About halfway up, twist your torso to one side – spreading your elbows wide will help you to balance.

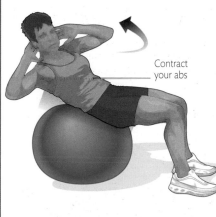

Contract your abs

3 Pause at the top of the movement, then lower and untwist your upper torso to return to the start position. Switch sides.

## 57 **PLANK FROM** KNEES

The plank is a simple move that trains your abdominals and spinal extensors as they work to maintain your raised position. You benefit from improved core strength, tighter abdominals, and a stronger back, all of which improve posture.

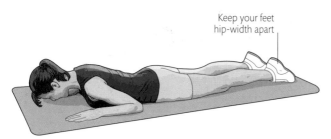

Keep your feet hip-width apart

1 Lie face down on a mat with your arms bent, elbows close to your sides, and palms facing down. Keep your head slightly raised off the floor.

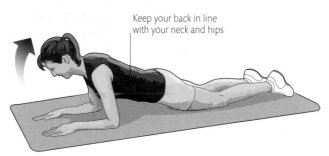

Keep your back in line with your neck and hips

2 Tighten your core and lift your abdomen, sliding your elbows forwards directly under your shoulders to raise your hips off the floor and create a straight line from your knees to your shoulders. Keep your shoulder blades wide and apart, and your spine in a neutral position. Hold this position for 15–20 seconds.

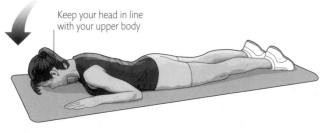

Keep your head in line with your upper body

3 Return to the start position and repeat 5 times, keeping your breathing regular throughout.

## 58 **PRONE** PLANK

This static floor exercise engages your core muscles, along with many of the major muscle groups of your upper and lower body, in order to maintain a fixed position. It can help to prevent lower-back problems or as part of your rehabilitation after a lower-back injury.

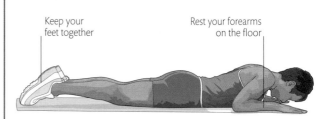

Keep your feet together

Rest your forearms on the floor

1 Lie face down on an exercise mat with your elbows by your sides and your hands alongside your head, palms facing the floor. Raise your head off the floor slightly. Rest the tips of your feet on the floor.

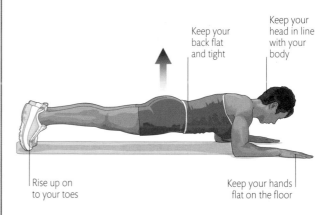

Keep your back flat and tight

Keep your head in line with your body

Rise up on to your toes

Keep your hands flat on the floor

2 Engaging your core and leg muscles, raise your body off the floor, supporting your weight on your forearms and toes, while breathing freely. Keep your head level. Hold the position for about 20 seconds.

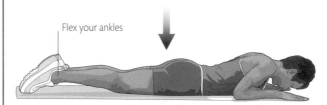

Flex your ankles

3 Gently lower your body back into the start position, and repeat as required.

## 59 SIDE PLANK (LEVEL 1)

This exercise works the muscles of your core, which support your spine. It is key in the rehabilitation of any injury to either your back or pelvis. The most basic form of this exercise is good for initial rehabilitation, and is a starting point for those who have not done it before or do not have sufficient core stability.

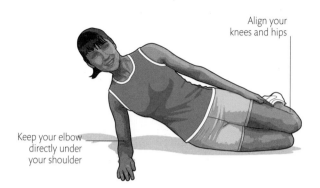

Align your knees and hips

Keep your elbow directly under your shoulder

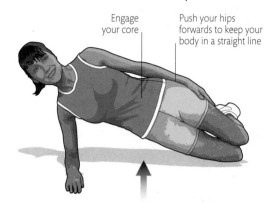

Engage your core

Push your hips forwards to keep your body in a straight line

1 Lying on your right side, prop yourself up on your right forearm and bend your knees so that your calves are at a right angle. Make sure that your right elbow is directly under your shoulder and in line with your hips. Rest your left arm along the side of your body.

2 Engage your abdominals and push down through your right elbow to raise your hips off the floor, making sure that you keep your ribcage elevated and your shoulder lowered. Hold for 8 seconds, then return to the start position for 2 seconds. Repeat as required, then switch sides.

## 60 SIDE PLANK (LEVEL 2)

This progression of the basic side plank exercise (»above) makes the muscles of your core work harder, as you are using them to stabilize your body, while supporting your weight on your arm and ankles.

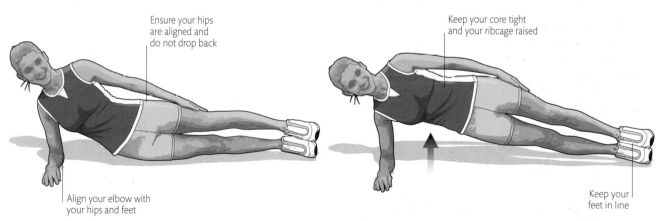

Ensure your hips are aligned and do not drop back

Align your elbow with your hips and feet

Keep your core tight and your ribcage raised

Keep your feet in line

1 Lying on your right side, prop yourself up on your right forearm. Extend your legs and keep your feet together. Make sure that your right elbow is directly under your shoulder and in line with your hips. Rest your left arm along your side.

2 Engage your abdominals and push downwards through your right elbow to raise your hips off the ground, ensuring you keep your ribcage elevated and your shoulder lowered. Hold for 8 seconds, then return to the start position for 2 seconds. Repeat as required, then switch sides.

## 61 **SWISS BALL** SIDE CRUNCH

This exercise improves your strength, core stability, and balance. It is quite advanced, so you should perform it under guidance, and only once you have mastered curl-ups on the ball (»p.186) and side crunches (»p.211).

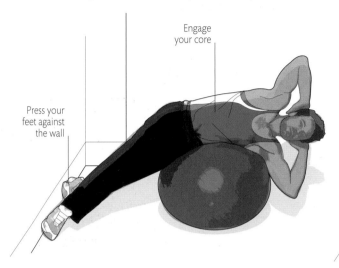

Press your feet against the wall

Engage your core

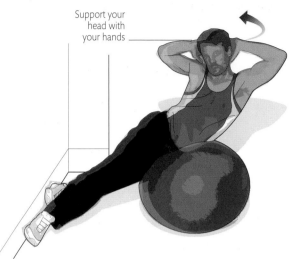

Support your head with your hands

1 Rest your left hip and side on a Swiss ball, pressing your feet against the wall for support, with your right leg in front of your left. Bend your arms at the elbows, with your hands touching the sides of your head.

2 Slowly raise your torso up to your right side, keeping the ball as still as possible by using the wall as a support. Hold this position for 2–3 seconds, then return to the start position. Repeat 10 times, then switch sides.

## 62 **SWISS BALL SIDE** CRUNCH WITH TWIST

This is an advanced exercise designed to improve strength, core stability, and balance. Perform it under guidance once you've mastered the easier exercises such as side crunches (»p.211), and curl-ups on the ball (»p.186).

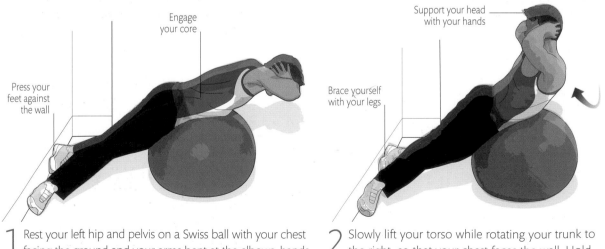

Press your feet against the wall

Engage your core

Support your head with your hands

Brace yourself with your legs

1 Rest your left hip and pelvis on a Swiss ball with your chest facing the ground and your arms bent at the elbows, hands touching the sides of your head. Press your feet against the wall for support, with your right leg in front of your left.

2 Slowly lift your torso while rotating your trunk to the right, so that your chest faces the wall. Hold this position for 2–3 seconds, then return to the start position. Repeat 10 times, then switch sides.

## 63 KNEELING SUPERMAN

This exercise strengthens the spinal extensor muscles and deep spinal stabilizers, which support your spine, and builds strength and stability in your core, lower back, and shoulders. It is a key movement for maintaining a healthy back, and an important rehabilitation exercise for a number of back conditions.

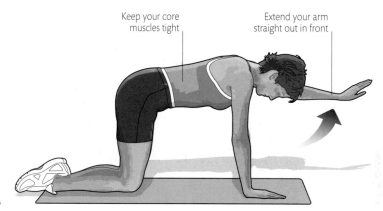

Keep your back in a neutral position

Align your head and spine

Keep your core muscles tight

Extend your arm straight out in front

1 Kneel on all fours, ensuring that your knees are aligned squarely under your hips. Keep your back straight and position your hands directly beneath your shoulders, pressing them flat on the ground and pointing forwards.

2 Engaging your core, raise one arm in front of you. Hold for 10 seconds and return to the start position. Repeat with your other arm.

### PROGRESSION – LEVEL 2

Raising a leg rather than an arm will demand more balance and control. Engage your abdominal muscles and lift your right leg behind you to hip height. Balance and hold for 10 seconds, then return to the start position. Be careful to keep your back straight and to not arch your spine. Repeat with your other leg.

### PROGRESSION – LEVEL 3

Combining an arm lift and a leg lift requires good strength and stability. Contracting your abs, simultaneously lift your right leg behind you to hip height and your left arm forwards to shoulder height. Hold for 10 seconds, then lower your leg and arm to the start position with control. Keep your body straight, and repeat with your other leg and arm.

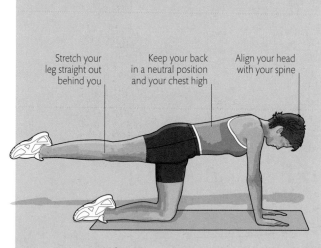

Stretch your leg straight out behind you

Keep your back in a neutral position and your chest high

Align your head with your spine

Do not twist your hips

Extend your arm straight out in front

## 64 MCKENZIE EXTENSION

This exercise helps to ease aches in your lower back, such as those caused by sitting for long periods of time. It is sometimes helpful in reducing pain if you have been diagnosed with a herniated disc (»p.70) or disc-related sciatica (»pp.46–49). You may feel some discomfort, but stop if you feel pain. Aim to perform 10 reps, several times a day.

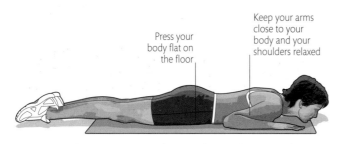

Press your body flat on the floor

Keep your arms close to your body and your shoulders relaxed

1 Lie face down on a mat with your hands flat on the floor and roughly level with your chin. Extend your feet, keeping your legs together.

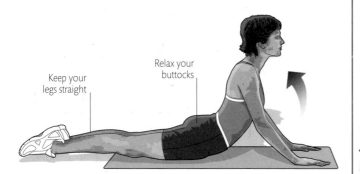

Keep your legs straight

Relax your buttocks

2 Pressing your hips against the mat and breathing out, lift your torso upwards slowly, using your arms for support. Raise your head and shoulders up as high as you can, keeping your lower back relaxed. Pause briefly at the top of the movement and use your arms to lower your torso back to the start position.

### VARIATION

If your injury means that one side of your back is more painful than the other, there is a useful variation of this exercise. While you are lying face-down on your stomach, as in Step 1, shift your legs towards your painful side before you extend your upper torso upwards.

## 65 LEG RAISE

This exercise strengthens your hip flexors and your core, and is a useful movement to help stabilize your pelvis and prevent lower-back problems. Ensure you use the muscles of your core and legs, rather than your back.

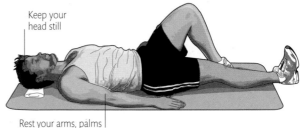

Keep your head still

Rest your arms, palms down, by your sides

1 Lie on your back with your head on a folded towel. Bend your left knee to relax your lower back, with your arms by your sides, hands palms-down, and your right foot pointing upwards.

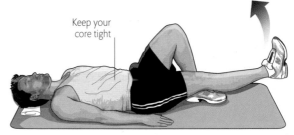

Keep your core tight

2 Keeping your knee straight, lift your right leg about 40cm (16in) off the floor (or higher as your muscles grow stronger) in a slow, fluid movement.

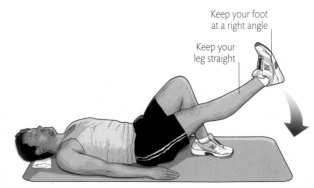

Keep your foot at a right angle

Keep your leg straight

3 Pause at the top of the movement for 3–5 seconds, then return to the start position, slowly and under control. Perform 15 reps, then switch legs.

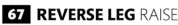

## 66 SIDE-LYING LEG RAISE

This exercise strengthens your gluteus medius muscles in your buttocks, which play a key role in pelvic stability and in the prevention of back problems. Use your core and leg muscles rather than your back.

## 67 REVERSE LEG RAISE

This exercise strengthens the gluteus maximus muscles in your buttocks. It promotes good pelvic stability and helps in the prevention and rehabilitation of lower-back problems. If your buttock muscles are weak, you may be tempted to use your back in the movement. You can prevent this by placing a pillow under your abdomen and pelvis.

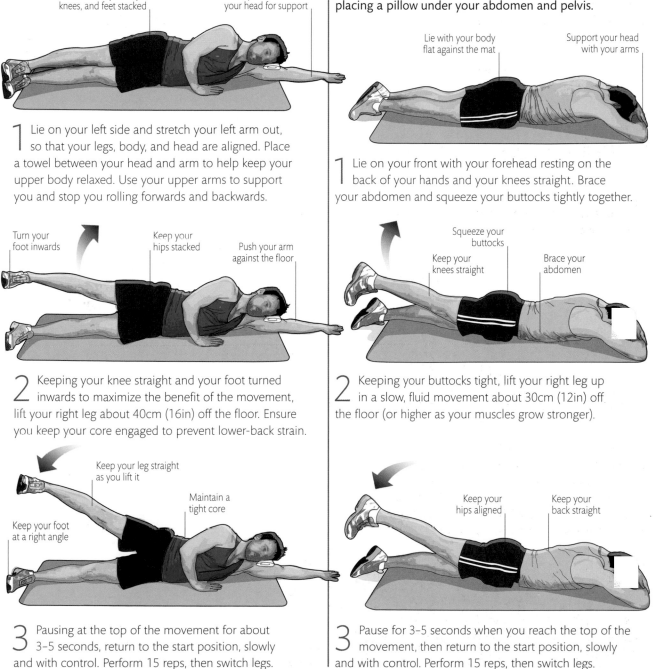

Lie with your hips, knees, and feet stacked

Extend your arm above your head for support

1 Lie on your left side and stretch your left arm out, so that your legs, body, and head are aligned. Place a towel between your head and arm to help keep your upper body relaxed. Use your upper arms to support you and stop you rolling forwards and backwards.

Turn your foot inwards

Keep your hips stacked

Push your arm against the floor

2 Keeping your knee straight and your foot turned inwards to maximize the benefit of the movement, lift your right leg about 40cm (16in) off the floor. Ensure you keep your core engaged to prevent lower-back strain.

Keep your leg straight as you lift it

Maintain a tight core

Keep your foot at a right angle

3 Pausing at the top of the movement for about 3–5 seconds, return to the start position, slowly and with control. Perform 15 reps, then switch legs.

Lie with your body flat against the mat

Support your head with your arms

1 Lie on your front with your forehead resting on the back of your hands and your knees straight. Brace your abdomen and squeeze your buttocks tightly together.

Squeeze your buttocks

Keep your knees straight

Brace your abdomen

2 Keeping your buttocks tight, lift your right leg up in a slow, fluid movement about 30cm (12in) off the floor (or higher as your muscles grow stronger).

Keep your hips aligned

Keep your back straight

3 Pause for 3–5 seconds when you reach the top of the movement, then return to the start position, slowly and with control. Perform 15 reps, then switch legs.

## 68 ISOMETRIC ADDUCTOR SQUEEZE

This is a key exercise for the rehabilitation of sacroiliac joint dysfunction (»p.44; 69), as regaining strength in your adductor muscles is essential for the treatment and prevention of lower-back pain.

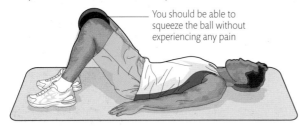

You should be able to squeeze the ball without experiencing any pain

1 Lie on your back with your pelvis in a neutral position, knees bent at a right angle, and feet flat on the floor. Place a medicine ball between your knees. Squeeze as hard as is comfortable, hold for 10 seconds, then relax to return to the start position. Repeat the movement as required.

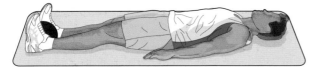

2 Place a medicine ball between your ankles. Lie on your back with your pelvis in a neutral position and keep your legs straight. Squeeze the ball between your ankles as hard as you can, hold for 10 seconds, and return to the start position. Repeat as required. This movement should not be painful.

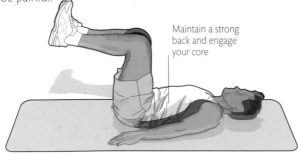

Maintain a strong back and engage your core

3 Lie on your back with your pelvis in a neutral position, and your hips and knees bent at right angles. Place a medicine ball between your knees. Squeeze as hard as is comfortable, hold for 10 seconds, then relax to the start position. Perform the necessary number of repetitions. You should not experience any pain when you squeeze the ball.

## 69 ADDUCTOR LIFT

A great exercise for strengthening your adductors. Weak adductors can lead to poor hip position and sacroiliac joint dysfunction (»p.44; 69). As your strength increases, you can use ankle weights to make it harder.

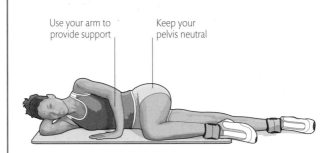

Use your arm to provide support

Keep your pelvis neutral

1 Lie on your right side with your hips stacked and your right arm bent under your head. Shift your weight forwards, using your left arm for balance. Bend your left leg to 90 degrees, with your left knee touching the floor. Keep your right leg straight. Breathe in.

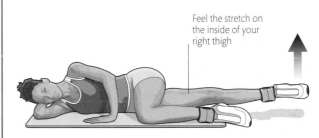

Feel the stretch on the inside of your right thigh

2 Keeping your arms and left leg in the same position, raise your right leg off the ground as high as you can, exhaling as you lift, then pause.

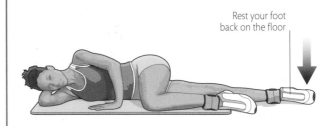

Rest your foot back on the floor

3 Return to the start position, inhaling as you lower your leg. Repeat as necessary, before switching sides to work your left leg.

## 70 BRIDGE

This exercise activates the large gluteal muscles of your buttocks and your hamstrings. It is an important core-stabilizing movement for the rehabilitation of numerous back problems, including sacroiliac joint pain (≫p.44; 69). There is a wide range of potential variations, making it a very versatile exercise. As your strength increases, you can try the single-leg bridge (≫below).

### VARIATION

This exercise can be varied by bending your knees further, or putting your feet on a Swiss ball. This adds a level of instability, making your core stabilizers work harder.

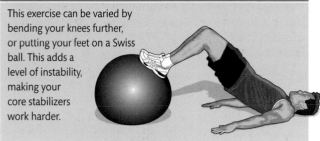

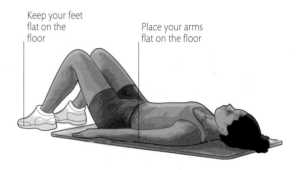

Keep your feet flat on the floor

Place your arms flat on the floor

Keep your knees in line with your pelvis and trunk

Maintain a straight back and do not arch your upper back

1 Lie on your back with your knees bent at right angles and your feet flat on the floor, hip-width apart. Keep your arms at your sides, with your palms facing down.

2 Engaging your core, slowly lift your buttocks off the floor until your body is in a straight line from your knees to your shoulders. Pause at the top, then reverse the movement to return to the starting position.

## 71 SINGLE-LEG BRIDGE

A development of the bridge (≫above), this exercise is useful for working the large gluteal muscles of your buttocks, your hip extensors, and your core. Because you are performing it on one leg, it forces you to control the rotation and tilt of your pelvis. It is important to ensure that you keep your hips level throughout.

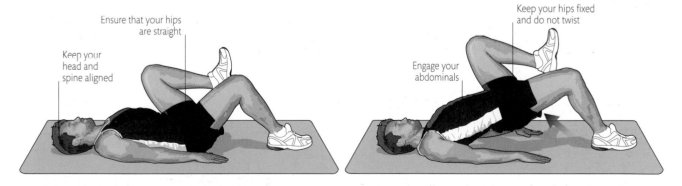

Ensure that your hips are straight

Keep your head and spine aligned

Keep your hips fixed and do not twist

Engage your abdominals

1 Lie on your back with your knees bent at 90 degrees, your feet hip-width apart, and your hands palms-down by your sides. Keeping your right foot flat on the floor, and your arms by your sides, raise your left knee up towards your torso until your thighs are at right angles.

2 Engaging the muscles of your abdomen and lower back, lift your buttocks until your hips are fully extended and your body is in a straight line from your lower knee to your shoulders. Hold this position, then reverse the movement to return to the start position, and switch legs.

## 72 LAT STRETCH

Specifically targeting the large muscles of your upper back, this simple stretch is a useful exercise for maintenance and rehabilitation for a range of back injuries.

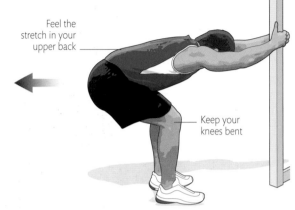

Feel the stretch in your upper back

Keep your knees bent

1 Stand facing an upright support that will take your weight. Grip the support with both hands and lean back, bending your knees. Push with your legs and pull with your arms.

## 73 QUAD STRETCH

This stretch works the quadriceps muscles at the front of your thigh, which enable you to straighten your knee. Because this stretch is performed in a standing position, it emphasizes good posture and balance.

Keep your head forwards and your spine neutral

Tilt your pelvis back slightly

1 Stand with your back to a firm table. Place your left foot on the table and, keeping your legs parallel, tilt your pelvis back slightly so you can feel the stretch in the front of your left thigh. Hold, lower, and repeat with your right leg.

## 74 HAMSTRING STRETCH 1

This is a simple general-purpose stretch that works all the muscles in your hamstrings, relieving the tightness that can stress your lower back. Stretch slowly and avoid "bouncing" at full extension.

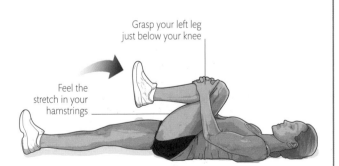

Grasp your left leg just below your knee

Feel the stretch in your hamstrings

1 Lie on your back with your legs extended. Bend your left knee. Pull gently on your left leg, bringing your knee towards your chest until you feel the stretch. Keep the back of your head on the floor. Relax and repeat with your right leg.

## 75 HAMSTRING STRETCH 2

This is another useful stretch for your hamstring muscles to help relieve tightness, which can cause pain in your lower back. Perform the stretch in a slow, controlled manner.

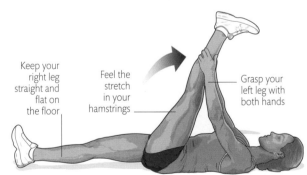

Keep your right leg straight and flat on the floor

Feel the stretch in your hamstrings

Grasp your left leg with both hands

1 Lie on your back with your legs extended. Lift each leg in turn, keeping your knee braced and your toes pulled back towards your body. If you are very flexible, try extending the stretch a little by pulling back on your leg.

## 76 LANCELOT STRETCH

This is a useful stretch if you suffer from stiffness around your spine, as it stretches your hip flexors and, in particular, your psoas muscle. Your psoas muscle is directly attached to your spine and it is important to keep it flexible.

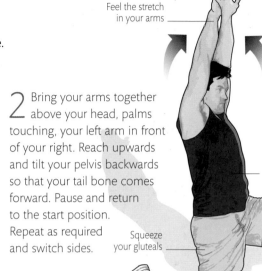

1 Stand with your feet shoulder-width apart and your hands on your hips. Lunge forward with your left leg, bending both legs so that your right knee and the top of your right foot are touching the floor. Keep your spine neutral and look straight ahead.

Look straight ahead

Bend your knee at a right angle

2 Bring your arms together above your head, palms touching, your left arm in front of your right. Reach upwards and tilt your pelvis backwards so that your tail bone comes forward. Pause and return to the start position. Repeat as required and switch sides.

Feel the stretch in your arms

Feel the stretch in your torso as you reach upwards

Squeeze your gluteals

## 77 ADDUCTOR STRETCH 1

Stretching your adductor or groin muscles is key to maintaining hip flexibility, and can help with lower-back pain.

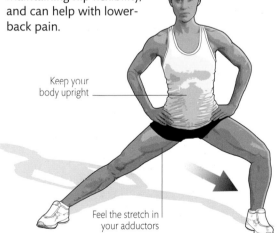

Keep your body upright

Feel the stretch in your adductors

1 Keep your body upright and put your hands on your hips. Bend your left leg so that your left knee is over your left foot, your right leg is extended, and your right foot is flat. Rock gently to the side. Relax and switch legs.

## 78 ADDUCTOR STRETCH 2

This version of the adductor stretch works more on the short adductor muscles of your groin. It is easy to perform, can be carried out almost anywhere, and forms a useful part of a general stretching routine.

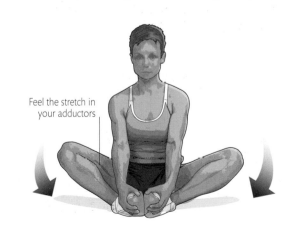

Feel the stretch in your adductors

1 Sit on the floor and take a firm hold of the tops of your feet. Bring your legs in close to your body, pressing the soles of your feet together. Push your knees gently down towards the floor as far as you can, and hold.

## 79 PIRIFORMIS STRETCH

This seated stretch is more advanced than the ITB foam roller stretch (»p.185) because you need greater flexibility in your hip joint to perform it correctly. It is useful for preventing or easing piriformis syndrome (»p.49), and is particularly important for those who exercise regularly.

1 Sit on the floor with your legs extended. Support yourself with your left hand behind you, and bend your left leg, crossing it over your right leg. Keep your left foot flat on the floor. Reach over with your right hand and gently press on the outside of your left knee until you can feel the stretch in the outside of your thigh. Hold briefly, then switch sides.

Feel the stretch here

## 80 CALF STRETCH

Tight calf muscles can cause a muscular imbalance by making your foot turn outwards and forcing your hip muscles to work harder. Your gait may become "flatter", which can lead to back pain.

Feel the stretch in your calf muscles

Push your heel into the floor

1 From a standing position, press your left hand against a wall and take a good step backwards with your right leg, keeping your feet hip-width apart. Bend your left leg forward, ensuring you keep your knee over your foot. Switch arms and repeat with your other leg.

## 81 CALF RAISE

This exercise helps to strengthen your calf muscles and improve your gait. It is important to avoid tight calf muscles, as they can put stress on the muscles of your lower back, and cause or aggravate pain in that area.

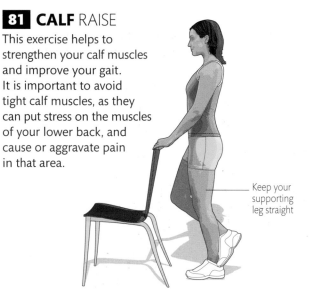

Keep your supporting leg straight

Keep your shoulders back

Engage your core

Raise yourself up on one leg

1 Stand on your left leg, with the toe of your right leg wrapped around the back of your left ankle. Support your body weight with your left leg, and rest your hands on the back of a chair. Breathe in.

2 Raise yourself up as high as you can go on to the ball of your left foot, breathing out as you do so. Pause briefly, then lower your heel back to the start position, breathing in. Repeat as required, then switch legs.

## 82 SINGLE-LEG STAND

This exercise is a good starting point for developing your balance in a weight-bearing position. It also improves control of your trunk and strengthens your buttock muscles, helping to improve your pelvic stability.

1 Pick a point on the wall in front of you and focus on it. Stand on one leg and tighten your buttocks and thighs all at the same time. Stand in front of a mirror if you need to check your posture and form are correct.

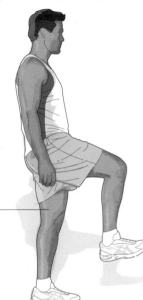

Contract the muscles in the buttock and thigh of your standing leg

### VARIATION

Once you can confidently perform a single-leg stand on a stable surface, try balancing on an Airex mat, wobble board (shown here), or Bosu ball to introduce an element of instability and make the exercise harder.

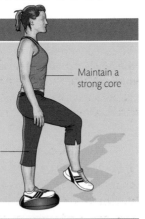

Maintain a strong core

Keep the knee of your standing leg firm but not locked

### PROGRESSION

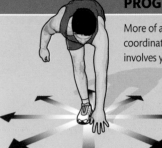

More of a challenge in terms of balance, coordination, and flexibility, this exercise involves you standing on one leg and touching the floor with your opposite hand at points around an imaginary clock face. If performed incorrectly, it can cause back injuries, so seek guidance before you try it.

## 83 WALL-SUPPORTED FOOT LIFT

This exercise strengthens the muscles of your feet and lower legs. It helps prevent flat feet and overpronation (»p.113), and improves your gait. It can help to prevent problems in your knees, hip, and back in the longer term.

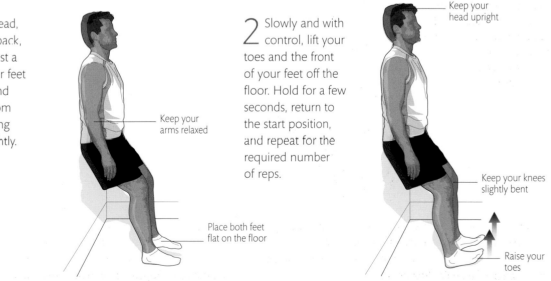

1 Rest your head, shoulders, back, and arms against a wall. Move your feet slightly apart and 30cm (12in) from the wall, bending your knees slightly.

Keep your arms relaxed

Place both feet flat on the floor

2 Slowly and with control, lift your toes and the front of your feet off the floor. Hold for a few seconds, return to the start position, and repeat for the required number of reps.

Keep your head upright

Keep your knees slightly bent

Raise your toes

## 84 SUPINE PELVIC TILT

This exercise helps with most types of acute lumbar pain by relieving pressure on the facet joints and gently stretching the muscles and ligaments of your back, strengthening your core and improving your posture. You should perform this exercise on the floor at first, but as you improve you can try it standing up.

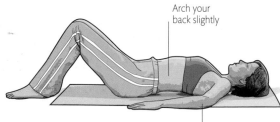

Arch your back slightly

Bend your elbows slightly

1 Lie on your back with your knees bent at a comfortable angle, your feet flat on the floor, your arms by your sides at a slight bend, and your lower back arched but relaxed.

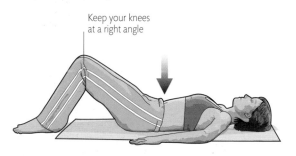

Keep your knees at a right angle

2 Gently press the small of your back into the floor and tilt your pubic bone upwards by tightening your abdominal and pelvic floor muscles. Hold for at least 6 seconds.

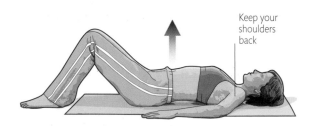

Keep your shoulders back

3 Relax and return to the start position, so that the small of your back is slightly arched once more. Repeat as required and relax.

## 85 KNEELING PELVIC TILT

This movement helps those with poor posture. Some experts recommend this as an alternative for the supine version of the exercise (»left) after the first trimester of pregnancy because it may interfere with blood supply to the foetus.

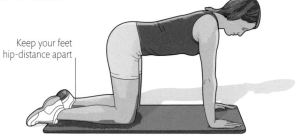

Keep your feet hip-distance apart

1 Kneel on a mat with your hands under your shoulders and your knees under your hips, keeping your back in a neutral position, and breathe in deeply.

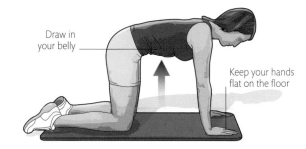

Draw in your belly

Keep your hands flat on the floor

2 Breathe out, pulling your abdominals in tight, and suck in your belly button towards your spine. With one fluid motion, reverse the curve in your lower back and tilt your hips.

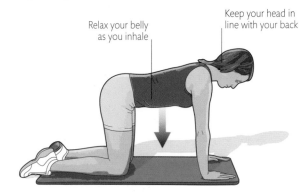

Relax your belly as you inhale

Keep your head in line with your back

3 Release and repeat for the required number of reps. Inhale and exhale as you perform the moves, feeling the pull and push of the movement deep within your core.

## 86 SEATED PELVIC TILT

It is harder to perform the pelvic tilt in an upright posture, either standing or sitting, but doing this exercise on a Swiss ball provides a helpful guide, as the ball will shift forwards slightly when you do the movement correctly.

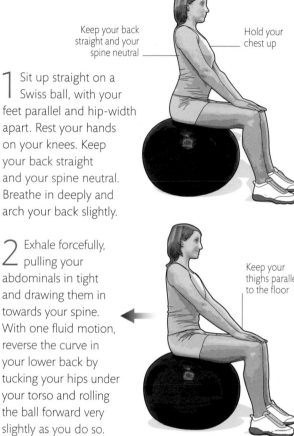

Keep your back straight and your spine neutral

Hold your chest up

1 Sit up straight on a Swiss ball, with your feet parallel and hip-width apart. Rest your hands on your knees. Keep your back straight and your spine neutral. Breathe in deeply and arch your back slightly.

Keep your thighs parallel to the floor

2 Exhale forcefully, pulling your abdominals in tight and drawing them in towards your spine. With one fluid motion, reverse the curve in your lower back by tucking your hips under your torso and rolling the ball forward very slightly as you do so.

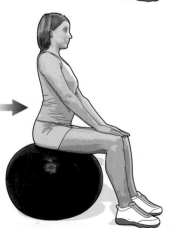

3 Hold the position for a few seconds, then release to return to the arched position in step 1. Repeat as required and relax.

## 87 PRONE BACK EXTENSION

This is a good maintenance exercise for the muscles of your lower back and core, but you should only attempt it if your lower back is free of pain. The only sensation you should feel while performing it is the muscles of your lower back tightening as they work.

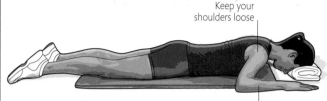

Keep your shoulders loose

Rest your forearms on the floor

1 Lie face down on a mat with a folded towel under your forehead to ensure proper alignment of your head and neck with your spine. Bend your arms and rest your forearms on the floor, palms down. Breathe in deeply.

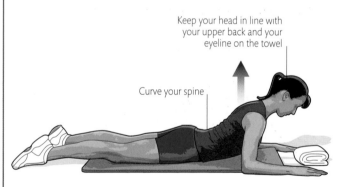

Keep your head in line with your upper back and your eyeline on the towel

Curve your spine

2 Engage your core and reach forwards with the top of your head to lengthen your spine, keeping your shoulders apart. Then, facing downwards, lift your head and shoulders off the floor, exhaling as you do so. Make sure that you do not use any strength from your arms.

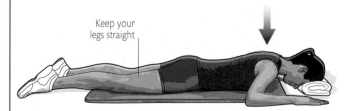

Keep your legs straight

3 Pause at the top of the movement, then inhale and slowly return to the start position without resting. Repeat as required.

## 88 STANDING BACK EXTENSION

This exercise gently arches your lower back, and it is useful for lumbar disc problems. You should perform it every couple of hours through the day. If it increases your pain, try the prone back extension exercise (»p.201) instead.

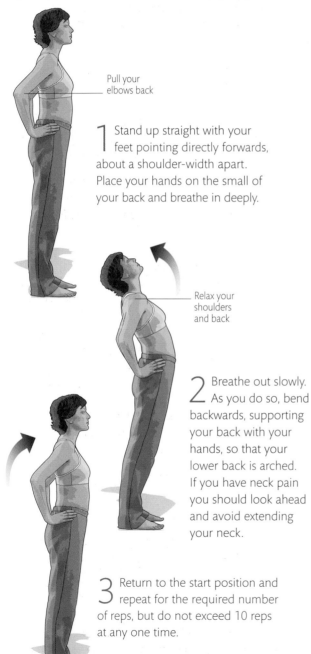

Pull your elbows back

1 Stand up straight with your feet pointing directly forwards, about a shoulder-width apart. Place your hands on the small of your back and breathe in deeply.

Relax your shoulders and back

2 Breathe out slowly. As you do so, bend backwards, supporting your back with your hands, so that your lower back is arched. If you have neck pain you should look ahead and avoid extending your neck.

3 Return to the start position and repeat for the required number of reps, but do not exceed 10 reps at any one time.

Keep your feet shoulder-width apart

## 89 KNEES-TO-CHEST STRETCH

This exercise helps if you have strained a facet joint (»p.68), and the surrounding muscles are tight and aching. However, you should proceed with caution if you know your pain is caused by a disc protrusion (»p.70).

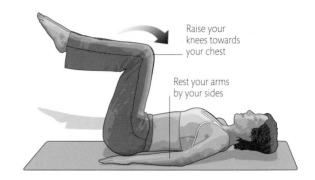

Raise your knees towards your chest

Rest your arms by your sides

1 Lie down and do a basic pelvic tilt (»p.200). Then draw your knees up towards your chest, keeping your lower back flat.

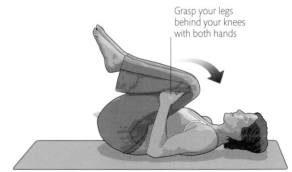

Grasp your legs behind your knees with both hands

2 Use your hands to help draw your knees closer to your chest. Keep your head on the floor.

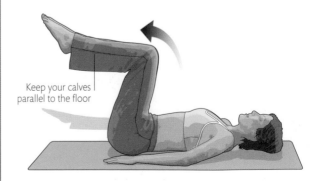

Keep your calves parallel to the floor

3 Let go of your thighs and return to the start position. Repeat for the required number of reps.

## 90 **SWISS BALL** BACK EXTENSION

This advanced exercise requires you to stabilize the full length of your body while increasing resistance (by placing your hands behind your head) and range of motion (the ball adds height to the lift).

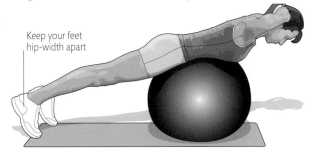

Keep your feet hip-width apart

1 Position your torso on a Swiss ball with your legs extended, and dig your toes into the mat. Alternatively, plant your feet against a wall. Rest your fingertips lightly at the back of your head and lengthen your spine. Breathe in.

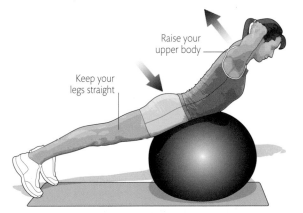

Raise your upper body

Keep your legs straight

2 Exhale as you squeeze your buttocks and slowly lift your torso to 45 degrees. Press your hips into the ball. Pause at the top, then inhale.

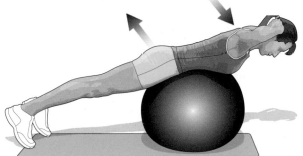

3 Slowly return to the start position without resting. Gradually build up the number of reps.

## 91 **BACK** ROTATION

This exercise improves general mobility and is particularly useful for relaxing the muscles of your back and pelvis. It also relieves facet joint pain (»p.68) by stretching the capsules and ligaments around the facet joints in your lower back: those on your left will be stretched as you drop your knees to the right, and vice versa.

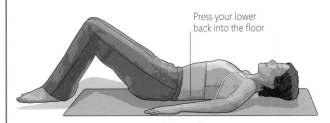

Press your lower back into the floor

1 Lie on your back with your knees bent, your feet flat on the floor and your arms by your sides, as for the pelvic tilt (»p.200). Press your lower back into the floor.

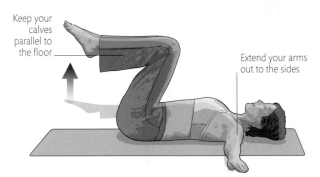

Keep your calves parallel to the floor

Extend your arms out to the sides

2 Keeping your knees together, lift them until they are above the middle of your abdominal region, and bring your arms straight out to your sides.

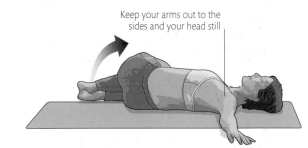

Keep your arms out to the sides and your head still

3 Let your legs flop over to the right as far as they will go. Breathe slowly and deeply, allowing your legs to drop a little further with each breath. Hold for as long as you can, then bring your legs back up and lower them to the other side. Repeat the movement as required.

## 92 FOUR-POINT SUPINE KNEE LIFT

This is a moderate-impact core-stabilizing exercise. It can be helpful for strengthening the deep muscles of your abdomen and your lower back, and can be a useful exercise for preventing pain in your lumbar region. To get the best results from the movement, keep the muscles of your core engaged throughout.

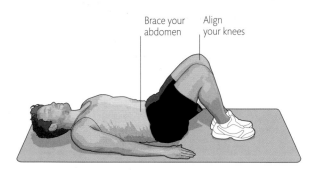

Brace your abdomen

Align your knees

1 Lie on your back and bend your knees, with your feet flat on the floor. Relax your shoulders and upper back, brace your abdomen, and keep your spine in a neutral position.

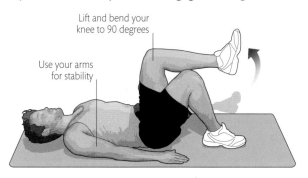

Lift and bend your knee to 90 degrees

Use your arms for stability

2 Keeping your abdomen braced, lift your left leg so that your hip and knee are at right angles. Keep your right foot firmly on the floor.

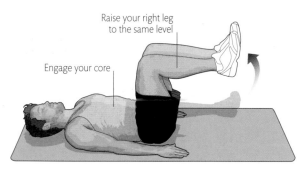

Raise your right leg to the same level

Engage your core

3 Still keeping your abdomen braced, lift your right leg until it is level with your left. Hold this position for a few seconds and use your arms to stabilize yourself.

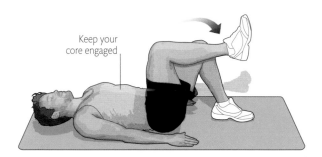

Keep your core engaged

4 Keeping your core engaged, slowly lower your left leg until your foot is flat on the floor.

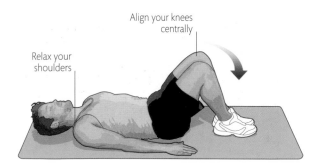

Align your knees centrally

Relax your shoulders

5 Now lower your right leg, returning to the start position. Repeat the exercise 5 times and then repeat the sequence beginning with your right leg.

### VARIATION

Once you can perform the basic four-point supine knee lift with confidence and you have improved the strength and stability in your abdomen and lumbar region, you can make the exercise harder by placing an air cushion (shown here) or Bosu board in the small of your back. Focus on maintaining stability in your torso and keeping the muscles of your core engaged. Try not to use your arms to keep you balanced.

Position the air cushion beneath your pelvis

## 93 **ISOMETRIC HIP** FLEXION

This exercise strengthens your deep abdominal muscles and hip flexors, and stabilizes your lower back. It can be used to treat sacroiliac joint dysfunction (»p.39; 69) and lumbar hypermobility (»p.56; 66).

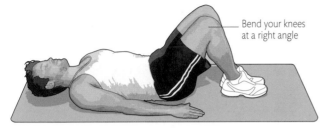

Bend your knees at a right angle

1 Lie on your back and bend your knees. Relax your shoulders and upper back, brace your abdomen, and keep your spine in a neutral position.

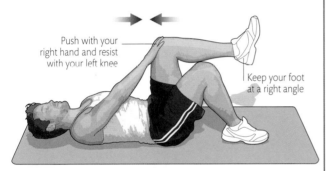

Push with your right hand and resist with your left knee

Keep your foot at a right angle

2 Place your right hand on your left knee. Push your knee and flex your hip simultaneously: the force of the push and flexion of the hip should be equal, so no movement will occur. Hold for 10 seconds.

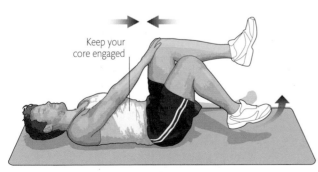

Keep your core engaged

3 Maintaining the resistance between your left knee and right hand, raise your right foot off the mat. Hold for 5 seconds, then relax and return to the start position. Perform the move 5 times, then change legs.

## 94 **SINGLE-LEG** ELONGATION

This exercise is used in the rehabilitation of facet joint and sacroiliac joint dysfunction (»p.68; 69); it also stretches the muscles of your lower back, and can help with three-curve scoliosis (»p.74). Perform this exercise only on the affected side.

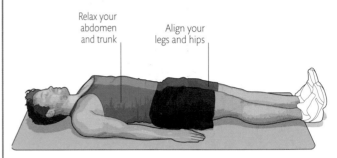

Relax your abdomen and trunk

Align your legs and hips

1 Lie on your back with your feet hip-width apart and your arms by your sides, palms down.

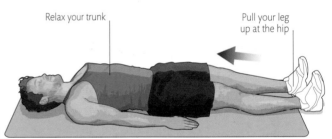

Relax your trunk

Pull your leg up at the hip

2 Keeping your arms by your sides, pull your unaffected leg up at the hip to shorten it.

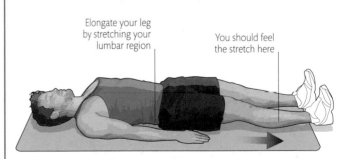

Elongate your leg by stretching your lumbar region

You should feel the stretch here

3 Now elongate the leg on your affected side by stretching the side of your lower back and your hip joint. Hold the position for 5 seconds, then relax. Repeat for 3 sets of 5 reps, only on this affected side.

## 95 PRONE KNEE BEND

This exercise is used to mobilize your femoral nerve and stretch tight muscles at the front of your hip and thigh. It can be useful for increasing the range of motion in damaged knee joints, and helps to prevent lower-back pain.

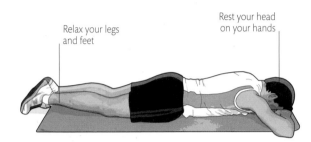

Relax your legs and feet

Rest your head on your hands

1 Lie face down on a mat. Bend your arms in front of you and rest your forehead on your hands. Relax your trunk and legs.

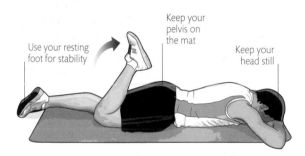

Use your resting foot for stability

Keep your pelvis on the mat

Keep your head still

2 Keeping your left leg flat on the mat, bend your right leg up as far as you can in a slow, relaxed motion. Ensure that you keep your hips still as you perform the movement.

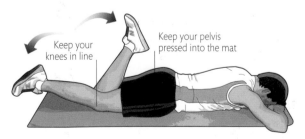

Keep your knees in line

Keep your pelvis pressed into the mat

3 Lower your right leg down and bend your left leg up simultaneously. Continue alternating legs, repeating 10 times for each leg, slowly and under control, then return to the start position.

## 96 SIDE GLIDE

This exercise was developed by physiotherapist Robin McKenzie to help acute lower-back pain due to disc problems that have shifted the pelvis to one side. Look in a mirror: if your right hip is more prominent, this exercise should help you pull your pelvis to the left and your trunk to the right. If your left hip is more prominent, do the exercise the other way round.

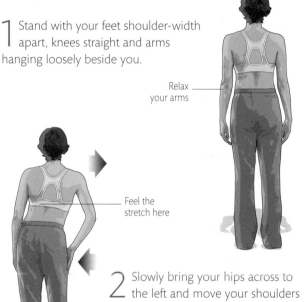

1 Stand with your feet shoulder-width apart, knees straight and arms hanging loosely beside you.

Relax your arms

Feel the stretch here

2 Slowly bring your hips across to the left and move your shoulders to the right, keeping them horizontal. This may cause twinges and the muscles will tighten up in resistance. Stop if the pain increases in your back or legs.

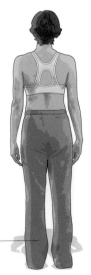

3 Relax and return to the start position. Repeat the sequence until you return to a neutral position with no lateral shift. Repeat 10 times every 2 hours. Once your tilt is corrected you can start prone (»p.201) or standing back extensions (»p.202).

Keep your legs straight and shoulder-width apart

## 97 STATIONARY LUNGE

Lunges are fantastic for the muscles of your buttocks and thighs, and can help to prevent lower-back problems, as these muscles all provide support to your back. Although you will feel the front of your thigh working first, the lunge is also strengthening your buttocks and the backs of your thighs, and helping to improve your hip mobility.

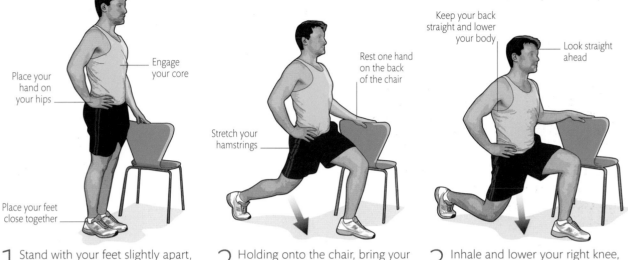

Place your hand on your hips

Engage your core

Place your feet close together

Rest one hand on the back of the chair

Stretch your hamstrings

Keep your back straight and lower your body

Look straight ahead

1 Stand with your feet slightly apart, your right hand on your hip, and your left hand resting on a chair back. Align your shoulders, hips, and feet.

2 Holding onto the chair, bring your left leg back, heel lifted, keeping your legs parallel. Keep your hips facing forward and your weight centred evenly.

3 Inhale and lower your right knee, with your left knee over your ankle. Exhale as you straighten your legs. Repeat as required, then switch sides.

## 98 FORWARD LUNGE

Once you are comfortable with the stationary lunge (»above), you can progress to this unsupported version of the exercise. This version of the lunge requires more balance as you do not have a chair to hold onto.

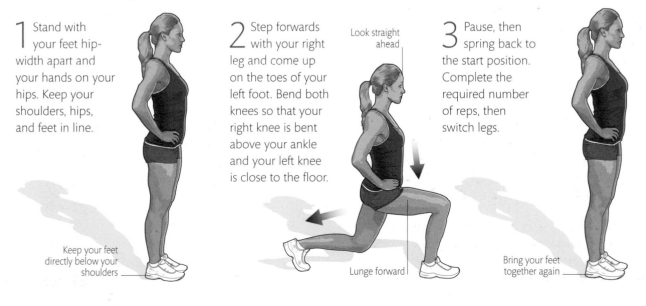

1 Stand with your feet hip-width apart and your hands on your hips. Keep your shoulders, hips, and feet in line.

2 Step forwards with your right leg and come up on the toes of your left foot. Bend both knees so that your right knee is bent above your ankle and your left knee is close to the floor.

Look straight ahead

3 Pause, then spring back to the start position. Complete the required number of reps, then switch legs.

Keep your feet directly below your shoulders

Lunge forward

Bring your feet together again

## 99 REVERSE LUNGE WITH KNEE LIFT

This exercise works the muscles in your thighs, buttocks, and shoulders, while also increasing your core stability. It helps with your flexibility and balance too, as the exercise requires you to centre your body weight on one leg for most of the exercise, while moving your other leg through a full range of movement. To make the exercise more difficult, try starting the movement from the raised knee position (**»Step 6**) without pausing in the middle.

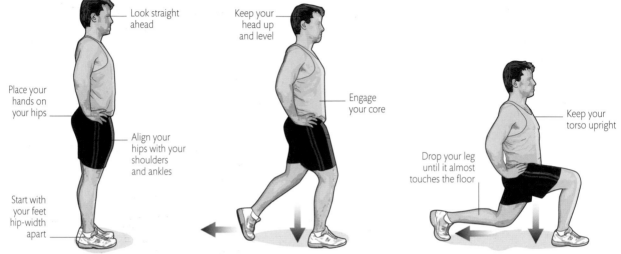

Look straight ahead

Place your hands on your hips

Align your hips with your shoulders and ankles

Start with your feet hip-width apart

Keep your head up and level

Engage your core

Keep your torso upright

Drop your leg until it almost touches the floor

1 Stand with your feet hip-width apart, your legs and back straight, and your hands on your hips.

2 Breathe in and lunge backwards with your left leg, taking your weight on your right leg as you do so, and bending your right knee slightly.

3 Continue the movement until you are in a full lunge position with your left knee almost touching the floor, or as far as you can comfortably go.

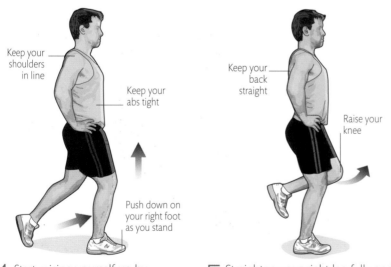

Keep your shoulders in line

Keep your abs tight

Push down on your right foot as you stand

Keep your back straight

Raise your knee

4 Start raising yourself up by straightening your right leg and pushing down on your right foot. Bring your left leg forwards at the same time.

5 Straighten your right leg fully and continue the forward movement with your left leg, pushing through your left knee.

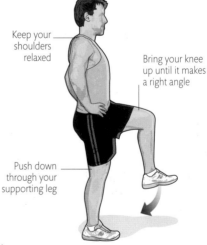

Keep your shoulders relaxed

Bring your knee up until it makes a right angle

Push down through your supporting leg

6 Push forwards and up with your left knee until it is at hip height and bent at a right angle. Pause and return to the start position. Repeat for the required number of reps, then switch legs.

## 100 HIP FLEXOR STRETCH

Your psoas muscles work as hip flexors and can shorten with prolonged sitting, creating a muscle imbalance. Stretching them reduces strain on your lower back.

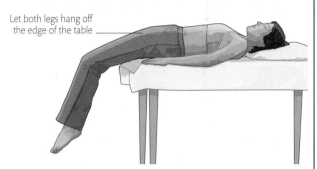

Let both legs hang off the edge of the table

1 Start by sitting on the edge of a firm padded table, with your legs hanging over the side. Then lie back and rest your head on a pillow or folded towel.

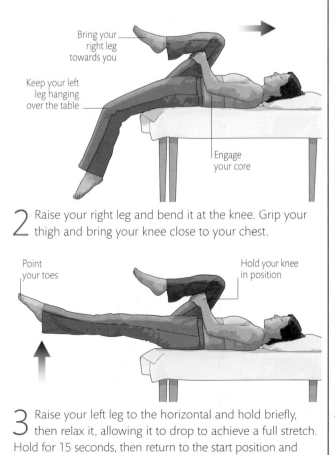

Bring your right leg towards you

Keep your left leg hanging over the table

Engage your core

2 Raise your right leg and bend it at the knee. Grip your thigh and bring your knee close to your chest.

Point your toes

Hold your knee in position

3 Raise your left leg to the horizontal and hold briefly, then relax it, allowing it to drop to achieve a full stretch. Hold for 15 seconds, then return to the start position and switch legs.

## 101 PSOAS LUNGE

This exercise is an adaptation of a standard lunge that focuses the stretch on your psoas muscle. The key to performing it is to keep your pelvis tucked underneath your torso.

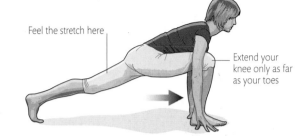

Feel the stretch here

Extend your knee only as far as your toes

1 Lunge your right leg forwards, and place your hands on either side of your right foot. Straighten your back leg, and press your left hip towards the floor.

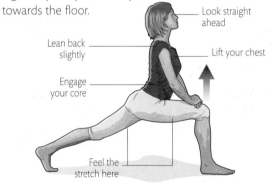

Look straight ahead

Lean back slightly

Lift your chest

Engage your core

Feel the stretch here

2 Tuck your hips underneath you and place both hands on your right thigh. Exhale, lift your chest, and look straight ahead of you.

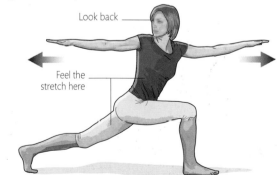

Look back

Feel the stretch here

3 Slowly reach your right arm behind you and twist your torso around, while reaching your left arm out in front of you, so that both arms are extended. Look back in the direction of the twist and hold briefly, then return to the start position. Repeat as required, and switch legs.

## 102 KNEELING HIP FLEXOR

This exercise will stretch your hip flexor muscles, which may be particularly tight if you spend a lot of time sitting down. Tight hip flexors can cause imbalances around your pelvis and lower back, leading to back pain. If you find your knees hurt during the movement, you can rest them on a cushion or soft pad.

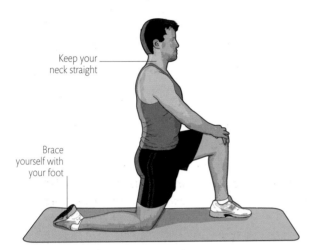

Keep your neck straight

Brace yourself with your foot

1 Kneel on your right knee, with your hands resting on your left knee for balance, so that your right knee is below your shoulders and your head is in line with your back. Keep your back straight.

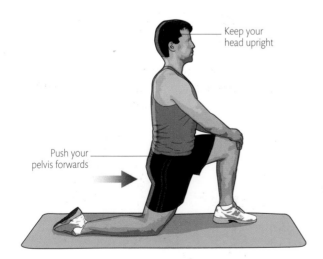

Keep your head upright

Push your pelvis forwards

2 Bring your left knee forward and feel the stretch in the thigh of your right leg, but don't extend your left knee over the front of your left foot. Hold the stretch for 15 seconds, relax, and switch sides.

## 103 PRONE ARM AND LEG LIFT

This exercise strengthens the muscles around your shoulders and along your spine, along with your buttocks and hamstrings. It is especially useful for people who can't kneel properly or have wrist problems and can't perform the kneeling superman exercise (»p.191).

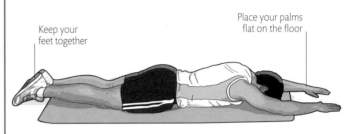

Keep your feet together

Place your palms flat on the floor

1 Lie face down with your forehead resting on the mat. Align your neck and head. Extend your arms in front of you with your palms facing down. Lengthen your torso by stretching your neck away from your body, and contract your abdominals.

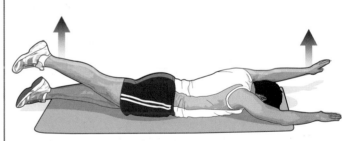

2 Keeping your head in line with your upper back, raise your left arm and your right leg 8–15cm (3–6in) off the floor. Hold the movement briefly.

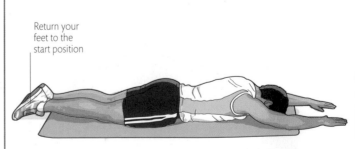

Return your feet to the start position

3 Lower your limbs slowly and with control, and return to the start position. Switch sides and continue to alternate sides until you have completed the required number of reps.

## 104 **OBLIQUE** CRUNCH

This exercise requires flexibility, stamina, and mobility. It can potentially aggravate some types of back pain, so seek guidance to ensure that it is right for you and that you are performing it with good technique.

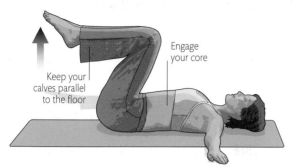

Keep your calves parallel to the floor

Engage your core

1 Lie on your back with your pelvis in a neutral position, your knees and hips bent at 90 degrees, and your arms outstretched at right angles to your body.

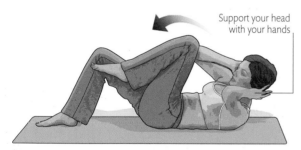

Support your head with your hands

2 With your hands held lightly to the sides of your head, simultaneously bring your left knee and right elbow together, planting your right foot firmly on the floor.

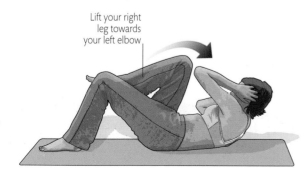

Lift your right leg towards your left elbow

3 Alternate the movement at a steady pace, ensuring that you curl up and rotate your trunk, and avoid pulling your head or neck. Complete the required number of reps before returning to the start position.

## 105 **SIDE** CRUNCH

Side crunches target the oblique muscles responsible for core strength and trunk stability. They can potentially aggravate some types of back pain, so consult your physiotherapist for guidance first.

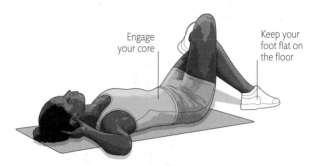

Engage your core

Keep your foot flat on the floor

1 Lie on your back with your pelvis in a neutral position, your left leg bent to 90 degrees, and your left foot firmly on the floor. Rest your right leg across your left knee, and place both hands at the base of your head.

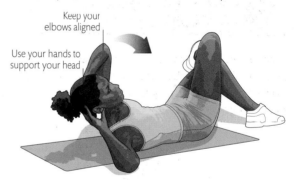

Keep your elbows aligned

Use your hands to support your head

2 Keeping your lower back pressed into the mat, lift your shoulder blades off the floor. Leading with your left elbow, curl your upper body towards your right knee.

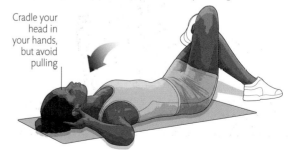

Cradle your head in your hands, but avoid pulling

3 Pause briefly, then return to the start position slowly and with control. Repeat until you have completed the required number of reps, then switch sides.

## 106 CHILD'S POSE

This yoga position gently stretches your spine, hips, thighs, and ankles. If you find the exercise uncomfortable, you can place a rolled-up towel between the back of your thighs and calves.

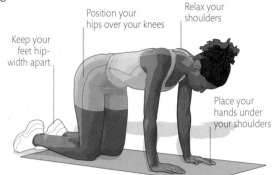

Keep your feet hip-width apart

Position your hips over your knees

Relax your shoulders

Place your hands under your shoulders

1 Kneel on all fours with your hands in line with your shoulders, your fingers pointing forwards, and your knees directly below your hips. Keep your back straight and your head in line with it.

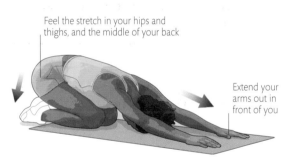

Feel the stretch in your hips and thighs, and the middle of your back

Extend your arms out in front of you

2 Keeping your hands in position, slowly lower yourself down onto your heels until your forehead touches the mat. Breathe in and out, and feel the stretch in your body.

### VARIATION

This exercise can also be performed with a slight variation to stretch the side muscles of your back. Instead of stretching your arms out directly in front of you, stretch them out diagonally, keeping them parallel as you do so. Hold the position for a few seconds, then repeat on the other side to fully benefit from the stretch.

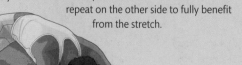

## 107 SWISS BALL ROLL-OUT

This advanced exercise builds stability and strength in your core muscles, as it makes your abdominals and lower back work together. It also strengthens your shoulders.

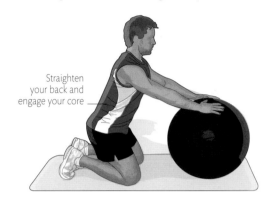

Straighten your back and engage your core

1 Kneel down, resting your hands and lower arms on the top of the ball. Ensure that your back is flat.

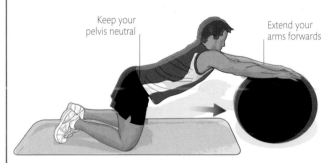

Keep your pelvis neutral

Extend your arms forwards

2 Roll the ball forwards by extending your arms, and follow it with your upper body as far as you can without arching your back. Use your abdominals to pull the ball back to the start position.

### VARIATION

Using a barbell instead of a stability ball is a high-level variation of this exercise, but should only be attempted once you have very good abdominal and spinal control. Kneel with your hands on the bar, shoulder-width apart. Keep your back flat as you roll the bar forward and use your abdominals to pull it back to the starting position.

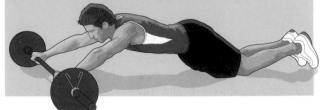

## 108 SIT-TO-STAND CHAIR SQUAT

Practising squats helps you develop the habit of using your hips and leg muscles instead of your back. This version is a good confidence-builder, as the chair or box provides a base and you do not have to squat too low.

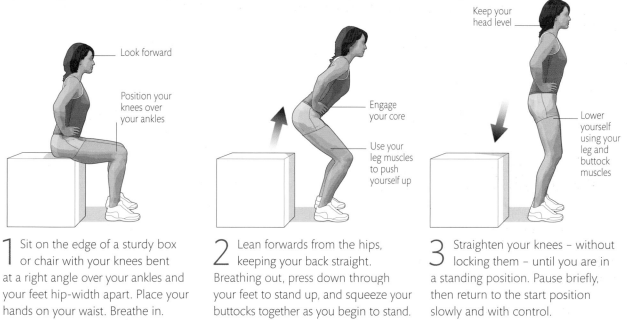

Look forward

Position your knees over your ankles

Engage your core

Use your leg muscles to push yourself up

Keep your head level

Lower yourself using your leg and buttock muscles

1 Sit on the edge of a sturdy box or chair with your knees bent at a right angle over your ankles and your feet hip-width apart. Place your hands on your waist. Breathe in.

2 Lean forwards from the hips, keeping your back straight. Breathing out, press down through your feet to stand up, and squeeze your buttocks together as you begin to stand.

3 Straighten your knees – without locking them – until you are in a standing position. Pause briefly, then return to the start position slowly and with control.

## 109 STAND-TO-SIT CHAIR SQUAT

This exercise is almost the reverse of the sit-to-stand version of the chair squat (»above). The arm movement differs slightly, in that your arms are outstretched in front of you, giving you a little more balance.

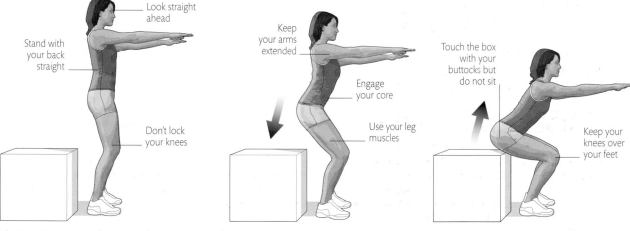

Look straight ahead

Stand with your back straight

Don't lock your knees

Keep your arms extended

Engage your core

Use your leg muscles

Touch the box with your buttocks but do not sit

Keep your knees over your feet

1 Stand in front of a sturdy box or chair with your feet hip-width apart, gently pressing your body weight down through your heels. Raise your arms in front of you and look straight ahead.

2 Pressing down through your heels, breathe in and bend at the knees, reaching back with your buttocks and lowering yourself towards the box. Keep your shoulders over your ankles.

3 Continue to bend at the knees until your buttocks touch the edge of the box, but do not sit down. Breathe out as you squeeze your buttocks and return to the start position.

# GLOSSARY

**Abductor** A muscle that functions to pull a limb away from your body. *See* Adductor.

**Active range of motion** During rehabilitation, the movements you are able to make yourself using muscle strength, as opposed to your *passive range of motion*.

**Acute (pain)** Pain that comes on suddenly but lasts only a short while and can be treated successfully. *See* Chronic.

**Adductor** A muscle that functions to pull a limb towards your body. *See* Abductor.

**Aerobic** A process that requires oxygen. Aerobic *metabolism* occurs during long-duration, low-intensity exercises, such as long-distance running and swimming. It is the opposite of *anaerobic*.

**Analgesic** A drug used to reduce pain.

**Anaerobic** A process that doesn't require oxygen. Anaerobic *metabolism* occurs during short-duration, high-intensity exercises, such as in some forms of intensive strength training. It is the opposite of *aerobic*.

**Antagonistic muscles** Muscles that are arranged in pairs to carry out flexion and extension of a joint; for example, one muscle of the pair contracts to move a limb in one direction, and the other contracts to move it in the opposite direction.

**Anterior** The front part or surface, as opposed to *posterior*.

**Barbell** A type of *free weight* made up of a bar with weights at both ends, which is long enough for you to hold with at least a shoulder-width grip. The weights may be permanently fixed or removable.

**Bone density** The amount of bone mineral in a given volume of bone.

**Brachialgia** Nerve pain in the arm.

**Cervical** Relating to the neck area.

**Chronic (pain)** Pain that persists for a long time and is often resistant to treatment. *See* Acute.

**Cognitive Behavioural Therapy (CBT)** A psychological approach that is used to explore and modify how your thoughts and beliefs influence your perception of pain and your situation.

**Cool-down** A period after completion of a training session that includes activities such as slow jogging, walking, and stretching of your major muscle groups. It is designed to help return your body to its pre-exercise state.

**Core** The central part of your body, mainly the stomach and lower-back muscles, but also including the pelvis, chest, and upper back.

**Core stabilizers** Deep trunk, abdomen, paraspinal, and *pelvic floor* muscles. These muscles provide support to your lower back.

**Corticosteroids** Hormones applied via injection, cream, or tablets, for example to reduce inflammation.

**CT scan** Stands for X-ray Computerized Tomography. This type of scan builds a three-dimensional picture of the body by taking two images and putting them together digitally.

**Diaphragm** The muscle that separates your chest cavity from your abdomen.

**Disc** A cushion-like pad that sits between each vertebra and acts as a shock absorber. Discs allow your spine to bend.

**Discography** A procedure that uses a special dye and X-rays to look at your spine and confirm or deny the disc(s) as the source of pain.

**Dumbbell** A type of *free weight* made up of a short bar with a weight at each end. It can be lifted with one hand.

**Dynamic exercise** Any activity in which your joints and muscles are moving.

**Erector** A muscle that raises a body part.

**Ergonomics** The study and design of devices and equipment that work in relation with the body to help prevent repetitive strain injuries.

**Extensor** A muscle that works to increase the angle at a joint – for example straightening your elbow. It usually works in tandem with a *flexor*.

**Facet joint** A small joint that connects each vertebra with the vertebra directly above and below it, providing stability to the spine.

**Flexor** A muscle that works to decrease the angle at a joint – for example bending your elbow. It usually works in tandem with an *extensor*.

**Form** The posture or stance used when performing exercises. Good or proper form makes the exercise more effective and helps prevent injury.

**Fracture** A break in a bone, ranging from minor cracks to serious breaks into separate fragments.

**Free weight** A weight – usually a *barbell* or *dumbbell* – not tethered to a cable or machine.

**Head** (of a muscle) The point of origin of a muscle.

**Herniated disc** When a portion of a spinal disc ruptures and bulges outside its normal position, and may press on the nerve roots of the spine.

**Hypermobile joint** A joint that is loosely held together because the *ligaments* are either naturally lax or have been overstrained (which can lead to instability).

**Hypomobile joint** A joint that moves less than it should. There are many reasons this can happen, including shortening of the muscles attached to, or crossing over, the joint.

**Inflammation** Swelling, pain, and redness of an area of the body as a response to a harmful stimulus.

**Isometric** A form of training in which you contract your muscles without moving your body or any limbs.

**Isotonic** A form of training in which your muscles work against a constant resistance, so that the muscles contract while the resistance remains the same.

**ITB (Iliotibial Band)** A tough group of fibres running along the outside of your thigh that primarily works as a stabilizer of the hip in standing, walking, and running.

**Lactic acid** A waste product of *anaerobic* respiration. It accumulates in your muscles during intense exercise and is involved in the chemical processes that cause muscular cramp.

**Lateral** Positioned towards the outside of your body. Movement in the lateral plane refers to a side-to-side movement.

**Ligament** A tough and fibrous connective tissue that connects your bones together at the joints.

**Lumbar** Relating to the lower-back area.

**Metabolism** The sum of all your body's chemical processes; it comprises anabolism (building up compounds) and catabolism (breaking down compounds).

**Mineral** Any one of many inorganic (non-carbon-based) elements that are essential for normal body function and that must be included in your diet.

**Mobility exercise** An exercise that helps you to maximize the movement of your joints.

**MRI (Magnetic Resonance Imaging)** A type of scan that reads the molecular structure of your body to form an image to aid diagnosis.

**Musculoskeletal** Affecting both the muscles and bones.

**Neuropathic** Relating to pain caused by abnormal processing of nerve signals due to damage or dysfunction.

**Neutral spine position** The most efficient posture in standing or sitting, or the mid-range position of a joint or region of the spine.

**Orthotics** A branch of medicine that deals with the design, manufacture, and fitting of orthotic devices to help support and rectify congenital or acquired problems in your limbs and torso. Orthotic devices include back and knee braces, and shoe insoles.

**Osteoarthritis** A degenerative disease in which the body suffers a loss of cartilage, leading to stiff joints.

**Pain-relief medication** This can be applied topically or administered by tablet or injection. Different medications have different functions, for example reducing pain by reducing inflammation, but all produce the result of limiting your experience of pain in the body.

**Passive range of motion** The movements a physiotherapist or helper is able to make with parts of your body while supporting their weight. *See* Range of motion.

**Pelvic floor** The area of muscle located in the lower part of the abdomen and attached to the pelvis.

**Plyometrics** Exercises that aim to improve the speed and power of movements by training muscles to contract more quickly and powerfully.

**Posterior** The back part or surface, as opposed to *anterior*.

**Proprioception** The term used to describe the information originating from joints, tendons, ligaments, and muscles that is sent to the brain to provide information about joint position, direction, and pressure.

**Range of motion (ROM)** A term used in physiotherapy, this is the movement a particular joint is capable of in every direction. Limited ROM means you are unable to use your joint as normal.

**Regimen** A regulated course of exercise and diet designed to produce a pre-determined result.

**Rehabilitation** The process of recovering fully from an injury, often with the assistance of professionals.

**Repetition (rep)** One complete movement of a particular exercise, from start to finish and back.

**Resistance training** Any type of training in which your muscles work against resistance. The resistance may be provided by a weight, an elastic or rubber band, or your own body weight.

**Rest interval** The pause between sets of an exercise that allows muscle recovery.

**Rupture** A major tear in a muscle, tendon, or ligament.

**Sacroiliac joints** The two joints located at the base of the back on either side of your spine between the sacrum and the ilia (hip bones).

**Sciatica** Nerve pain in the leg.

**Sensorimotor** Relating to processes and activities involving the communication between the brain and the muscles via the nerves.

**Set** A specific number of *repetitions*.

**Skeletal muscle** Also called striated muscle, this type of muscle is attached to your skeleton and is under voluntary control. Contracting your skeletal muscle allows you to move your body under control.

**Smooth muscle** A type of muscle found in the walls of all the hollow organs of your body which is not under voluntary control.

**Spinal stenosis** Narrowing of the spinal canal due to bony spurs developing on the vertebrae which protrude into the spinal canal.

**Sprain** An injury sustained by a *ligament* that is overstretched or torn.

**Stabilizers** Small muscles close to the spine which hold the vertebrae or spinal region in alignment for static posture or while dynamic movements are being performed.

**Static exercise** An exercise in which you hold one position – for example pushing against an immovable object.

**Strain** An injury to muscle fibres caused by overstretching.

**Swiss ball** A large, inflatable rubber ball used to promote stability during exercise. Also known as an exercise ball.

**Tear** A rip in, for example, a muscle.

**Tendinopathy** Painful *tendons*, often resulting from overuse while doing repetitive actions.

**Tendon** A type of connective tissue that joins your muscles to your bones, so transmitting the force of muscle contraction to your bones.

**Thoracic** Relating to the chest and back between the neck and lumbar regions.

**Torticollis** An acute stiff and painful neck which makes turning your head sideways difficult and painful. It is often triggered by lying or falling asleep in an awkward position. Also known as "wry neck".

**Traction** A technique used to straighten or realign bone fractures into a permanent position, or to relieve pressure on the spine and skeletal system.

**Warm-up** A series of low-intensity exercises that prepares your body for a workout by moderately stimulating your heart, lungs, and muscles. These normally involve a combination of *dynamic exercises* and low-intensity cardiovascular work.

**Whiplash** An injury in the neck area following an acceleration-deceleration force, usually as the result of an indirect impact.

**Wobble board** Circular in shape with a flat top and hemispherical underside, this piece of equipment is used to promote good balance, and to improve your *core* stability.

# USEFUL ADDRESSES

## UK and EIRE

**Age UK**
York House
207–221 Pentonville Road
London N1 9UZ
Tel: 0800 107 8977
www.ageuk.org.uk

**Arthritis Foundation
of Ireland**
1 Clanwilliam Square
Grand Canal Quay, Dublin 2
Tel: 01 661 8188
www.arthritisireland.ie

**Arthritis Research UK**
Copeman House, St Mary's Gate
Chesterfield
Derbyshire S41 7TD
Tel: 0300 790 0400
www.arc.org.uk

**Back Care**
16 Elmtree Road
Teddington
Middlesex TW11 8ST
Tel: 020 8977 5474
www.backpain.org

**Body Control Pilates Association**
35 Little Russell Street
London WC1A 2HH
Tel: 020 7636 8900
www.bodycontrol.co.uk

**British Acupuncture Council**
63 Jeddo Road
London W12 9HQ
Tel: 020 8735 0400
www.acupuncture.org.uk

**British Institute of
Musculoskeletal Medicine**
PO Box 1116
Bushey
Hertfordshire WD23 9BY
Tel: 020 9421 9910
www.bimm.org.uk

**British Pain Society**
Third Floor, Churchill House
35 Red Lion Square
London WC1R 4SG
Tel: 020 7269 7840

**Chartered Society
of Physiotherapy**
14 Bedford Row
London WC1R 4ED
Tel: 020 7306 6666
www.csp.org.uk

**General Chiropractic Council**
44 Wicklow Street
London WC1X 9HL
Tel: 020 7713 5155
www.gcc-uk.org

**General Osteopathic Council**
Osteopathy House
176 Tower Bridge Road
London SE1 3LU
Tel: 020 7357 6655
www.osteopathy.org.uk

**Institute for Complementary
and Natural Medicine**
Can-Mezzanine
32–36 Loman Street
London SE1 0EH
Tel: 020 7922 7980
www.i-c-m.org.uk

**Irish Society of Chartered
Physiotherapists**
Royal College of Surgeons
Saint Steven's Green, Dublin 2
Tel: 01 402 2148
www.iscp.ie

**Manipulation Association of
Chartered Physiotherapists**
PO Box 6759
Westbourne, Dorset BH4 0DA
Tel: 01202 706 161
www.macpweb.org

**National Ankylosing
Spondylitis Society**
Unit 0.2, One Victoria Villas
Richmond, Surrey TW9 2GW
Tel: 020 8948 9117
www.nass.co.uk

**National Osteoporosis Society**
Camerton
Bath, Somerset BA2 0PJ
Tel: 01761 471 771
www.nos.org.uk

**National Register of Hypnotherapists
and Psychotherapists**
First Floor, 18 Carr Road
Nelson, Lancashire BB9 7JS
Tel: 01282 716 839
www.nrhp.co.uk

**Organisation of Chartered
Physiotherapists in Private Practice**
Physio First, Minerva House
Tithe Barn Way, Swan Valley
Northampton NN4 9BA
Tel: 01604 684 960
www.physiofirst.org.uk

**Pain Concern UK**
1 Civic Square
Tranent, East Lothian EH33 1LH
Tel: 01875 614 537
www.painconcern.org.uk

**Posturite UK**
The Mill
Berwick
East Sussex BN26 6SZ
Tel: 0845 345 0010
www.posturite.co.uk

**Royal Association for
Disability and Rehabilitation**
12 City Forum, 250 City Road
London EC1V 8AF
Tel: 020 7250 3222
www.radar.org.uk

**Society of
Orthopaedic Medicine**
4th Floor, 151 Dale Street
Liverpool L2 2AH
Tel: 0151 237 3970
www.somed.org

**Society of Teachers of the
Alexander Technique**
1st Floor, Linton House
39–51 Highgate Road
London NW5 1RS
Tel: 020 7482 5135
www.stat.org.uk

**The Total Back Care Centre**
505 Hagley Road
Smethwick
West Midlands B66 4AX
Tel: 0121 434 5670
www.totalbackcare.co.uk

# AUSTRALIA

**Australian Acupuncture
and Chinese
Medicine Association**
PO Box 1635
Coorparoo DC
QLD 4151
Tel: 07 3324 2599
www.acupuncture.org.au

**Australian Feldenkrais Guild**
Tel: 1800 001 550
www.feldenkrais.org.au

**Australian Orthopaedic
Association**
Level 12
45 Clarence Street
Sydney
NSW 2000
Tel: 02 8071 8000
www.aoa.org.au

**Australian Osteopath
Association**
Suite 4
11 Railway Street
Chatswood
NSW 2067
Tel: 1800 467 836
www.osteopathic.com.au

**Australian Physiotherapy
Association**
Level 1
1175 Toorak Road
Camberwell
VIC 3122
Tel: 03 9092 0888
www.physiotherapy.asn.au

**Australian Society
of Teachers of the
Alexander Technique**
PO Box 405
Beechworth
VIC 3747
Tel: 1300 788 540
www.alexandertechnique.org.au

**Australian Traditional
Medicine Society**
PO Box 1027
Meadowbank
NSW 2114
Tel: 02 9809 6800
www.atms.com.au

**Chiropractors'
Association of Australia**
2/36 Woodriff Street
Penrith
NSW 2750
Tel: 02 4731 8011
www.chiropractors.asn.au

**Royal Australian
College of
General Practitioners**
1 Palmerston Crescent
South Melbourne
VIC 3205
Tel: 03 8699 0414
www.racgp.org.au

**Shiatsu Therapy
Association of Australia**
PO Box 248
Surrey Hills
VIC 3127
Tel: 03 9890 5701
www.staa.org.au

# INDEX

# ACKNOWLEDGMENTS

## AUTHORS' AND PUBLISHER'S ACKNOWLEDGMENTS

The authors would like to acknowledge the valuable contributions of learned colleagues of The British Institute of Musculoskeletal Medicine and the International Spine Intervention Society for their collective years of experience and study in diagnosis and management of spinal pain. The authors would also like to extend their grateful thanks to their patients.

The authors and publishers would like to thank the following people and organizations for their generous help in producing this book.

**For modelling:**
Emily Hayden; Eva Hajidemetri; John Tanner; Annie Hajidemetri; Gareth Jones; Scott Tindall; Mary Paternoster; Sam Bias Ferrar; Anne Browne; Chris Chea; Louise Cole; Sarah Cookson; David Doma; Amanda Grant; Michelle Grey; Anouska Hipperson; Elizabeth Howells; Christopher James; Gunilla Johansson; Megan Lolls; Zoe Moore; Sean Newton; Caroline Pearce; Yasmin Phillips; Jamie Raggs; Lucy Shakespeare; Rufus Shosman; William Smith; Kirsty Spence; Sheri Staplehurst; and Sally Way.

**For use of facilities:**
Dr Eric Ansell at 999 Medical and Diagnostic Centre.

**For equipment:**
Paul Margolis of Margolis Office Interiors Ltd (www.margolisfurniture.co.uk) for supplying the ergonomic chair.

**For reference photography:**
Nigel Wright, XAB Design; Gillian Andrews; Keith Davis; Phil Gamble; Eva Hajidemetri; Cobalt ID; Russell Sadur; and Graham Atkins-Hughes.

**For illustrations:**
Philip Wilson; Debbie Maizels; Phil Gamble; Mark Walker; Debajyoti Dutta; Mike Garland; Darren R. Awuah; and Jon Rogers.

**For additional material and assistance:**
Dr. Sue Davidson; Scarlett O'Hara; Nicky Munro; Hugo Wilkinson; Joanne Clark; Margaret McCormack; Scott Tindall; Derek Groves; Glen Thurgood; Len Williams; and the British Weightlifting Association (BWLA).